Cash's Textbook of Orthopaedics and Rheumatology for Physiotherapists

CASH'S TEXTBOOK OF ORTHOPAEDICS AND RHEUMATOLOGY FOR PHYSIOTHERAPISTS

edited by
PATRICIA A. DOWNIE FCSP

introduced by
Professor B. T. O'Connor MS, MchOrth, FRCS, FRACS
Robert Jones Professor of Orthopaedics in The University of Birmingham at The Robert Jones and Agnes Hunt Orthopaedic Hospital, Oswestry

faber and faber LONDON·BOSTON

First published under this title in 1984
by Faber and Faber Limited
3 Queen Square London WC1N 3AU
Reprinted 1988 and 1990
Typeset by Wilmaset, Birkenhead
Printed in Great Britain by
Redwood Burn Ltd, Trowbridge, Wiltshire

Previously published as part of *Cash's Textbook of Medical Conditions for Physiotherapists* 1951, 1957, 1965, 1971, 1976, 1979 and *Cash's Textbook of Physiotherapy in Some Surgical Conditions* 1955, 1958, 1966, 1971, 1977, 1979

British Library Cataloguing in Publication Data

Cash, Joan E.
  Cash's textbook of orthopaedics and rheumatology for
  physiotherapists.
  1. Orthopedia   2. Physical therapy   3. Rheumatism
  I. Title   II. Downie, Patricia A.
  617'.3'0024616   RD731

  ISBN 0–571–13268–5

Contents

Contributors

Mrs C.E. Apperley MCSP
Senior Physiotherapist
Robert Jones and Agnes Hunt Orthopaedic Hospital
Oswestry SY10 7AG

G.J. Benke FRCS, FRCS(Ed)
Consultant Orthopaedic Surgeon
Good Hope District General Hospital
Sutton Coldfield B75 7RR

Miss J.A. Bentley MCSP, ONC
Superintendent Physiotherapist
Robert Jones and Agnes Hunt Orthopaedic Hospital
Oswestry SY10 7AG

Mrs P. B. Butler MSC, MCSP
Research Physiotherapist
Orthotic Research and Locomotor Assessment Unit
Robert Jones and Agnes Hunt Orthopaedic Hospital
Oswestry SY10 7AG

Mrs V. Draycott MCSP, ONC
Senior Physiotherapist
Robert Jones and Agnes Hunt Orthopaedic Hospital
Oswestry SY10 7AG

G.A. EVANS MB, BS, FRCS, FRCS(orth)
Consultant Orthopaedic Surgeon, Children's Orthopaedic Unit
Robert Jones and Agnes Hunt Orthopaedic Hospital
Oswestry SY10 7AG

J.A. Fowler BA, MCSP, DipTP, MBIM
Principal, School of Physiotherapy
The Royal Liverpool Hospital College
Liverpool L7 8XN

Mrs E. Goss MCSP
Senior Physiotherapist
Robert Jones and Agnes Hunt Orthopaedic Hospital
Oswestry SY10 7AG

Miss J. Hickling FCSP
Formerly Superintendent Physiotherapist i/c Manipulation Unit
St Thomas' Hospital, London SE1 7EH

Miss S.H. McLaren FCSP, DiPPE
Formerly Superintendent Physiotherapist
The Hermitage Rehabilitation Centre
Chester-le-Street, Co Durham DH2 3RF

Dr A. G. Mowat MB, FRCP(Ed)
Clinical Lecturer in Rheumatology, University of Oxford
Consultant Rheumatologist, Nuffield Orthopaedic Centre, Oxford

J.P. O'Brien MB, BS, PhD, FRCS(Ed), FACS
Director, Department for Spinal Disorders, Institute of Orthopaedics
Robert Jones and Agnes Hunt Orthopaedic Hospital
Oswestry SY10 7AG

G.K. Rose OBE, FRCS
Honorary Consultant Orthopaedic Surgeon *and* Director of the
Clinical Gait Assessment Laboratory
Robert Jones and Agnes Hunt Orthopaedic Hospital
Oswestry SY10 7AG

E.R.S. Ross FRCS, FRACS
Consultant Orthopaedic Surgeon
Wythenshawe Hospital, Manchester

M. Rutter, BA, Dip Visual Communication
One Ash, West Lane
Chester-le-Street, Co Durham DH3 3HL

J. Stallard BTech, CEng, MIMechE
Deputy Director, Orthotic Research and Locomotor Assessment
Unit
Robert Jones and Agnes Hunt Orthopaedic Hospital
Oswestry SY10 7AG

Mrs M.E. Tidswell BA, MCSP, ONC, DipTP
Principal, Oswestry and North Staffordshire School of Physiotherapy
Robert Jones and Agnes Hunt Orthopaedic Hospital
Oswestry SY10 7AG

Dr D.J. Ward MB, FRCP
Consultant Rheumatologist
Robert Jones and Agnes Hunt Orthopaedic Hospital
Oswestry SY10 7AG

Miss P.M. Wood MCSP, DipTP
Principal, School of Physiotherapy
Withington Hospital, Manchester M20 8LR

Introduction

This book has been completely revised and has much new information from surgeons, physicians and physiotherapists working in the field of neuromuscular-skeletal disorders. Although primarily written for those in the physiotherapy profession, much of the information will be useful to both nurses and doctors who meet orthopaedic problems.

The Institute of Orthopaedics, Oswestry is proud of its staff who were the major contributors to this book and expresses its best wishes for successful practice to all who read or browse through this book which is the drawing together of two vast subjects from two previous titles into a composite text.

Brian T. O'Connor
MS, MChOrth, FRCS, FRACS
Robert Jones Professor of Orthopaedics
in
The University of Birmingham
at
The Robert Jones and Agnes Hunt
Orthopaedic Hospital
Oswestry

Editor's Preface

More than 30 years have passed since Joan Cash wrote *Physiotherapy in Medical Conditions* and *Physiotherapy in Some Surgical Conditions*. At first she wrote them herself seeking advice from medical and physiotherapy colleagues. As medicine and surgery became more specialised, as well as technical, she invited additional contributors to share their expertise in these two books.

Joan Cash recognised the growth of specialisation and from chapters in the original titles she developed first, *Neurology for Physiotherapists* and, then, *Chest, Heart and Vascular Disorders for Physiotherapists*. Now I, too, have felt the need to rationalise the present medical and surgical textbooks. They have both continued to grow haphazardly, with overlap and idiosyncratic division. It seemed logical that the orthopaedic, fracture and rheumatology chapters could come together, and so this title is born.

This has not been an easy volume to assemble and I am conscious of omissions and failures! Some of the chapters are technical and academic, others reflect the absolute practical approach by physiotherapists to their patients. Some are heavily referenced, others are not. Different approaches to the same problems are clearly evident, indicating the importance for the physiotherapist to understand the rationale of different treatments and then to apply what she considers is best for the individual patient, after consultation with the doctor.

What I hope I have done is to provide a solid background to that area of medicine which has, in the past, been described as 'carpentry on the human body'. While nuts, bolts and plates may indeed be used, and saws, files and levers are stock in trade instruments, the patient on whom these are used is a human being who requires an understanding approach. Some orthopaedic patients require little or no physiotherapy, but others require it over many months and, in some cases, years. This applies to the rheumatology patient also, and orthopaedic surgery is inextricably bound up with many of them: it is for this reason that a large section of the book is devoted to the clinical and physiotherapeutic management of those with a rheumatological disorder.

Readers will note that many of the contributors are from the Robert Jones and Agnes Hunt Orthopaedic Hospital, Oswestry. Why so? First, when I devised this volume I wanted the contributors to be fully aware of the needs of students as well as trained therapists. Oswestry has a School of Physiotherapy, an Institute of Orthopaedics and a Department of Rheumatology – it seemed the perfect answer. Secondly, I admit it was a personal choice. I have long admired the pioneering role of Dame Agnes Hunt who started the cripples' home at Baschurch in 1900, and then interested Robert Jones, a Liverpool orthopaedic surgeon, to become the honorary surgeon to it. I have recently re-read the *Heritage of Oswestry*, a private publication which describes the development of the hospital from its inception as the cripples' home to the world renowned centre it is today. There is an interesting mention of the beginning of the School of Physiotherapy:

> It is interesting to record that in 1918 Dame Agnes Hunt started what was then a Massage School with one Swedish Masseuse and three young ladies who were to combine this work, if they so desired, with a Housekeeping course, to take six months to complete. This School was taken over by Miss Dalton, who remained with the Hospital until 1945, and increased the course to one of 15 months.

In the early days, orthopaedics revolved round bone tuberculosis, osteomyelitis, rickets, bone-setting, etc; later it was poliomyelitis and the devastations of war injuries; today it is joint replacement, bone transplants, biomechanical assessments, etc. In all this Oswestry has been in the forefront of teaching generations of surgeons, nurses and allied professionals.

It is invidious to select individuals for acknowledgement, but on this occasion I must. Professor Brian O'Connor, the present Robert Jones Professor of Orthopaedics at Oswestry, has been enthusiastic, helpful and persuasive as the needs demanded and I am most grateful. Mr Gordon Rose OBE, FRCS has been a respected adviser to physiotherapists for many years and I count it an honour that he has provided four chapters for this book as well as advising on others. From myself as editor, and for all the prospective readers, I extend to him our sincere thanks. Miss Winifred Cannell was Principal of the School of Physiotherapy based at Oswestry when this book was devised; she organised the Oswestry contributors, discussing content and timing, and in her well-earned retirement she has acted as the local co-ordinator. I am most grateful to her.

As in a previous title I accept full responsibility for including two chapters from Miss Sandy McLaren. They will be controversial to some purists, but they do show so clearly how enjoyment can be used to conquer the fear which so often hinders final restoration to activity.

I cannot forget the artists and photographers who have provided the many contributors with illustrative matter – I thank them all, but particularly the Photographic Department at Oswestry for many superlative pictures. Audrey Besterman, as ever, has laboured diligently on new drawings as well as providing a most helpful 'touching-up' service; for all of which I am indeed appreciative.

Without the great pioneers we should not, today, be able to provide so much skilled help to the physically disabled (the cripples of a past era), and in such a book as this it is right that we honour the memory of them: Hugh Owen Thomas, Robert Jones, Agnes Hunt, Gathorne Girdlestone, Rowley Bristow, George Perkins, Reginald Watson-Jones to name but a few. In my edition (the fourth) of *Fractures and Bone Injuries* by Reginald Watson-Jones there is a dedicatory quotation which sums up the gratitude we owe them and which we must never forget:

> They, whose work cannot die, whose influence lives after them, whose disciples perpetuate and multiply their gifts to humanity, are truly immortal.

P.A.D., 1983
London

Chapter 1

The Mechanics of Lower Limb Orthoses

by J. STALLARD, BTech, CEng, MIMechE

INTRODUCTION

It is well known that mechanics are based on Newton's three Laws of Motion (Williams and Lissner, 1977a). Contrary to popular opinion, engineers do not constantly recite these to themselves and it is not suggested that therapists should either! However, Newton's 3rd Law is not only easy to remember, it is also self-evident and of great benefit to those who wish to have an elementary understanding of the subject. 'To every action, there is an equal and opposite reaction.' What this means is that unless there is *resistance*, there cannot be *force*. If you pull with a force of 10 Newtons, then something must oppose that pull with the same force.

FORCE

Force is the physical action which tends to change the position of a body in space. Some confusion exists about the units in which force can be expressed. Many different units have been used over the years, but the one which has been adopted as an International Standard is the Newton (N). An appropriate way of remembering the magnitude of 1N is to think of it as approximately the force which one apple (from which Newton developed his ideas!) exerts at rest under the influence of gravity. Thus a lightweight man would weigh between 600–800N.

In orthotics, force derives from two main sources: muscles and gravity. These can combine with other mechanical systems to produce force from stored energy (springs etc) or from inertial reaction, which will be discussed in more detail later.

Since force always acts along a straight line it may be represented graphically by a line, the length of which is proportional to the *magnitude* of force, the *direction* of which corresponds to that of the force, the start of which represents the *point of application* of force. Drawing this line (a vector) is a convenient way of indicating the effect of a force applied to a mechanical system. The application of force by a therapist on the lower limb of a patient (Fig. 1/1a) can be represented vectorally (Fig. 1/1b), as can the reaction (the equal and opposite force of the leg on the hand (Fig. 1/1c)).

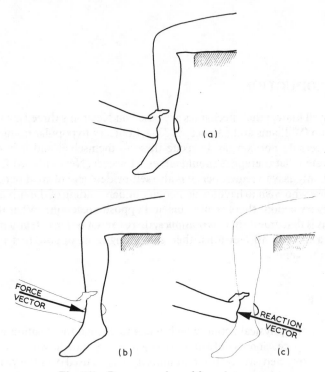

Fig. 1/1   Representation of force by a vector

Since the weight of the body is in effect a force acting vertically downwards, it too can be represented vectorally by a line from the centre of mass of the body (Fig. 1/2).

MOMENTS

A force system is rarely simple since it is frequently a combination of forces, and because secondary effects (most commonly moments) also

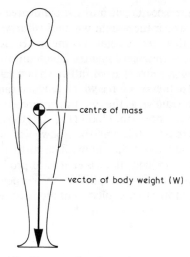

Fig. 1/2   Force acting through the centre of mass

occur. In order to gain some understanding of the problems that result, it is convenient to examine the problem of an unstable knee caused by extensor paralysis. Every therapist knows that with the knee fully extended the lower limb can support the weight of the body even when it is muscularly deficient (Fig. 1/3a). They further know

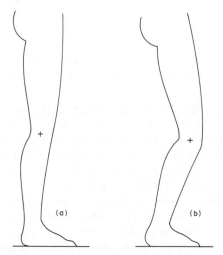

Fig. 1/3   Knee in (a) extension; (b) flexion

that when this same knee is put into a small degree of flexion (Fig. 1/3b), it collapses under the weight which it is carrying. The reason this happens is that the weight of the body acting vertically downwards produces a *moment* about the knee – the direction of which changes when the knee moves from full extension into flexion.

A *moment* is the action of a force which tends to cause rotation of a body about a point (known as the fulcrum or moment centre). When giving passive movements to the elbow (Fig. 1/4) the therapist applies a force some way from the fulcrum (the elbow joint) in order to cause the forearm to rotate about the elbow. The further away from the fulcrum the force is applied, the easier it is to produce the turning effect. A *moment* is *force* (F) multiplied by the perpendicular *distance* (L) from the line of force to the fulcrum or moment centre (Fig. 1/4).

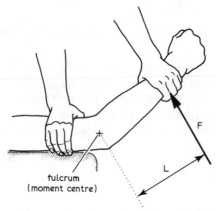

Fig. 1/4 Turning moment about the elbow joint. Applying passive movements to the elbow. Moment=F×L

In Fig. 1/5a the moment produced about the knee from the shoe (the weight which acts vertically downwards) is 10N×40cm=400Ncm. However, this ignores the weight of the shank of the lower limb, which is itself heavy and very significant. In order to understand the turning effect of the shank it is necessary to know where its centre of mass is located. *Centre of mass* is the point at which the mass of a body is considered to be concentrated and is the point of perfect balance (Williams and Lissner, 1977b). Figure 1/5b shows the same leg without the boot, with the centre of mass marked at 18cm horizontal distance from the knee centre and the weight of the shank indicated as 50N. In the position shown the shank produces a moment

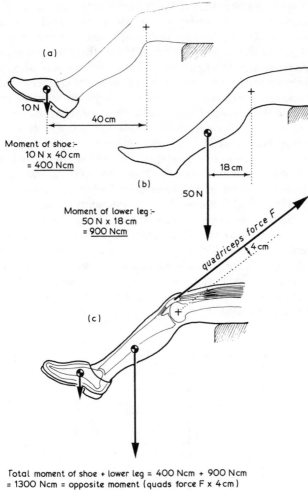

(a)

10 N

40 cm

Moment of shoe :-
10 N x 40 cm
= 400 Ncm

18 cm

(b)

50 N

Moment of lower leg :-
50 N x 18 cm
= 900 Ncm

quadriceps force F

4 cm

(c)

Total moment of shoe + lower leg = 400 Ncm + 900 Ncm
= 1300 Ncm = opposite moment (quads force F x 4cm)

$$\therefore F = \frac{1300 \text{ Ncm}}{4 \text{ cm}} = 325 \text{ N}$$

Fig. 1/5 Balancing a moment about the knee with the quadriceps muscle

of 900Ncm (i.e. 50N×18cm). Thus the overall effect when the shoe is
worn is shown in Figure 1/5c and the total moment about the knee is
the summation of the two effects, which gives a moment of 1300Ncm.

To keep the leg stable in that position it is necessary to provide an
equal and *opposite* moment, and this is achieved by the quadriceps
acting through the patellar tendon. From Figure 1/5c it can be seen

that the moment arm of the patellar tendon is only 4cm, and by simple mathematics we can determine that in order to produce the balancing moment of 1300Ncm, the force with which the quadriceps must pull is 325N (i.e. 325N×4cm=1300Ncm). Notice that the comparatively small moment arm through which the quadriceps acts demands a much greater force than the combined action of the boot and leg weight acting through their respective much greater moment arms.

Care must be exercised with units when considering moments. *Force* units, e.g. Newton (N) and *moment* units, e.g. Newton centimetres (Ncm), are different and must *not* be confused.

To return to the unstable knee: it can be seen that the line of force of the body-weight, which acts vertically downwards from the centre of mass, passes in front of the knee centre when the knee is fully extended (Fig. 1/6a). This produces an extending moment which is resisted by the posterior capsule thus maintaining the knee in extension. With the knee in flexion, the line of force passes behind the knee centre, thus producing a flexing moment (Fig. 1/6b). If the quadriceps are not active, or are insufficiently powerful to balance that flexing moment, then the knee will collapse. The greater the degree of knee flexion, the larger the moment arm and the less likely the quadriceps are to cope.

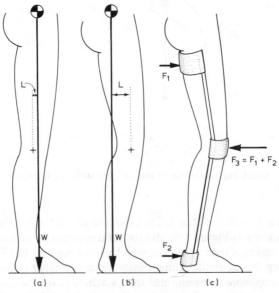

Fig. 1/6   Balancing a moment about the knee with a caliper

The orthotic solution to an unstable knee is almost axiomatic, and a long-leg caliper is universally fitted to the flail knee (Fig. 1/6c). What is perhaps less well known is the mechanical effect of this device. The cliché 'three-point fixation' is oft repeated, and is true enough, but it obscures to many people the real effect. Newton's 3rd Law will reveal everything. 'To every action there is an equal and opposite reaction.' When a fixed flexion deformity occurs it is inevitable that a knee-flexing moment will be produced, the magnitude of which will rise as the degree of flexion deformity increases. Without a caliper, a flail knee with flexion deformity has an unbalanced flexing moment applied to it which is equal to body-weight (W) multiplied by the perpendicular distance (L) from the knee (Fig. 1/6b). When the orthosis is applied it resists this unbalanced moment by producing an *equal* and *opposite* moment through *three-point fixation* (Fig. 1/6c). Anyone who has ever broken a stick over their knee will understand how this is effective in producing a 'bending' effect (Fig. 1/7).

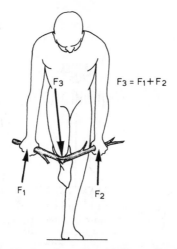

$$F_3 = F_1 + F_2$$

Fig. 1/7   The bending effect of three-point fixation

If it can be arranged that the line of force acting at the knee passes directly through its centre, then clearly no moment would be applied. When a long-leg caliper is fitted to an unstable knee with a full range of movement, it is set so that negligible moments are produced about the knee. In this situation the orthosis is merely a stabilising device and only small forces occur between the leg and the orthosis.

INTERFACE PRESSURE

One difficulty which can occur with a caliper is high interface pressure at the knee or, less often, at the thigh band.

Pressure is the intensity of loading applied to a particular area (Fig. 1/8). A large load concentrated on a small area will give very high pressure. Increasing the area, or decreasing the load, is the only way in which pressure can be reduced. With any type of bracing it is advisable to minimise the applied loads as far as possible, and at the same time spread them over the greatest possible area. It is for this reason that, for example, thigh bands on calipers should be made as broad as is practical.

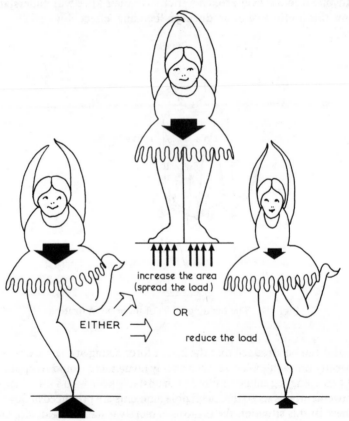

increase the area
(spread the load)

EITHER

OR

reduce the load

Fig. 1/8   Pressure: the distribution of load

To reduce pressure further, the forces F_1, F_2 and F_3, required to achieve stabilisation of the knee, can be minimised by increasing to a maximum the moment arm through which F_1 and F_2 act (Fig. 1/6c). Moments are a product of both force and moment arm, and increasing or decreasing one has the opposite effect on the magnitude of the other to maintain the same moment. Thus it is in the interest of the patient to locate the thigh band as high as possible since this will decrease not only F_1 but also F_3, because (as indicated by Newton's 3rd Law) $F_3 = F_1 + F_2$. Figure 1/9 gives a comparison of forces for different application points on a long-leg brace.

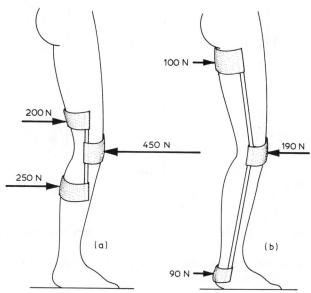

Fig. 1/9   The beneficial effect of long lever arms

Another well-known fact is that 'the higher the degree of knee flexion deformity, the larger the forces required to support the leg'. Once it is understood how the unbalanced moment about the knee centre is developed, then the reason becomes obvious. As was stated earlier, the line of body-weight from the centre of mass passes behind the flexed knee centre (Fig. 1/10a). With larger flexion deformities the moment arm from knee centre to line of action of force increases (Figs. 1/10b and c). Even though nothing else changes (body weight must stay the same) this increases the flexing moment about the knee in

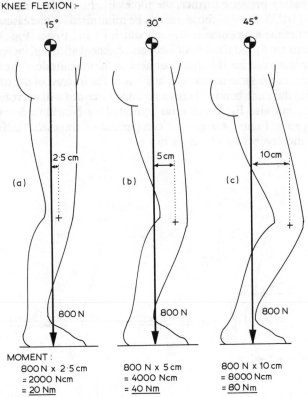

KNEE FLEXION :-

15°   30°   45°

2·5 cm   5 cm   10 cm

(a)   (b)   (c)

800 N   800 N   800 N

MOMENT :
800 N x 2·5 cm   800 N x 5 cm   800 N x 10 cm
= 2000 Ncm   = 4000 Ncm   = 8000 Ncm
= 20 Nm   = 40 Nm   = 80 Nm

Fig. 1/10 The increase in bending moment with increasing knee flexion

proportion with the increased moment arm, and a consequent increase in stabilising forces occurs.

RESOLUTION OF FORCES

Patients who use calipers frequently need also to use crutches. These have two primary functions:
1. To improve stability by increasing support area.
2. To provide a means of propulsion through ground reaction forces.

In both of these functions it is necessary for the crutch to apply forces to the ground, and this is generally done through the handle along the axis of the crutch. During ambulation the crutches are always sloping, which means that the applied forces are never perpendicular relative to the ground. The implication of this is that there must be a proportion of the overall force which acts *vertically* and a further proportion which acts *horizontal* with the ground (Fig. 1/11). Provided that the magnitude and direction of the force along the crutch axis is known, it is possible to determine these two 'components' of that force by simple manipulation of its vector representation. This is done by dropping a perpendicular line from the 'top' end of the vector and drawing a horizontal line from the other end (Fig. 1/11). The point of intersection of these two lines will show their magnitude – the direction of force being indicated by following the 'component' vectors around from the top to meet the other end of the overall force vector.

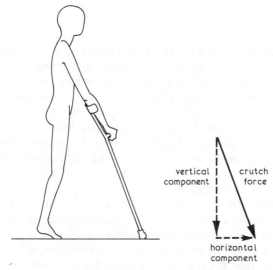

Fig. 1/11   The resolution of crutch force

Friction

From Newton's 3rd Law it can be seen that for a horizontal component of crutch force to exist, there must be an *equal* and *opposite* force. This comes from the friction between the crutch tip and the floor surface. Without this frictional opposing force the crutch would slide on the floor surface and fail to fulfil its function. *Coefficient of friction* describes the frictional properties which exist between two surfaces (Fig. 1/12). Clearly it is in the patient's interest that crutches should resist slipping, and so the tips are made from a high friction material such as rubber.

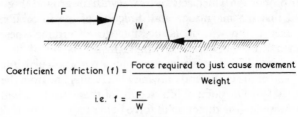

$$\text{Coefficient of friction } (f) = \frac{\text{Force required to just cause movement}}{\text{Weight}}$$

$$\text{i.e. } f = \frac{F}{W}$$

Fig. 1/12 Coefficient of friction

STABILITY

Stability, which crutches can help to provide, is vital for any form of ambulation, an activity which requires both intrinsic and extrinsic stability. *Intrinsic stability* prevents the human body (which is a multi-segmental structure) from collapsing under itself. Where muscular deficiency exists – for example a flail hip or knee – then orthotic assistance in the form of three-point fixation is required. In the static situation, *extrinsic stability* ensures that an intrinsically stable body does not topple over. This means that the centre of mass, when projected vertically downwards, must be contained within the support area of the body.

An illustration of three forms of extrinsic stability can usefully be gained from the study of a cone (Fig. 1/13). On its point a cone will require only tiny movements sideways to take the centre of mass outside the support area. This is known as *unstable equilibrium*. When lying on its side, the cone may be rolled and the centre of mass then follows the support area so that it takes up a new position of equilibrium: this is known as *neutral equilibrium*. However, when a

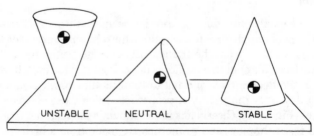

Fig. 1/13 Stability: conditions of equilibrium

cone which is standing on its base is tilted it will drop back to its original position, as long as the centre of mass does not pass outside the support area. This is known as *stable equilibrium*. Once the centre of mass goes beyond the outside edge of the cone it loses its stable equilibrium and falls on to its side.

WALKING AIDS

Walking aids fall into three categories and can perform a number of functions.

CATEGORIES
1. Sticks
2. Crutches
3. Frames

FUNCTIONS
1. Provision of increased extrinsic stability
2. A means of exerting propulsive forces
3. Part of the intrinsic stabilisation system

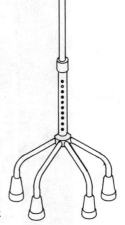

Fig. 1/14   A quadropod stick

Sticks

Sticks give the lowest level of assistance and in most cases provide a degree of increased *extrinsic stability* by enlarging the support area. They also enable some injection of *propulsive force* by reacting against the ground through the arm (or arms).

The tripod and quadropod sticks are a special case (Fig. 1/14): because of their multi-point ground contact, they can resist rotation about their vertical axis. Patients who have difficulty with rotational instability around the hips find that these particular aids can be of great assistance. In addition to their rotational reaction they also have some resistance to forward or side thrust and this enhances the provision of *extrinsic stability*.

Crutches

Crutches provide support across at least one joint in the arm. There are three main types: axillary, Canadian and elbow crutches (Fig. 1/15). Axillary and Canadian crutches cross both the wrist and elbow joints, and give patients a greater level of stability. In contrast elbow crutches cross only the wrist joint, and as such they, of the three main types, least enhance patient stability.

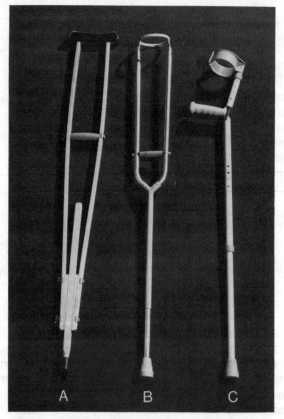

Fig. 1/15   Crutch types: A. axillary; B. Canadian; C. elbow

Crutches are usually grounded at points further from the body than are sticks, and because of this give larger support areas. This, coupled with better arm stabilisation, means that they provide a higher level of *extrinsic stability* (Fig. 1/16).

For patients who use long-leg calipers and have no hip control (e.g.

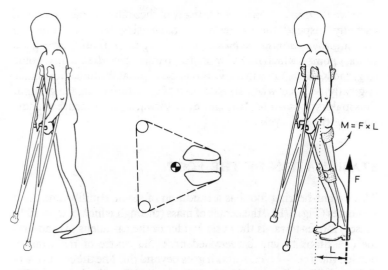

Fig. 1/16 (*left*) The support area provided by crutches. The extrinsic stabilisation is improved with crutches because of the increased support area

Fig. 1/17 (*right*) Stabilising flail hips with crutches. M=moment; F=force; L=length

paraplegics with lesions at lumbar-1 level and above) crutches form an important part of the *intrinsic stabilisation* system. By leaning forward to support themselves on the crutches they ensure that the applied forces produce an extending moment about the hips (Fig. 1/17). This condition must be satisfied at all times for such patients. It is a difficult feat and explains why so few paraplegics are able to ambulate with long-leg calipers.

In addition to providing stability, crutches enable patients to exert *propulsive forces*. The most common means of achieving this is for the arms to pull against the crutches – the equal and opposite reactive forces being the crutch tip/ground interface friction. It is essential for patients to have intact latissimus dorsi muscles if they are to generate these forces, for it is the arms pulling towards the body under their influence which cause the crutch to react against the ground.

Frames

The third category, namely frames, comes in a variety of forms (pulpit frames, Rollators, etc). They all provide a large support area for improved *extrinsic stability*. Since many of these also enable patients to partially 'suspend' themselves in the frame using their arms, they can also improve *intrinsic stabilisation*. All types of frame have good contact points, which make it possible to inject *propulsive forces*. Some (e.g. the Rollator) also incorporate wheels so that frictional resistance is greatly reduced when support points are lifted from the ground, thus making it easier to push the device forward to commence the next phase of the gait cycle.

STABILISATION OF THE FOOT

The weight-bearing foot has a condition of stable equilibrium. As it supinates (Fig. 1/18), the centre of mass (through which body-weight passes) moves towards the outer border of the calcaneus (3) and fifth toe (2). Stability will be retained until the centre of mass moves outside the line 3–2. As soon as it goes beyond this line the condition of stable equilibrium is lost, because the moment from body-weight (W) immediately changes from being corrective into one which wants to increase supination. The sudden loss of balance which then occurs has been experienced by most people.

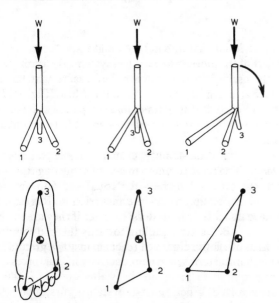

Fig. 1/18 Stability of the foot in supination. 1=great toe; 2=fifth toe; 3=calcaneus; W=body-weight

Limited range in the subtalar joint means that this does not normally occur in pronation. However, in the rheumatoid foot the centre of mass can move outside the line 3–1 (Fig. 1/18) if the disease is in an advanced stage. When this happens an orthosis of the type shown in Figure 1/19 is necessary if the patient is to walk. As can be seen from the diagrammatic representation (Fig. 1/19a), the resolution of forces tends to pull the strap down the outside iron and pull the foot (represented by the cone) towards the iron. Thus in order to make the orthosis work effectively it is necessary to put a loop on the outside iron (Fig. 1/19b) to provide the *equal* and *opposite* force to the vertical component and a wedge in the shoe to oppose the horizontal component of the strap force.

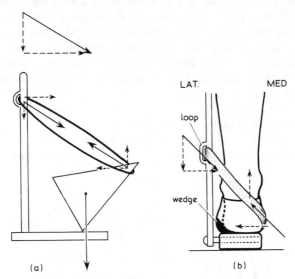

Fig. 1/19   Stabilising the pronated foot

DYNAMIC FORCES

One of the aims of a lower limb orthosis is to enable patients to walk. This is, in mechanical terms, a dynamic activity in that forces over and above those required to maintain the status quo (i.e., the 'static' situation) are involved. When a change of state occurs, such as starting to walk from standing still or changing speed and direction when walking, extra force is required to bring that about. While it is possible to determine the magnitude of these increased forces, given the various parameters, the mathematics can be complex and it is really only necessary for therapists to understand the effect of dynamic situations.

During walking, the centre of mass rises and falls and also sways from side to side. This implies that the body is accelerated upwards and downwards and from side to side. The force required to raise the body upwards is over and above that of body-weight, and in order to permit the body to fall back again the force of the body on the ground must be less than body-weight. Swaying of the body sideways is brought about by small side-thrust forces on the ground.

Thus it can be seen that the ground forces involved in walking are quite complex. The forces are monitored by a force platform (force plate). This is a flat rigid plate, set flush into a walkway, which registers components of force applied to the top surface. The use of force platforms during the last 40 years has established the levels and patterns of the various components of ground reaction force for normal walking. For convenience, ground reaction force is split into three components:

the vertical (Fz)

horizontal in line of walking (Fy)

horizontal at right angles to line of walking (Fx).

Typical patterns for normal steady pace walking are shown in Figure 1/20.

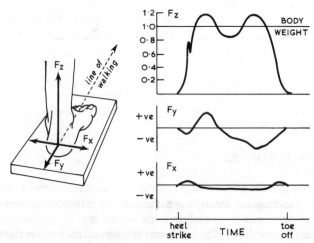

Fig. 1/20   Ground reaction forces in walking. Fz=vertical; Fy=horizontal in line of walking; Fx=horizontal at right angles to line of walking

Notice that Fz (the vertical component) rises to approximately 1.2 body-weight just after heel strike, drops to around 0.8 body-weight at mid-stance and rises again at the end of single stance phase – once again to approximately 1.2 body-weight. For running, a different pattern of Fz emerges and the force on the lower limb can rise to almost 3×body-weight (Fig. 1/21).

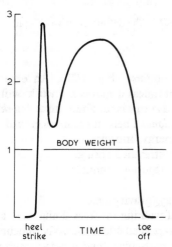

Fig. 1/21   Vertical ground reaction force in running

In the normal leg, these dynamic forces put greater demands on the bones, tendons and muscles. However, with a braced lower limb, the orthosis also has to bear the increased burden. Many patients perform swing-through gait when wearing calipers and this introduces forces greater than those experienced in reciprocal ambulation (Stallard et al, 1978a; 1980). The design of orthotic devices must reflect the need to withstand the extra forces involved in the dynamic activities which are undertaken by patients.

WORK DONE AND ENERGY

One of the reasons for treating patients by physical therapy or orthotics is to enable them to get some work done. In mechanics the term 'work done' has a very specific meaning and it involves moving bodies. *Work done* is the *force* applied to a body multiplied by the *distance* through which the body moves under the influence of and in

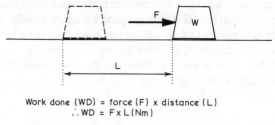

Work done (WD) = force (F) x distance (L)
∴ WD = F x L (Nm)

Fig. 1/22   The definition of work done

the direction of that *force* (Fig. 1/22). An object can be pushed extremely hard, but unless it moves no 'work' will be 'done'.

On the other hand *energy* is the ability to do '*work*' and has the same unit (Nm) as *work done*. There are many forms of energy:

Biochemical energy (muscles)
Stored energy (stretched springs)
Kinetic energy (motion – momentum)
Heat
Potential energy (gravity), etc.

Clearly the act of walking involves doing *work* and expending the various forms of *energy* available to the body (biochemical, kinetic and potential energy in particular), and it is the interchange of *energy* to *work done* which is at the heart of mechanical *dynamic* systems. The *efficiency* with which we move is the *ratio of work done to energy expended*.

INERTIAL FORCES

Any object tends to retain the mechanical state in which it finds itself. This *resistance to change* is known as *inertia*, and dynamic forces are required to overcome this effect. When running to catch a bus, it takes an effort to slow down and stop. That is because of the momentum of the running body and its inertia. To every action, Newton states, there is an equal and opposite reaction, and the reactive effect to forces applied to overcome inertia is known as *inertial reaction*. This effect is an integral and important part of walking. At the end of swing phase for example, the hip extensors apply a decelerative force on the swing leg, and this in turn produces an inertial reaction on the trunk which pulls it forward in space.

Any orthosis applied to the lower limb will alter the dynamics of walking. The increase in weight of the 'lower limb system' will obviously increase its inertia and so affect the inertial reaction. Long-leg braces prevent knee flexion, and this limits the ability of the patient to 'smooth out' the rise and fall of the centre of mass during walking. Thus the amount of energy required to walk will be increased and the overall efficiency of ambulation decreased.

CONCLUSION

Much research is being done to establish more efficient forms of walking for the heavily handicapped. Orthotics can play a major part in this, and a number of devices have been developed within the Robert Jones and Agnes Hunt Orthopaedic Hospital, Oswestry to enable the paralysed to walk more effectively (Davies and Lucas, 1977; Rose, 1979; Rose et al, 1981; Stallard et al, 1978b).

Attention to detail by therapists can improve the efficiency of their patients. Careful consideration should be given to orthotic devices and walking aids. Even the type of crutch used to perform swing-through gait can affect the efficiency of the patient. Dounis et al (1980) and Sankarankutty et al (1979) showed that Canadian crutches are the most efficient for swing-through gait. Hopefully, future research by therapists and workers from other disciplines will enable patients to ambulate with increasing effectiveness.

REFERENCES

Davies, J.B. and Lucas, D. (1977). The Salop Skate. *Physiotherapy*, **63**, 4, 112–15.

Dounis, E., Stevenson, R.D. and Wilson, R.S.E. (1980). The use of a portable oxygen consumption meter (Oxylog) for assessing the efficiency of crutch walking. *Journal of Medical Engineering and Technology*, **4**, 6, 296–8.

Rose, G.K. (1979). The principles and practice of hip guidance articulations. *Prosthetics and Orthotics International*, **3**, 37–43.

Rose, G.K., Stallard, J. and Sankarankutty, M. (1981). Clinical evaluation of spina bifida patients using hip guidance orthosis. *Developmental Medicine and Child Neurology*, **23**, 30–40.

Sankarankutty, M., Stallard, J. and Rose, G.K. (1979). The relative efficiency of 'swing through' gait on axillary, elbow and Canadian crutches compared to normal walking. *Journal of Biomedical Engineering*, **1**, 55–7.

Stallard, J., Sankarankutty, M. and Rose, G.K. (1978a). Lower-limb vertical ground reaction forces during crutch walking. *Journal of Medical Engineering and Technology*, **2**, 4, 201–2.

Stallard, J., Rose, G.K. and Farmer, I.R. (1978b) The ORLAU Swivel Walker. *Prosthetics and Orthotics International*, 2, 35–42.

Stallard, J., Dounis, E., Major, R.E. and Rose, G.K. (1980). One leg swing through gait using two crutches. *Acta Orthopaedica Scandinavica*, 51, 71–7.

Williams, N. and Lissner, H.R. (1977a). *Biomechanics of Human Movement*, ch 2, p 10. W.B. Saunders Co, Philadelphia.

Williams, N. and Lissner, H.R. (1977b). *Biomechanics of Human Movement*, ch 2, p 8. W.B. Saunders Co, Philadelphia.

BIBLIOGRAPHY

American Academy of Orthopaedic Surgeons (1975). *Atlas of Orthotics: Biomechanical Principles and Applications*. C.V. Mosby Co, St Louis.

Brunnstrom, S. and Dickinson, R. (1977). *Clinical Kinesiology*, 3rd edition. F.A. Davis Co, Philadelphia.

Carlsoo, S. (1972). *How Man Moves*. William Heinemann Limited, London.

D'Astrous, J.D. (ed) (1981). *Orthotics and Prosthetics Digest*. Edahl Productions, Ottawa.

Day, B.H. (1972). *Orthopaedic Appliances*. Faber and Faber, London. (Out of print; available in libraries.)

Department of Health and Social Security (1980). *Classification of Orthoses*. HMSO, London.

Frankel, V.H. and Burstein, A.H. (1970). *Orthopaedic Biomechanics*. Lea and Febiger, Philadelphia.

Freeman, M.A.R. (1973). *Adult Articular Cartilage*. Pitman Medical, London.

Frost, H.M. (1973). *Orthopaedic Biomechanics*. Chas Thomas, Springfield, Illinois.

Kennedy, J.M. (1974). *Orthopaedic Splints and Appliances*. Baillière Tindall, London.

McCollough, N.C. (1978). Orthotic management in adult hemiplegia. *Clinical Orthopaedics*, (131), 38.

Murdoch, Geo. (ed) (1976). *The Advance in Orthotics*. Edward Arnold (Publishers) Limited, London.

Rehabilitation Engineering Centre, Moss Rehabilitation Hospital. *Lower Limb Orthotics – A Manual*. Temple University, Drexel University, Philadelphia.

Rose, G.K. (1980). Orthoses for the severely handicapped – rational or empirical choice? *Physiotherapy*, 66, 3, 76–81.

Stewart, J.D.M. (1975). *Traction and Orthopaedic Appliances*. Churchill Livingstone, Edinburgh.

Tohen, Z.A. (1973). *Manual of Mechanical Orthopaedics (Prosthetics and Orthotics)*. Chas Thomas, Springfield, Illinois.

Williams, N. and Lissner, H.R. (1977). *Biomechanics of Human Movement*. W.B. Saunders Co, Philadelphia.

Chapter 2

Biomechanics of Gait

by G.K. ROSE, OBE, FRCS

Because Newton's laws apply to everything and everyone, dead or alive, the failure to appreciate the application of mechanical principles to the study of human activities, both normal and pathological, leads to a naïve assessment of the situation. This in turn can make therapy either ineffectual and time wasting or, in the worst circumstances, positively dangerous. The living organism will respond somewhat differently from a mechanical device to these laws because it has the capacity both for some element of self-repair and for a much higher level of internal control and adjustment than is found in inanimate mechanisms.

Locomotion includes both animate and inanimate mobility. Gait is that part of locomotion used by animals with limbs. Bipedal gait provides the evolutionary advantages of relative elevation of eyes and other sense organs and the freeing of the fore limbs to evolve and develop manual skills. Unlike wheels it can cope with a wide variety of terrains and requires no special surfaces to move on, although some are easier than others. It is a complex co-ordinated process with a rich nervous control feedback and it is highly *redundant*. The word redundant in this context means that there are many overlapping mechanisms with slight differences capable of doing similar tasks. The loss of one or several of these mechanisms, therefore, does not bring the organism to a standstill, but progressively reduces the available options in the way walking can be achieved. Similar reductions occur when the effectors are abnormal, as with weakness or paralysis of muscles, reduction in joint movement with deformity and pain.

FUNCTIONS OF THE LEGS
1. Supports of the elevated body and sense organs.
2. Agents of propulsion. On the level this is much over-estimated.

The pattern of muscular activity is mainly shock absorbing rather than propulsive and it does not increase to any extent with an increase in speed (Fig. 2/1). Furthermore, study of the reactive forces on the ground will show that push-off does not exist during this activity.

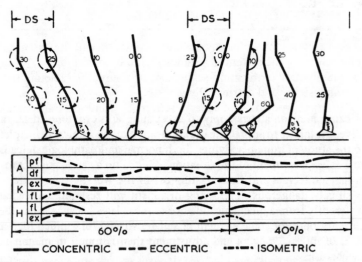

Fig. 2/1   Joint movements during a gait cycle. *Note* that two-joint muscles such as hamstrings can act isometrically while the knee joint is moving into flexion. DS=double stance; A=ankle, K=knee, H=hip; pf=plantar flexion, df=dorsiflexion, ex=extension, fl=flexion

3. Most important is the pattern of joint movement to minimise both the rise and fall and the sideways excursion of the body centre of mass, and this reduces the energy cost of walking which is of overriding importance to the human organism. This has a remarkable capacity to use instinctively the available options in the most efficient way. A subject set to walk on successive days under similar circumstances will reproduce speed and cadence to within 1 per cent. In pathological situations a limp may for that individual be the lowest energy-cost gait, and in these circumstances all efforts to train the patient to walk otherwise will fail.

4. Absorption of the shock of impact of each foot in turn, thereby reducing joint wear. This is achieved by eccentric contraction of muscles.

5. The overall raising of the centre of mass, e.g. going upstairs or a hill.

6. Assorted activities from wrestling to cosmetic display.

In considering the components involved in walking, one way to classify is to divide these into two sets which have been named:

Components of locomotion

Components of gait.

COMPONENTS OF LOCOMOTION

These are mandatory for any form of locomotion and the absence of one will bring the system to a standstill. They consist of:

1. Stabilisation of the multi-segmented structure, the skeleton, both intrinsically and extrinsically.
2. Internal production of energy from muscle and the transmission and modification of this energy through the skeletal segments to the point of external reaction with the contact surface.
3. Appropriate control system, with both redundancy and feedback.

Considering these components in more detail, salient points to be noted are:

1. That for *extrinsic stability* the support base may be divided as in Figure 2/2. It will be seen that when displaced, provided the centre of mass does not go beyond one foot when the displacing force is removed the body falls back on to the full support. This is what happens in walking (Fig. 2/3). It saves energy and when the 'fall back' occurs some inertial energy is available to help the rock on to the other foot.

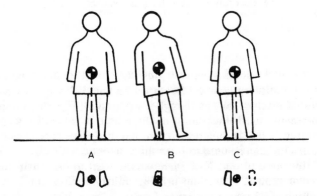

Fig. 2/2   A. A static stable standing position with centre of mass within the support area of the two feet. B. Static stable position with one-foot support area. Clearly not as assured as (A). C. Dynamic stable position – not in itself stable, but will fall back to stable position (A)

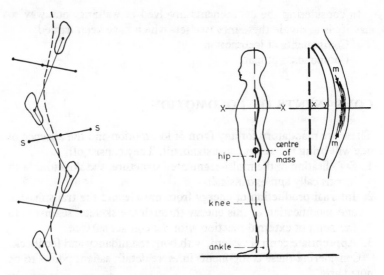

Fig. 2/3 (*left*) The dotted line is the path of the centre of mass. *Note* that it does not go over each foot as this assumes support. S–S is the shoulder line and moves in the opposite direction to the pelvis.

Fig. 2/4 (*right*) Considered as a solid body the average centre of mass of the human body is just in front of sacral vertebra 2. It is fallacious, however, to use a vertical line drawn through this to consider the mechanics of other joints. Apparently at line X–X there is a flexion moment x–y (shown in the enlarged section). If this were the case, in order to maintain this posture, continuous activity of the erector spinae at this level m–m, would be necessary, but in fact this is not shown on EMG

When considering *intrinsic stability* it is often not appreciated that a multi-segmented structure like the skeleton must not be treated mechanically as though it was a solid. Figure 2/4 shows a commonly used illustration of the centre of mass of a standing subject. A line is then drawn through this and it is then said that such a line can be used to show the moments about various joints. If this were true at X-X there would need to be activity in the erector spinae. This is not present and the explanation is shown in Figure 2/5 where the general centre of mass is off-set from the topmost book. This does not fall, for the balance of this book depends only on the relationship of its centre of mass to its support area. When applied to the body it will be seen that one bone

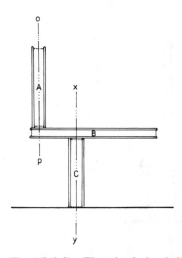

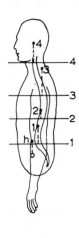

Fig. 2/5 (*left*)   Three books in a balanced stable position. The general centre of mass line x–y is irrelevant when considering the stability of the 'joint' between books A and B. The centre of mass of A lies in line o–p, it is within the support area of A which is therefore stable on B

Fig. 2/6 (*right*)   Considering balance stability about any joint, it will be clear from Fig. 2/5 that the only relevant centre of mass is that of all the portion of the body above that joint. Lines h1, 2, 3 and 4 correspond to hip, lumbo-sacral, thoraco-lumbar, mid-thoracic and mid-cervical articulations, and it will be seen that the centre of mass of the relevant portion of the body is above their respective articulations. Therefore, although the human spine is curved, each segment, is in fact, balanced on the one below it, and requires no muscular effort to support this. It does require muscle activity to maintain the balance

balances on the other, the minimal injection of controlled muscular activity being made as is necessary to maintain this (Fig. 2/6). The overall saving of energy is illustrated well by Figure 2/7. Furthermore, in different postures the position of the centre of mass changes considerably and may be well outside the body (Fig. 2/8). In this situation, of course, continuous muscle activity would be necessary to maintain the posture. It will be observed that the ankles have plantar flexed moving the body backwards in order to keep extrinsic stability, the basis of a well-known party trick.

2. The ground reaction rises upwards through the contact area, and this can be expressed as the *vector*, a line which represents the direction of a force and by its length the amount. Figure 2/9 shows a single such vector displayed at heel strike and the relationship of

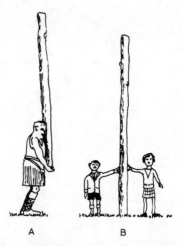

A   B

Fig. 2/7 The energy saving of muscle used to balance as opposed to support. The energy required to hold the caber in A is clearly much greater than in B, particularly if the children have a controlled feedback to act quickly and promptly before the caber has tilted more than very slightly

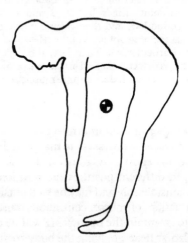

Fig. 2/8 The location of the centre of mass outside the body in this position. It is possible in modern techniques of high jumping that the body goes over the bar and the centre of mass below it. To keep extrinsic stability by moving the centre of mass over the feet the buttocks go backwards. Hence the impossibility of bending forward like this and remaining stable with heels against the wall

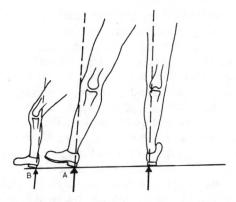

Fig. 2/9 Vector of ground reaction in two planes. *Note* that in this particular case (A) it passes in front of the knee joint and causes an extending moment which stabilises without muscle action. If the knee was flexed (B) due to a contracture the moment will be flexing. In the transverse plane the vector passes through the medial compartment of the knee which is normal

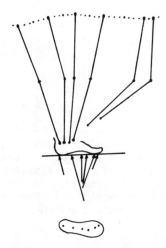

Fig. 2/10 Ground reaction vectors as the foot moves through the stance phase. Note the rise and fall of the hip joint and hence the body centre of mass. *Note* also that the foot is here represented in the mid-stance position to avoid confusion. It is not in this position for the first and last three 'stick' diagrams. The pathway of the vectors along the foot is shown but this does not correspond with pressure under the sole (see text)

this to all joints of the leg and trunk determines the mechanical interrelationship of gravitational and muscle forces about each joint. Figure 2/10 shows the vectors throughout a single stance phase in one plane (they do, of course, vary in the other plane). It will be seen that they move along the foot and alter their relationship to the knee, and therefore, the moment about it, at a time when this also is moving in space.

3. Energy is primarily produced by muscle. The modification of this energy within the segments has been called the 'flux' of energy and is an important concept. It changes through potential, kinetic and inertial forms. For example, the elevation of the body during the first half of stance produces the potential energy storage which is released as kinetic energy during the second half, and then translated into a momentum which assists the next uphill part of stance (Fig. 2/11). The swing leg will have a stored potential energy as the foot comes off the ground. As it swings forwards this becomes kinetic and then as the leg comes to a standstill in space, the inertial energy drags the body forward and this provides an important contribution to propulsion.

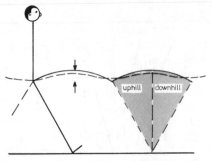

Fig. 2/11 Vaulting action of stance leg considered as a non-articulated limb. *Note* the large rise and fall and jerky acceleration/deceleration produced compared with the normal relatively smooth sinusoidal curve with much less amplitude. This makes clear the 'uphill' phase which requires the injection of energy, largely returned in the downhill, and spilling over to the next uphill as an inertial contribution

COMPONENTS OF GAIT

It is not necessary to have all these in order to maintain movement. They consist of:

1. *Flexion-extension action of the swing leg* (or legs in certain types of

assisted gait, e.g. 'swing-through') which is a compound pendulum, and fundamentally obeys the same laws applicable to this. It has a natural harmonic motion which can be modified by muscle activity. As seen in Figure 2/1, normal flat walking requires very little such activity and it has been demonstrated that in a compound pendulum model with thigh, shank and foot constrained to correspond with the limit of the leg joints the resultant movement of all 'joints' when it was swung closely resembled those in normal walking (Mena et al, 1981). To maintain this movement requires minimal energy, and it is, therefore, related to the optimum individual cadence. The average adult male leg has a harmonic motion of 76 beats per minute, and it is no coincidence that this is the optimally adopted cadence. This leg is carried forward in space by pelvic motion of both horizontal rotation of the pelvis and by:

2. *The vaulting action of the stance leg.* This imposes a rise and fall of the body centre of mass. With a straight leg as in a long-leg caliper this moves as shown in Figure 2/11 and will accelerate and decelerate in a jerky manner. The components of gait are used to smooth out this movement path to an optimum amplitude in all planes and to minimise the acceleration/deceleration change. Of these, the knee has the most profound effect and complete loss of movement here will cause a rise in energy consumption of about 25 per cent (Fishman et al, 1982).

3. *Horizontal rotation of the body at hips and trunk* (normally) and/or at floor/footwear surface (pathologically). The pelvis rotates forward about the stance hip as this goes through the flexion-extension phase. A relative internal rotation of this hip occurs with an external rotation of the swing hip. The effect of this pelvic movement is to increase the forward movement of the subject in space and will increase the stride length by up to 20 per cent.

A contrary rotation, associated with arm movement, will occur in the spine and has an important energy conserving function.

4. *One foot clearance to avoid frictional loss of energy.* It is achieved by a combination of several factors:

(a) Those indicated in (2) and (3) above. Relative shortening of a leg clearly occurs with knee bending as it does with plantar flexion of the contra-lateral foot. Horizontal rotation forward of the pelvis with the stance leg also shortens leg length.

(b) Abduction of the hip of the swing leg occurs in association with adduction of the stance hip combined with stance leg subtalar movement. This produces a lateral movement of the pelvis away from the swing leg. This shifts the body centre of mass towards but not over the stance foot (see Fig. 2/3) and is yet another example of energy exchange or flux.

As one foot is raised the body centre of mass moves over the other foot-support area storing a minimum of energy to produce foot clearance during swing phase, and when this is terminated the system returns to the stable double-foot stance without a further energy contribution by the subject. Shortening of one leg by circumduction may be used in pathological situations, but is only employed when there is no alternative as it adversely moderates the pendulum action.

5. Spinal movements to supplement or replace those in the legs.
6. The inertial contribution of arm movement.

The study of gait is subdivided into: (1) kinematics; (2) kinetics and (3) estimation of total energy cost.

KINEMATICS (ALSO CALLED KINESIOLOGY)

This is the study of the harmonious structure of the pattern of movement in locomotion, analysed in terms of time, space, velocity and acceleration. The basis of this study from the point of view of the clinician is the pattern of angular movement, and the control of this.

A complete gait cycle from the point of view of a single plane can be

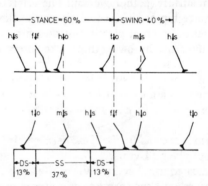

Fig. 2/12   hs=heel strike; ff=foot flat; ho=heel off; to=toe off; ms=mid-swing; DS=double stance; SS=single stance. Sub-divisions of the phases of walking commonly used to describe the events which occur. *Note* the relationship of events in one leg with the other, and that twice in each phase of walking double stance occurs when both touch the ground, and share the load in varying degrees

represented by Figure 2/12 and can easily be memorised by the 'rule of three' for the stance phase:

(a) The hip moves through one full range.

(b) There are two knee flexions, the initial on heel strike which is shock absorbing and modifies the pathway of the centre of mass of the body. Extension then occurs to be followed by a second flexion prior to toe off which then increases during initial swing to allow the foot to go through.

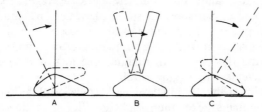

Fig. 2/13 The three rockers, heel (A), ankle (B) and toe (C). *Note* that the shank moves forward during all rockers and also downwards in (A) and upwards in (C)

(c) The three rockers at the ankle-foot complex (Perry, 1967) (Fig. 2/13). These comprise the heel, ankle and toe rocker and it is the ankle rocker which is responsible for the major forward progression of the limb in space as one would anticipate. Because it is furthest from the trunk, a small angular deviation here achieves a relatively large movement forward of the body. The heel rocker is concerned with shock absorption, partly because of the eccentric contraction of the dorsiflexors of the foot which lower this smoothly to the ground, as opposed to the foot slap

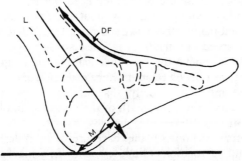

Fig. 2/14 Demonstrates the moment (M) about the contact area of the heel and deceleration of foot slap by dorsiflexors (DF)

generated by the ground reaction moment about the ankle joint when these muscles are paralysed (Fig. 2/14).

This is combined with the shock absorption effect of arch fall through the plantar aponeurosis, and with the calcaneo-contact articulation. The toe rocker is concerned with shear-stress relief, with the advancement of the leg in space and with the smooth transition from stance to swing phase. The average stance phase occupies some 60 per cent of the total cycle of stance and swing. As in the adult the complete cycle averages about 1000 milliseconds, therefore, one stance phase takes 600 milliseconds, and emphasises the problem of direct observation of the many changes which are occurring both simultaneously and sequentially during this period. In running, the total is reduced to 600 milliseconds with jogging at 700.

During swing, the hip flexes with extension of the knee and the foot maintains the optimum slight dorsiflexion to allow clearance. At heel strike the knee is commonly slightly flexed ready for the primary shock-absorbing flexion of stance.

It is a definition of walking that a double-limb support occurs. This happens twice during each stance phase and occupies about 13 per cent (i.e. 130 milliseconds) of the total phase commencing at heel strike for this period and ending after a similar period at toe off. In running and jogging there is a 'float' period with no limb support.

Cadence is the frequency of succession of right and left steps. The stride length is the distance moved in one walking cycle and may be measured between two heel strikes of one leg. Clearly if the subject is to travel in a straight line both stride lengths must be equal. Step length is the distance by which one foot advances beyond the other. While optimally these are equal they need not be so and one can indeed be either zero or negative without any deviation of the body path. The combination of cadence and stride length determine speed. To increase speed one tends to increase stride length rather than cadence as this retains the smoother gait. Stride length is plainly limited by lack of pelvic rotation, knee extension and ankle rocker, but it is less apparent, initially, that limited extension of one hip produces reduction in step length of the other leg and hence stride length of both.

Movements in the other planes have already been dealt with apart from longitudinal rotation of limb segments. In general at heel strike the internal rotation of the limb occurs beginning at the hip and progressively increasing distally. It continues during stance with associated pronation of the foot until heel rise then supination commences and the leg begins to externally rotate. The range of rotation is relatively small, the tibia moving compared with the floor through some 15 degrees – 7 degrees internally and 8 degrees externally – but the shock-absorption function is of considerable importance.

Muscular activity in walking as determined by electromyography can only indicate the phases of muscular activity and not strength at this time. Therefore, this activity comes into the ambit of kinematics. These are illustrated in Figure 2/1 for level walking and are presented in two different ways. This represents a consensus of findings by various investigators among whom there can be quite wide differences because of the age and general build of the subjects used. While this information must not be regarded as absolute for every patient, it does illustrate the general principles agreed by all investigators.

Note should be taken of the concentric and eccentric activities and of the relatively short duration of muscular activity, again saving energy. This relates to the ability of the body to stabilise the joints in relationship to the vectors (see Fig. 2/9). If this becomes impossible, commonly due to joint contractures, then the muscles will need to function perhaps continuously which is tiring, or if, as in a neurological condition, the muscle is very weak or absent it will mean that the patient cannot walk without an orthosis.

Again the movement in the other planes must not be forgotten: knowing that the stance hip abducts one can deduce that the abductors will here be acting eccentrically stabilising the hip under the influence of gravity and this indeed proves to be the case.

It is important to realise that the testing of muscle power in the recumbent position, quite apart from its relative inaccuracy, does not necessarily imply a direct relationship to function. For example, the flexors of the hip may appear relatively weak but when the patient is upright all that these are required to do is to assist the pendulum activity of the leg; thus the usefulness of the weak muscles may be considerable.

KINETICS

Kinetics is the study of the forces that produce or change motion. It is, therefore, concerned with the mechanical stresses on the body both internal and external.

The primary source of mechanical energy is muscle and although the use of this is minimised, some is inevitably required as is the resultant mechanical stress on the bones and joints about which it acts.

Externally we live in a gravitational field and we need both to resist and to use this. The solution to the problem of maintaining intrinsic stability, resisting the gravitational force which makes us tend to collapse in a heap, has been indicated as the avoidance of continual muscular activity to provide support, and the achievement of this by the balancing of one bone on another which uses muscle only as a control mechanism. During walking where a joint is off-set from the mid-line, as is the hip, it is difficult to get the centre of mass of the body completely above the joint in the coronal plane. One has also to consider the force on the joint itself. Figure 2/15 shows the moments about a hip. The forces are BW=body-weight and AM abductor muscles. If BW balances AM to hold the hip in one position, and in this example b=2a, then AM=2BW and the total load on the hip 3BW. This can be reduced in a number of ways:

1. By reducing diet. For every pound (lb) reduction the load on the hip is decreased by three pounds (lbs).
2. By shortening the moment arm (b) – moving the trunk further over the hip.
3. By using a walking stick in the other hand: pressing down on this pushes upwards on the body and again reduces BW.

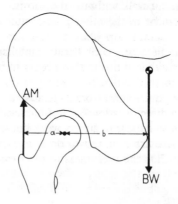

Fig. 2/15 Compressive force on the hip joint. BW=body-weight; AM=abductor muscles; ab=moment arm

The other external force is the ground reaction and we measure this by means of a force platform (force plate). This is a sophisticated electronic and apparently quite immovable plate which when walked upon will measure the stresses to which it has been submitted in all

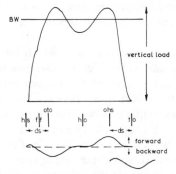

Fig. 2/16 hs=heel strike; ff=foot flat; oto=other toe off; ho=heel off; ohs=other heel strike; to=toe off; ds=double stance
Normal force platform patterns. The characteristic double peak vertical load during stance is seen above, while below the event markings is the pattern of fore and aft reaction of the platform. During the second double-stance phase this pattern for the other foot can be seen to largely cancel the resultant force from the first

planes and produces results as shown in Figure 2/16. It is from these results that the vectors already referred to can be calculated. From these and from the relationship with the various joints, the forces about these joints can be calculated and the results used in the design of prostheses, both external and internal, and of orthoses.

Knowledge of these makes clear the dynamic stabilisation which can occur in the leg while walking and allows this to be carried out even with, for example, a completely paralysed quadriceps muscle (Fig. 2/9). It will be seen that the vector has a moment about the knee joint which resists flexion; provided gait is adjusted to maintain this beneficial moment during the whole of stance no problems are encountered in maintaining stability in the knee despite the absence of an extending muscle. Difficulty is encountered, however, when going down a slope away from the subject and it is in these circumstances only that the knee-stabilising caliper, although worn all the time, actually functions.

To return to the question of 'push-off', it will be seen that at the end of the stance the ground is pushing forwards on the foot in the horizontal plane which suggests that the foot is pushing backwards. From the point of view of one leg this is true but it does not imply the need for any energy to be developed in the leg any more than does a similar ground reaction from the spokes of a wheel. Furthermore, as in the main at this time there is a double stance, it will be observed that there is an equal and opposite reaction in the other leg and the result, therefore, is that the legs do not at this time contribute any resultant backward push.

As the foot is the part of the leg to which the ground reaction is applied it is important to give brief consideration to this, and firstly to note that the vector of ground reaction is a mathematical expression of the resultant of the forces in all planes. The path of the point of application of this as it moves forward along the foot is often expressed in diagrams such as Figure 2/10. This must not be regarded as giving any direct indication of the forces on the sole of the foot, as in the shod patient it can be seen to exist at one time at a point where no contact is made with the foot, between the sole and heel. The stress under the sole of the foot can be divided into pressure (vertical loading) and shear (the horizontal). The sole is designed to tolerate quite high levels of these, but problems arise if these are exceeded.

Pressure is force per unit area and deformities of the foot which reduce the area of application can greatly increase the pressure. Similar results will be produced by increase in force. Walking at a moderate pace the inertial effect of forward movement will raise the force applied to an average of $1\frac{1}{3}$ body-weight which would again be increased if the moment around the heel at contact is not moderated by the mechanism of controlled plantar flexion already indicated. This is further enhanced by the active dorsiflexion of the great toe which, working through the plantar aponeurosis, raises the medial arch of the foot and this is then lowered by the eccentric action of extensor hallucis longus on contact (Fig. 2/17) (Hicks, 1951).

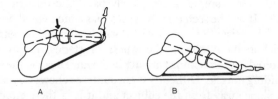

Fig. 2/17   The great toe automatically extends just before heel strike. This tightens the plantar fascia as it is connected through the sesamoid to the base of the proximal phalanx. In turn, this raises the arch by flexion at the navicular-cuneiform joint as shown in A. In B the long extensor has gradually lowered the great toe at foot flat, lowering the arch and absorbing shock

Shear is equally important and indeed many serious problems of ulceration of the foot, as in spina bifida, cannot be solved unless this is eliminated. The normal mechanism is the provision of the specialised fibro-fatty subcutaneous tissue under the heel and metatarsal heads. With the skin in contact with the ground and therefore stationary, this allows a forward rolling of the calcaneus on heel contact and of the metatarsal heads at the toe rocker (Fig. 2/18) (Rose, 1958; 1962; 1982).

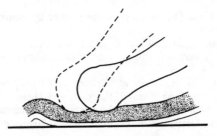

Fig. 2/18 At toe rocker the first metatarsal head rolls forward in the fibro-fatty tissue while the skin remains still in contact with the ground, thus absorbing shear. A similar mechanism occurs at heel strike in the so-called calcaneo-contact articulation

CONCLUSION

Gait is an extremely complex function, and studies even of small parts have occupied many whole books. Both the understanding and the observation of gait require very considerable study if it is to be understood. It is important to remember that each patient has a complex feedback computerised control system, and where disagreement arises between a patient and the rules a physiotherapist has been taught, it is wise to give consideration to the situation in the light of the general principles here indicated. Recently, a patient with an osteoarthritic hip fiercely resisted the instruction to use her stick in the hand opposite to the hip. (In general this advice is correct, for pressure downwards on the stick will then assist the abductors of the affected hip and relieve the pressure on the hip joint.) In this particular case, however, she had a marked adduction deformity and her overriding need was to maintain extrinsic stability which she could only do by using the stick in the same hand. It was little gain to her to diminish the pressure on her hip joint if she fell over!

REFERENCES

Fishman, S. et al (1982). *Metabolic Measures in the Evaluation of Prosthetic and Orthotic Devices*. Research Division, College of Engineering, New York University.

Hicks, J. H. (1951). The function of the plantar aponeurosis. *Journal of Anatomy*, 85, 414.

Mena, D., Mansour, J.M. and Simon, S.R. (1981). Analysis and synthesis of human swing leg motion during gait, and its clinical applications. *Journal of Biomechanics*, 14, 12, 823.

Perry, J. (1967). *The Mechanics of Walking. A Clinical Interpretation*. In *Principles of Lower-Limb Bracing* (Perry, J. and Hislop. H.J. (eds)), pp 9–32. American Physical Therapy Association, Washington, USA.

Rose, G.K. (1958). Correction of the pronated foot. *Journal of Bone and Joint Surgery*, 40B, 674.

Rose, G.K. (1962). Correction of the pronated foot. *Journal of Bone and Joint Surgery*, 44B, 642.

Rose, G. K. (1982). *Pes Planus*. In *Disorders of the Foot* (Jahss, M.H. (ed)). W.B. Saunders Co, Philadelphia.

BIBLIOGRAPHY

Basmajian, J.V. (1978). *Muscles Alive*. Williams and Wilkins Co, Baltimore.

Broer, M. (1973). *Efficiency of Human Movement*. W.B. Saunders Co, Philadelphia.

Brunnstrom, S. (1972). *Clinical Kinesiology*. F.A. Davis Co, Philadelphia.

Higgins, J.R. (1977). *Human Movement, An Integrated Approach*. C.V. Mosby Co, St Louis.

Wells, K.F. and Luttgens, K. (1976). *Kinesiology. Scientific Basis of Human Motion*. W.B. Saunders Co, Philadelphia.

Chapter 3

Applied Gait Assessment

by P.B. BUTLER, MSc, MCSP

The mandatory components of locomotion and the components of gait have been examined in Chapter 2. It is now proposed to extend this concept further to see how the therapist may approach gait assessment and the techniques that are available. The process of gait assessment may be divided into three stages:

1. The gait itself is examined and analysed.
2. One or more theories are formulated to explain particular features of the patient's gait and a solution is proposed. This is probably the most important stage. Full consideration must be given to all the implications of the proposal, a point which will be considered in greater depth in a later example. The solution may include therapy, surgery or orthotic prescription.
3. In the experimental stage the solution is put into practice.

This process takes the form of a flow diagram, so that ideally the analytical process will continue until a satisfactory end-point is reached (Fig. 3/1). This may be achieved almost immediately by, for example, the provision of a walking aid, or may involve a much longer time-scale if extensive therapy is required.

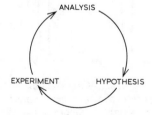

Fig. 3/1   Flow diagram of gait assessment

COMPONENTS OF GAIT ASSESSMENT

There are four main areas involved in gait assessment:
    Kinematics: monitoring gait patterns
    Kinetics: measurement of forces
    Electromyography: monitoring muscle activity
    Efficiency: monitoring performance, for example by speed and
    heart rate.

PRELIMINARY ASSESSMENT

Analysis of a patient's gait should first be put into its context. A careful
history will reveal what the patient finds to be his major problems, the
duration and degree of his signs and symptoms, particularly pain, and
the effect of these on his lifestyle. All aspects of mobility thus become
a part of gait assessment and will include rising from sitting and
climbing stairs. It is important to discover the patient's own solutions
to his problems, as these can give valuable guidance about profitable
areas of experimental solutions.

EXAMPLE 1
A patient stated that she found walking easier when carrying her
shopping bag in the right hand. Examination revealed weak right hip
abductors and a positive Trendelenburg sign. Carrying a weight in the
right hand brought the centre of mass of the trunk, head and arms
towards the hip joint without the compensatory body sway otherwise
involved (Fig. 3/2).

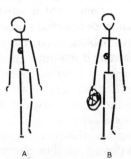

A   B

Fig. 3/2   A. Mid-stance right leg. Weak right hip abductors. Compensatory
body sway used to bring centre of mass of head, arms and trunk over right hip.
B. Mid-stance right leg. Weight of shopping bag eliminates compensatory
movement

Following the functional history the patient is examined in recumbency and the range of movement of the limbs and spine recorded, together with sensory status and proprioception, muscle power and tone and degree and type of pain. It should be remembered that the range of movement during walking can often differ considerably from that found in examination of the patient.

Equally important is examination in standing. The posture may be observed together with the effect of the upright position on muscle tone or weakness. The patient is asked to stand first on one leg and then on the other, revealing problems of balance and control, or of isolated muscle weakness. A note is made of the walking aids used. Inspection of the shoes – the uppers, inside and soles – can give many useful clues about walking patterns.

Gait assessment continues using each of the four aspects as appropriate for each patient.

KINEMATICS

This is the study of the *gait patterns* and *geometry* of walking. The key to this is observation, which is made easier and more successful by a visual recording of the gait. This recording serves two functions: first, it permits detailed analysis at the time of assessment and, second, it provides a permanent record for later comparison, perhaps at intervals of one year or more.

Visual recording

There are two common methods of visual recording, namely video and film. The most successful in a clinical environment is video, as it permits immediate replay. Thus the three stages of assessment can take place immediately and the effect of an experimental solution such as a walking stick or orthosis can be seen. Film has the advantage, as does high-speed photography, of avoiding the acceleration blur of the swing leg but if film is used it will require processing before viewing and the immediacy of the results is lost. Recent advances in high-speed video eliminate acceleration blur. Video has the further advantage in that being an electronic system it allows other electronically monitored physiological or physical data to be mixed directly for display on the video screen, for example, the ground reaction force.

Both video and film may be replayed in slow motion so permitting a more detailed and accurate assessment than by observation alone.

These visual recording methods do require equipment which can be expensive and will still require careful observation to be successful. Many therapists will not have access to visual recording equipment. They will need to develop expertise in gait analysis while the patient is walking at normal speed, and to do so quickly for patients who have a low exercise tolerance.

Written records

It is essential to note findings in gait analysis for future reference and this may be done in written form, by some diagrammatic means, or by a graphical notation such as Benesh Movement Notation (McGuinness-Scott, 1982).

Observation of the patient

Observation and analysis should be made in three planes – sagittal, coronal and horizontal (overhead) – although often it will be possible to use only the first two. The patient should be observed from the right and left lateral view, from the front and from behind and if possible from overhead. Close-ups can provide much specific information, and the therapist without visual recording facilities should be prepared to look closely at particular joints, walking alongside the patient if necessary.

Initial analysis

When commencing the analysis it is helpful first to make an overall judgement about the gait which can provide many clues.

EXAMPLE 2

A 10-year-old girl presented with an uncertain, hesitant appearance when walking barefoot and a happy confidence when in shoes. She had bilateral tightness of the tendo calcaneus and so did not have the option of putting her heel to the ground when walking barefoot (Fig. 3/3a). She thus had a small support area with consequent decrease in balance and confidence. The heel height of her shoes (which she had chosen herself) compensated exactly for the tightness of her tendo calcaneus, resulting in a steady confident walk with increased step length (Fig. 3/3b).

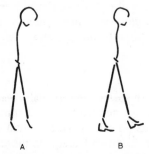

A	B

Fig. 3/3 A. Toe-stepping gait caused by tight tendo calcaneus. B. Heel
height of shoes compensates for tightness of tendo calcaneus

Further analysis

There are three main aspects to be considered when analysing gait:
1. The sequence in which events occur.
2. The range of movement of the joints.
   (1 and 2 will encompass the components of gait.)
3. Closely associated with these is the timing in which events occur.

Thus in the lateral view the sequence of events which form one
stride can be noted (see Fig. 2/12, p. 52) and the positions of the arms,
head, trunk and legs observed. A simple example of disturbed
sequence is the patient who has a toe strike before putting the foot flat,
and then goes to toe off. Inspection of range of motion during walking
will reveal such abnormalities as a flexion deformity. A deformity in
one joint almost always creates a compensatory movement in another
joint in the same plane. For example, a fixed flexion deformity at the
knee will result in flexion at the hip during walking to keep the centre
of mass over the base of support (Fig. 3/4). Similarly a fixed flexion

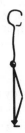

Fig. 3/4 Fixed flexion of knee with compensatory flexion of hip to keep
centre of mass over base of support

deformity at the hip will result in a flexed knee. This highlights an important aspect of gait assessment, namely that of isolating cause from effect, and correct interpretation will lead to successful recommendation.

EXAMPLE 3a
A boy of 12 years with spastic cerebral palsy was noted to walk on his toes with grossly hyperextended knees. Examination showed that he had bilateral tight tendo calcaneus, a normal range of knee flexion with slight hyperextension and adequate musculature. Gait analysis showed that his problems were twofold:

1. A control problem imposed by his cerebral palsy giving imbalance between his dorsal and plantar flexors and causing him to have an equinus. The plantar flexors contracted so limiting his range of movement.
2. This limited ankle range gave a mechanical problem of joint movement pattern.

The fixed equinus caused abnormal moments which pushed the knee into hyperextension (Fig. 3/5a). Surgery to elongate the tendo calcaneus overcame the problem and the boy was able to obtain a more normal gait with a reduction of knee stress (Fig. 3/5b).

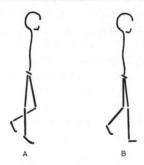

A   B

Fig. 3/5   A. Fixed equinus causing abnormal moments and pushing knee into hyperextension. B. Elongation of tendo calcaneus overcomes this problem and a more normal gait results with a reduction of knee stress

EXAMPLE 3b
A 7-year-old boy with muscular dystrophy presented with a similar problem at first view. He had a toe-stepping gait with tightness of the tendo calcaneus, normal knee range but weak quadriceps muscles. However, this child's problems were very different from the preceding case, being (1) the limited range of movement at his ankle

and (2) stabilisation of a multi-segmented structure (the leg) because of weak musculature.

Elongation of the tendo calcaneus had been considered, but the necessity of considering all the implications of a solution is shown very clearly here. This child was using the mechanical effect of his equinus to produce an extending moment to stabilise his knee during stance phase and so compensate for his quadriceps weakness. If this facility were removed by tendon elongation, it is very probable that he would not then have sufficient knee stability to walk at all. This child required careful follow-up to ensure that he did not develop knee flexion deformity.

EXAMPLE 4

An elderly man with an arthritic right knee and severely restricted flexion was noted to walk with circumduction of the right leg in swing phase and lateral tilting of the trunk to the left. He had elected to compensate in this way for his inability to clear the right foot from the ground by the normal knee flexion (Fig. 3/6a). Another patient with a similar problem – an ankylosed right knee in a man of 35 years following a road traffic accident – opted to use increased plantar flexion of the left ankle to clear the right leg (Fig. 3/6b). The elderly man found that he was more stable using circumduction than rising on to his toe and with his slower gait the method he adopted was more energy efficient. The younger man preferred the cosmesis of rising on to his toe and accepted the slight increase in energy cost. Each patient will instinctively make use of the available options in his own preferred way.

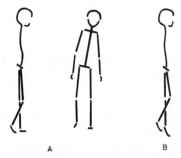

A   B

Fig. 3/6   A. A fixed flexion deformity at the right knee prevents normal swing-through. Circumduction and lateral tilt are used to compensate for loss of knee flexion and to clear the foot. B. Fixed knee flexion in this patient is compensated by increased plantar flexion

Observation of the anterior and posterior views will reveal such problems as increased lateral trunk sway and deformities of the hip, knee and subtalar joint in the coronal plane. Width of base can be noted.

EXAMPLE 5

A lady with long-standing rheumatoid arthritis complained of pain in the left knee on weight-bearing. Gait analysis showed an abnormal range of motion. There was laxity of the medial collateral ligament with joint instability giving a deforming moment about the knee at mid-stance (Fig. 3/7a). Examination had shown this deformity to be fully correctable, and an orthotic solution was proposed. An orthosis applying three-point-fixation held the knee in correct alignment, and pain was reduced on weight-bearing (Fig. 3/7b).

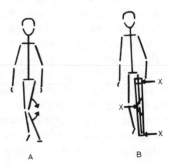

Fig. 3/7 A. Left mid-stance. Instability of the knee gives a deforming moment about the knee. B. Left mid-stance. An orthosis applying three-point fixation (xxx) holds the knee in the correct position

The overhead view provides additional information about horizontal rotations to that obtained from the other views.

EXAMPLE 6

A child with cerebral palsy wore out his shoes in one month on the antero-medial aspect of the uppers. Examination revealed an absence of external rotation and extension at the hips and limited internal rotation. Gait analysis in shoes showed:
1. a control problem imposed by the cerebral palsy with muscle imbalance at the hips leading to muscle contractures; and
2. this resulted in a reduced range of motion at the hips with no

extension or external rotation possible and subsequent effect on pelvic movement.

Barefoot, the child found walking slow and difficult with a short step length. Normally the hip externally rotates in swing phase (Fig. 3/8a), and internally rotates in stance. This child had no external rotation and so the hip was already in internal rotation as the foot grounded with no further pelvic movement available (Fig. 3/8b). The only way that the pelvis could complete rotation was by rotation at the foot/ground interface. The shoes were assisting gait because of the reduced friction between shoe and ground compared with foot and ground. The penalty was wear of the shoes which was difficult to eliminate if the child was to continue to walk.

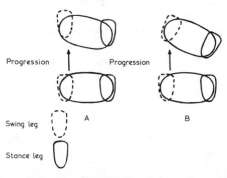

Fig. 3/8 A. Normal situation. Pelvis viewed from above. The swing leg externally rotates at the hip and the stance leg internally rotates. B. Child with cerebral palsy and little rotation at the hips. No external rotation available and the swing leg grounds in slight internal rotation. No further internal rotation available and pelvis completes rotation at the foot/ground interface

It is useful to take measurements of particular features of gait, such as abnormal joint angles. Step and stride length can be measured providing valuable follow-up information.

A simple and convenient method of measuring step length is to stick paint-soaked felt pads to the patient's shoes. Two rectangles of orthopaedic felt approximately 1.5cm×1cm are stripped of the surface felt until 2–3mm thick. This provides an absorbent surface for the paint. Washable water colour is used, a different colour for right and left shoes. The pads are stuck to the *front* edge of the heel (Fig. 3/9) and not on the posterior edge which may cause the patient to slip. The patient walks across a washable floor or length of paper. A

Fig. 3/9 To show optimal position of paint soaked pads for measuring step length. On *heels* if heel strike obtained; on *lateral border* if no heel strike

distance of at least 6 metres (20ft) permits the patient to get into a normal stride and to exclude the last few decelerating steps, the middle section being measured.

The time taken for the events of one stride will supply further information on the nature of the patient's problems. It includes comparison of the duration of swing and stance phase on each leg. Thus a patient with a painful hip may present with a pain-avoiding (antalgic) gait and have a shorter stance phase on the affected leg.

KINETICS

This is measurement of the *forces* involved in walking. There are two types of force to be considered:
1. The external forces such as the ground reaction force.
2. The internal forces of the body, such as individual muscle forces which are, at present, largely unquantifiable during gait.

Ground reaction force

The ground reaction force can be measured, and force platforms (force plates) are used to monitor both the horizontal and vertical components. The patient walks over a force platform, set flush into a walkway, and the components of force, which are equal and opposite to that exerted by the patient, are registered. A vector of this ground reaction force can then be constructed (Fig. 3/10).

In example 5 (p. 68), the lady with an unstable rheumatoid knee will have a ground reaction vector as in Figure 3/11b with a large valgus-deforming moment acting about the joint. The effect of the orthosis can also be seen (Fig. 3/11c). This is an extreme example, but even subtle changes in force can result in the ground reaction vector passing to one side or the other of the joint centre, so changing the

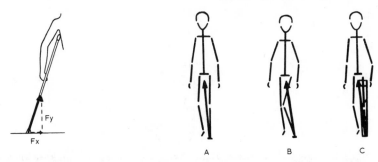

Fig. 3/10 Ground reaction vector to a crutch. Fy=vertical component; Fx=horizontal component

Fig. 3/11 A. Normal ground reaction vector mid-stance left leg. (*Note*: Vector passes slightly medial to knee joint axis.) B. Instability of the knee. Left mid-stance. Large deforming moment about the knee. C. Orthosis controls knee instability and a normal vector results

direction of the moment. Such changes may be apparent to the experienced eye without the use of force monitoring but there will be many occasions when the changes are detected only with this type of instrumentation, particularly for the beginner in such studies.

Reference back to the two cases involving hyperextended knees (examples 3a (p. 66) and 3b (p. 66)) will show how important monitoring ground reaction force can be. In example 3a, the boy with spastic cerebral palsy, the vector was seen to pass well in front of the knee (Fig. 3/12a) which produced a very large knee-extending moment so causing abnormal stresses in the knee. However, despite apparently similar kinematics, example 3b, the boy with muscular

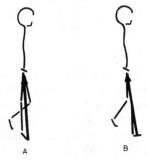

Fig. 3/12 A. Vector passes in front of knee producing a large knee-extending moment. B. Post-surgery. Vector passes through knee joint

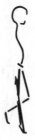

Fig. 3/13   Boy with muscular dystrophy. Vector passes through knee joint centre. Surgery could cause vector to pass behind knee and muscles are not strong enough to counteract this

dystrophy, had a vector which passed through the centre of the knee thus eliminating any moment (Fig. 3/13). In his case, surgery would almost certainly have caused the vector to pass behind the knee joint centre, thus producing a knee-flexing moment which his weak quadriceps would have difficulty in opposing.

The therapist should be aware of the forces involved in gait and their possible effects, although their measurement and interpretation is a specialty.

ELECTROMYOGRAPHY

This is a rapidly expanding field in which *muscle activity* is monitored during joint movement and walking. Again it is a specialised area and requires instrumentation. It is possible to monitor the phasic activity of various muscles and discover which muscles work in stance or swing phase and at which parts of the phase. This can then be related to the kinematic and kinetic data, for example to determine which muscle group is causing a particular movement or abnormal vector.

EXAMPLE 7
Assessment of a young man with early muscular dystrophy showed that he had a typical myopathic posture, with fixed flexion deformities of 15 degrees at the knees and 10 degrees at the hips with weakness of hip and knee extensors (Fig. 3/14a). Because of the weakness of his extensors this patient needed to place the vertical plane of the centre of mass of his head, trunk and arms through or behind his hip joints. He attempted to achieve this by extending his spine, although his flexion contractures made it more difficult. His ground reaction vector

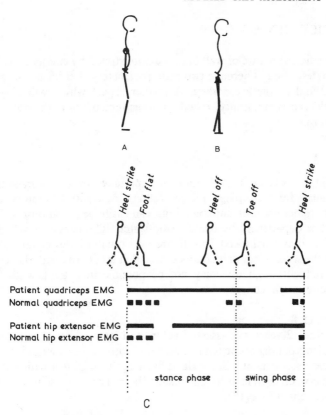

Fig. 3/14 A. Typical myopathic posture. Extension of spine to place vertical plane of centre of mass of head, trunk and arms near hip joints. B. Vector passes in front of hips. C. Electromyographic studies showed extensor muscle action in all phases of gait in this patient

showed that, despite his extended spine, the origin of the vector was forward on his feet and the vector passed in front of his hip, thus producing a hip flexing moment (Fig. 3/14b). Electromyographic studies of his hip extensors and quadriceps confirmed that he did not quite succeed in placing the vertical plane of the centre of mass behind the hip axis. He therefore needed and demonstrated considerable extensor muscle action during all phases of gait (Fig. 3/14c). Follow-up of this patient included ensuring that his hip and knee flexion contractures did not increase, as this could prevent his walking.

EFFICIENCY OF GAIT

The efficient nature of walking, as demonstrated by energy cost, has been described. There are two main parameters of efficiency of gait, *speed* and *energy expenditure*. A further aspect which will also be considered is endurance, based on measurements of both speed and heart rate.

Speed

Speed is easily calculated from the time taken to walk a measured distance, for example 6 metres (20ft). In a gait laboratory this measurement will be automated but can easily be accomplished in a ward or department by using a stop-watch. The patient is asked to walk at his normal speed. Results are more reliable if timings are taken after the second length is completed, so that familiarity with the test is ensured, although this may not be possible in patients with low exercise tolerance.

EXAMPLE 8

A girl of 12 years was assessed before and after calcaneal osteotomy with lengthening of the tendo calcaneus, with a seven-month interval between assessments. She walked five lengths of 20 feet with a short rest between each length. The results showed an increase in speed of 46 per cent (Fig. 3/15).

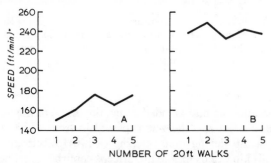

Fig. 3/15 A. Pre-operative speed over 5 walks. B. Postoperative speed over 5 walks

Heart rate

Heart rate has been shown to be a reliable parameter of energy expenditure (Astrand and Rhyming, 1954; Rowell, Hayler and Wang,

1964) and to increase linearly with work load at submaximal levels (Bengtsson, 1956; Bradfield, Paulos and Grossman, 1971; Poulsen and Asmussen, 1962; Wahlund, 1948). It is preferable in a clinical context than assessment of energy expenditure by oxygen uptake, which usually involves wearing a nose-clip and breathing through a mouthpiece with collection of expired air. Heart rate is not a quantitative method of energy cost and indeed at this time no reliable or reproducible method exists. When combined with speed and cadence (number of steps per minute) it provides a useful baseline in gait assessment.

Factors other than energy expenditure can affect heart rate, the most notable being emotional stress. It is recognised, however, that this diminishes markedly when work is undertaken (Astrand and Rhodahl, 1970). The effects of both emotional stress and other factors, such as ambient temperature, which affect heart rate, can also be diminished by careful control of the environment in which tests are performed.

There are a number of methods of monitoring heart rate, and these are given below in decreasing order of complexity. It should be noted that the confidence that can be placed in the results decreases with each method, for the given reasons.

1. *Telemetry of electrocardiogram.* Surface chest electrodes can be used to obtain a signal, and telemetry of this signal means that the apparatus need not be restricting on the patient or involve a trailing cable (Khan, Thomasson and Rose, 1975; Stallard et al, 1978). This is the most reliable method of obtaining information for patients who are walking.

2. *Lightweight beat to beat pulse meters.* These can be worn by the patient and readings taken during gait. This measurement is liable to prove difficult and readings will be more easily made when the patient has stopped walking. However, recording of pulse rate in connection with work should take place during work, or, as in this case, at the instant that the patient stops walking.

3. *Monitoring of recovery rate.* This may be done manually or using either of the previous two methods. In the same individual the correlation coefficient between the pulse rate during submaximal work and $1-1\frac{1}{2}$ minutes after the work may be high and has been shown to be $r=0.96$ (Astrand and Rhodahl, 1970). Thus although the reliability of this measurement is less because the patient is no longer walking, it can provide a useful guide if no other method is available.

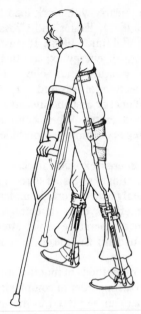

Fig. 3/16 Hip-guidance orthosis (hgo). This can provide effective low energy reciprocal, as opposed to swing-through ambulation with crutches for patients with spinal cord lesions of L1 and above

EXAMPLE 9

A patient was prescribed a hip-guidance orthosis (hgo) (Fig. 3/16) (Rose 1979), as an interim learning device, after which it was considered that he would graduate to knee-ankle-foot orthoses (KAFOs or long-leg calipers) only. The change to KAFOs was monitored carefully over a series of weekly assessments, starting with an initial assessment in an hgo, in which heart rate was monitored by telemetry (Fig. 3/17a). When the patient's performance had reached a plateau, assessment showed that ambulation was costing 10 beats per minute (bpm) more than with an hgo (Fig. 3/17b). Inclusion of speeds on these two tests made a more complete measure of efficiency. It is clearly seen that he walked 20 per cent slower in KAFOs. On this basis a decision was taken to return him to a hip-guidance orthosis.

Endurance

Monitoring speed and heart rate can provide useful information in the less heavily handicapped patient. If a patient with near normal

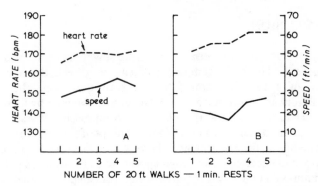

Fig. 3/17 Monitoring heart rate: A. Trial 1: Hip-guidance orthosis (hgo) and crutches. B. Trial 2: (3 months later) Knee-ankle-foot orthoses (KAFOs) and crutches

exercise tolerance is requested to walk continuously, a more representative picture of his problem may emerge.

EXAMPLE 10

Two comparative trials were made of a patient walking consecutive 80-feet lengths until tired, one without orthoses and one after $5\frac{1}{2}$ months' practice with bilateral plastic below-knee fixed ankle orthoses. The improvement in both speed, heart rate and distance walked is shown (Fig. 3/18).

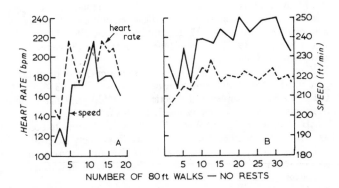

Fig. 3/18 Monitoring endurance: A. Trial 1: No orthoses. B. Trial 2: (6 months later) Bilateral ankle-foot orthoses (AFOs). Endurance test showed improvement in speed, heart rate and total distance walked

CONCLUSION

Many of the patients seen by a therapist will benefit from gait assessment. The more complex problems may need the help and advice of a gait laboratory, but in both these and the more straightforward cases much useful data can be obtained by following the preceding guidelines. It is necessary to approach gait assessment in an organised manner, and retain the concept of analysis, formation of hypothesis and experiment. There is no substitute for thought, practice and experience, and what appears to be the solution with the first impression may well require further assessment and analysis.

REFERENCES

Astrand, P.O. and Rhyming, I. (1954). A nomogram for calculation of aerobic capacity (physical fitness) from pulse rate during submaximal work. *Journal of Applied Physiology*, **7**, 218.

Astrand, P.O. and Rhodahl, K. (1970). *Textbook of Work Physiology.* McGraw Hill, New York.

Bengtsson, E. (1956). The working capacity in normal children evaluated by submaximal exercise on the bicycle ergometer and compared with adults. *Acta Medica Scandinavica*, **154**, 91–109.

Bradfield, R.B., Paulos, J. and Grossman, L. (1971). Energy expenditure and heart rate of obese high school girls. *American Journal of Clinical Nutrition*, **24**, 1482–8.

Khan, A., Thomasson, H. and Rose, G.K. (1975). A method for assessing the physiological cost of doing work in handicapped children. *Developmental Medicine and Child Neurology*, **17**, 6, Supplement 35, 159–60.

McGuinness-Scott, J. (1982). *Benesh Movement Notation.* Chartered Society of Physiotherapy, London.

Poulsen, E. and Asmussen, A. (1962). Energy requirements of practical jobs from the pulse increase and ergometer test. *Ergonomics*, **5**, 33–6.

Rose, G.K. (1979). Principles and practice of the hip guidance orthosis. *Prosthetics and Orthotics, International*, **3**, 1, 37–43.

Rowell, L.B., Hayler, H.L. and Wang, Y. (1964). Limitations to prediction of maximal oxygen uptake. *Journal of Applied Physiology*, **19**, 919.

Stallard, J., Rose, G.K., Tait, J.H. and Davies, J.B. (1978). Assessment of orthoses by means of speed and heart rate. *Journal of Medical Engineering and Technology*, **2**, 1, 22–4.

Wahlund, H. (1948). Determination of physical working capacity; physiological and clinical study with special reference to standardisation of cardio-pulmonary functional tests. *Acta Medica Scandinavica Supplement*, **215**, 132, 1–78.

BIBLIOGRAPHY

Carlsoo, S. (1972). *How Man Moves*. William Heinemann Limited, London. *See also* Bibliography on page 60.

Chapter 4

Footwear

by G.K. ROSE, OBE, FRCS

While the earliest records of the human race, both pictorial and written, represented man as shod it must be remembered that a very large proportion of the world's population at this time goes barefooted over rough terrain without, apparently, grave disadvantages. The specialised tissues, both skin and subcutaneous, of the sole of the foot readily undergo hypertrophic changes to provide the necessary toughness and insensitivity to allow walking in these circumstances.

It is important to recognise that not every thickening of the skin as seen on the normally shod foot is the cause of problems and requires to be removed but can be a useful adaptive protective change to pressure resulting in a satisfactory function. The wearing of foot covering almost from the beginning served many functions, ranging from protection against mechanical and thermal traumata through to decorative and social purposes, such as indicating status (in Egypt Princes had always to appear unshod in the presence of the Pharaoh), or so limiting walking capacity to indicate that the owners were so rich as to have no need to indulge in this vulgar practice. Elevating the heel occurred in the 15th century and shoe heels have varied in height and style since. Sometimes heel elevation was combined with a raise of the sole (the patten) (Fig. 4/1) to elevate the foot above the contamination of the street; but often it was confined to the heel to make the wearer look taller and to give a stiffer, more upright, posture.

Only fairly recently were left and right boots made, and an even more recent change has been the considerable decline in the use of firm boots which provide protection for the ankle. It is not always realised that the subtalar joint is level with the upper border of a man's shoe (see Fig. 4/5) and this therefore exerts no control over this joint nor the ankle directly. Partly because of this, tilting alterations to the outside of the shoe will often have little effect on the foot itself.

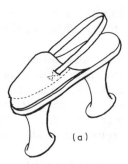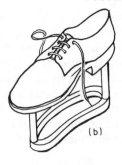

Fig. 4/1 (a) Mediaeval patten often put over other footwear. (b) Modern metal patten used now almost exclusively to lengthen the good leg when the other is treated for Perthes' disease with an elongated patten-ended caliper

Another development which has occurred in recent years has been the introduction of man-made materials and consequently a revolution in manufacturing processes. The basic requirement still remains: a *last*. This is a wooden or plastic positive which dictates the exact shape, size and fit of the shoes built upon them. Emphatically it has to be understood that a last is not a cast. It might be thought that if a careful weight-bearing plaster cast was made of the foot and a shoe then constructed upon this that it must be a perfect comfortable fit, but this is far from the case as the following allowances have to be made:

1. Alteration of foot shape in walking – the normal rise and fall of the arches combined with supination and pronation which occurs with every step.
2. That the shoe itself varies in shape during walking. This is particularly so in the area of the creases over the base of the toes.
3. That 'suspension' must be provided. This term is used by prosthetists to indicate the measures taken to prevent an artificial leg falling off during the swing phase. In the shoe this requires a narrowing of the back to grasp the heel area, and some form of hold over the forefoot without deforming the foot. This also reduces the tendency of the foot during stance to push forward initially and then backwards and so avoids blistering.
4. That allowance has to be made for growth in children.
5. The manufacturer endeavours to provide shoes which will be a safe, acceptable, non-deforming fit for as wide a range of people as is possible of each size, making allowance for the variations which occur in length and width.

Last making is, therefore, both a science and an art, but no-one has yet produced that much sought design of the fashion world in which the inside is larger than the outside!

On the last, the orthodox method is to stretch leathers of varying characteristics to produce the upper with some stiffening in the toe and in the heel to prevent it being trodden down, combined with an appropriate lining. The parts of the upper are stitched together and this is then stitched to the sole which is stiffened with a metal or wooden strip running from the area where the heel is added forward to the tread.

In the modern mass-produced shoe, while some stitching may be used in the uppers (although even here with synthetic materials an appearance of stitching may be moulded on) the heel and sole components are either cemented to the upper, or are moulded directly in position bonding with the upper during this process. From the point of view of shoe alterations the important difference is that whereas previously it was possible to take the shoe partly to pieces and insert, for example, a caliper heel socket and then reconstruct the shoe, this cannot now be done particularly as the heel may be found to be of a honeycomb structure. It has imposed on the orthotist a need to study modern adhesive techniques and in this case to cut off the heel and then to cement on another of solid construction.

The advent of man-made materials focussed attention on an important aspect of shoe construction, namely the need to allow for the escape of perspiration. Investigation shows that a leather sole allows a negligible proportion of sweat to escape through it, so that there is, in this respect, no disadvantage in replacing leather by the longer-wearing modern plastics. Perhaps the largest proportion of moisture is removed from the shoe by the air sucked in and expressed around the foot during the various phases of walking. A very moderate proportion passes through a leather upper. Importantly, however, the amount lost by all these methods does not equal that produced, so that at the end of a day the shoe is wetter than in the morning – and frequently this does not completely disappear by the next morning. Ideally, therefore, no pair of shoes should be worn on successive days. The early man-made materials were completely impervious to water, but later developments have improved this situation although they do not equal leather. Particularly impervious are those shoes with a high shine which is produced by coating them with a secondary plastic layer. Similarly, these materials may provide good thermal insulation and heat discomfort is a common complaint of patients with rheumatoid arthritis who are provided with moulded plastic shoes, although many tolerate this because of other advantages. Another factor with these materials is that the creases produced inside the shoe can be sharper and harder than those of leather and this can cause problems.

In considering shoe modifications in the medical field these can be classified as regards their function as follows:

1. *Intrinsic*: designed to cause some change in posture and/or mechanical stresses within the foot.
2. *Extrinsic*: designed to cause optimum distribution of mechanical stresses on the outer surfaces of the foot. These can be sub-divided into (a) *encasement*, in general the area of the upper and (b) *inevitable*, those under the sole of the foot which cannot be avoided in the act of walking. These can be further sub-divided into (i) pressure stress and (ii) shear stress.

Intrinsic

Two very different situations occur here:

(A) The mobile postural deformity, e.g. the hypermobile pronated (flat) foot.
(B) Deformity rigid in one or more planes, e.g. in inversion the spasmodic valgus, or in several planes the rheumatoid pronated foot.

The important difference is the degree of interface pressure between the foot and the orthosis used. In (A), once the unstable foot (see Fig. 7/19, p. 135) is placed in the stable position which will occur when the orthosis is put on, the body-weight passes through the bony architecture of the foot when the force applied by the orthosis is very slight (see Chapter 7). In (B) the situation is very different and there may be a substantial force at the interface either due to muscle spasm resisting correction or to the fact, as in the rheumatoid foot, that a large proportion of body-weight is applied here. The best that can be done in such circumstances is to diminish the pressure by increasing, as far as possible, the area of application remembering that pressure equals force/area. To some extent the patient may diminish the problem by walking slowly as this diminishes the vertical load deriving from body-weight. In cases of muscle spasm, either discomfort or the corrective effect of the orthosis will sometimes increase the spasm and the hindfoot can then be forced out of the shoe.

It can be seen that it is important in these circumstances to ask oneself whether the device is corrective or supportive; if it is corrective, what is the degree of resistance to correction and what force will then have to be applied. If it is supportive, how badly is the foot deformed and, therefore, what support will be required, but in both circumstances to estimate whether the interface pressure can be tolerated by the patient.

Extrinsic

Encasement has already been dealt with in considering the relationship between a cast of the foot and a last.

In *pressure stress* the load is optimally distributed over the largest area and in this respect it can be seen that the broad print of a 'flat foot' is much less likely to cause trouble than the relatively small area of a cavus foot (Fig. 4/2). Where, in the sole of any foot, there is a very

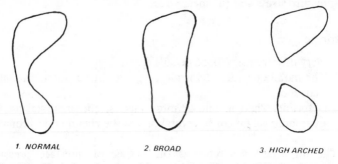

1. NORMAL   *2. BROAD*   *3. HIGH ARCHED*

Fig. 4/2 Variations in area of force application with different foot types

local prominence, as will occur with a clawed toe where the tightening of the plantar fascia forces the corresponding metatarsal head through the sole tissue, it is customary to try and diminish the pressure from this area by the use of an insole on which is mounted a leather-covered foam metatarsal dome or bar of varying softness (Fig. 4/3). This should only be used where the pressure is relatively minor, or as a temporary measure in more severe cases, for as time goes on the pressure of the dome itself, particularly if very firm, will cause atrophy of the tissues on which it presses with a consequent hollow which will accommodate the dome; the relief is lost and an even more difficult situation than the original arises. The highly specialised fibro-fatty tissues in the sole of the foot are a valuable component of gait and should be preserved with respect. For a localised single area of pressure, surgery is a preferable option. Where considerable and permanent loss of this tissue has occurred a modern thermo-plastic closed-cell foam such as Plastazote which can be heated and then stood upon to produce a perfect replica of the underside of the foot can be the best solution. It must have beneath it a second undeformed layer of the same material, for the deformation of the first layer will have flattened the foam cells at the point of maximum pressure, and in severe cases this will 'bottom out'.

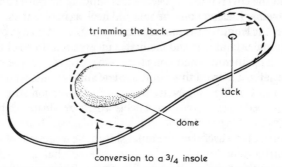

trimming the back

tack

dome

conversion to a 3/4 insole

Fig. 4/3 Leather-covered sorbo metatarsal dome on a full insole. For comfort the corrective placing of the dome is important and, as it is usually too far forward, trimming of the back as shown on the dotted line is a useful final adjustment. As pressure in the metatarsal area is often accompanied by some clawing of the toes a full insole can press these against the toe cap and produce discomfort. Either a three-quarter insole should be ordered or the full insole cut as indicated. In all cases of modification the resultant insole needs then to be anchored by a single tack through the heel area

Excellent as this procedure is, in the most difficult cases such as the neuropathic ulcers of spina bifida or leprosy, they will not heal unless shear is also removed, and to do this it is necessary to provide a substitute for the subcutaneous tissue to allow the foot to roll forward. This is done by the provision of an absolutely rigid rocker sole. Unfortunately the commonly provided metatarsal bar is quite useless for this function as it is necessary that the contour should be as shown in Figure 4/4.

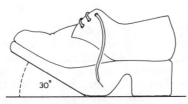

30°

Fig. 4/4 The mandatory sole contour to avoid both pressure and shear stress under the fore-foot. The sole must be absolutely rigid

Heel and sole height

The heel height is something on which advice is often sought from the physiotherapist. Research has shown that in a nylon stocking with a heel height of two and a quarter inches or less, the friction between the shoe and the covered foot prevents this slipping forward and causing toe problems. Raising both the sole and heel, as in recent shoe design, increases the length of the moment arm from the outer edge of the heel to the subtalar joint axis and facilitates inversion injuries of the ankle joint both ligamentous and bony (Fig. 4/5). Conversely the wider the heel the safer it is from this point of view and patients who have had such injuries, liable as they are to recurrent inversion strain, can be greatly helped by the provision of heels which are 'floated out'. Figure 4/6 shows three types of these which are progressively more efficient; (C) is particularly useful on the inner side in the treatment of pronated feet. Furthermore it has to be remembered that if a support is provided within a shoe this cannot function unless it is itself supported (Fig. 4/7).

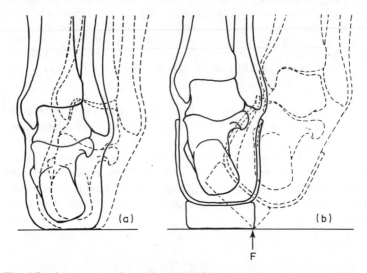

Fig. 4/5 Antero-posterior radiographs of the ankle (a) barefoot, and (b) in a shoe; normal posture in complete lines and supinated into the unstable position in broken lines. The instability only slightly increases in the barefoot position owing to the outward role of the calcaneo-contact articulation. In a shoe the movement of the ankle in space is greatly increased as is the moment arm about the fulcrum F. These radiographs were taken in a man's shoe and with very considerable increase in heel height the adverse forces increase proportionately. (Diagrammatic representation)

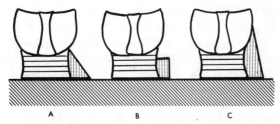

Fig. 4/6 Various types of 'floated out' heel

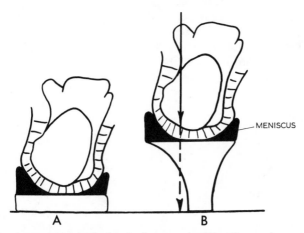

Fig. 4/7 Any support applied to the foot must itself be adequately supported as in A. In B the heel meniscus is ineffective because the body-weight will simply enforce rotation about the narrow heel

It is a common experience that patients with a short leg who are provided with a raised boot to compensate for this, will soon abandon it if the raise is substantial (one or more inches). Small raises are produced by appropriate additions to the sole and the heel up to three quarters of an inch. Above this it is usual to insert a layer beneath the upper, running from the front to the back of the boot. Sometimes this is given up because of the weight which can be now overcome by the use of appropriate plastics; often it is given up because the shoe is thereby rendered rigid without an adequate compensatory curvature of the sole contour which should be tapered from just behind the metatarsal heads of the toe (called confusingly in the footwear trade, toe spring) and this enables the normal 'toe rocker' (see Fig. 2/13c, p. 53) to be used.

For the patient with rheumatoid arthritis modern plastics enable shoes to be made from a plaster cast which can accommodate quite considerable deformities. Inherent disadvantages of this have been indicated and it is now becoming the practice to provide shoes of this construction made from standard lasts. Increased depth is usually provided to accommodate insoles. At the same time particular attention is paid to the fastening which should be of a simple type, commonly using 'touch and close' material (Velcro).

Chapter 5

Bone and Joint Pathology

by G.J. BENKE, FRCS, FRCS(Ed)

A knowledge of the normal structure and function of bones and joints will help towards a clearer understanding of the pathological changes which can occur. For such details reference should be made to standard anatomy and physiology textbooks.

While being strong and resilient, bone is a very active tissue. This will become clearer later in the chapter with the description of some of the principal metabolic diseases. Bones are so structured that they can fulfil three essential mechanical functions:

1. They provide support through their rigidity.
2. They give protection to vital structures as seen in the skull, chest, spinal canal and pelvis.
3. They provide a strong system of levers, linked by joints, which are able to withstand the strong forces of muscle pull required to maintain various postures and produce locomotion.

Bone is a specialised form of connective tissue. There are two types:

(a) *Cancellous bone* which is formed of a meshwork of trabeculae. Its honeycombed appearance gives the impression of weakness, but it is, in fact, very strong. The trabeculae are laid down in such a way as to enable the bone to withstand the compressive and tensile stresses to which it is exposed. This is clearly shown in the neck and head of the femur (Fig. 5/1).

(b) *Compact bone* (cortical bone) has a much more solid appearance, although microscopically it consists of systems of fine interlinked canals and spaces.

The shafts of long bones are mainly formed of compact bone which is thicker in the mid-shaft region and is designed to withstand bending stresses. They have a central cavity called the medullary canal. This reduces the weight of the bone without significantly weakening it.

Bones are surrounded by a vascular fibrous periosteum except where the surface is covered by articular cartilage. The inner layer of

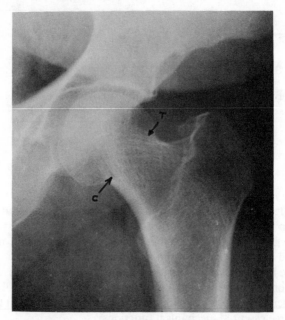

Fig. 5/1 Trabecular pattern of the femoral neck. The medial compression (C) and lateral tension trabeculae (T) are demonstrated radiographically

this membrane contains the osteogenic (bone-forming) cells called osteoblasts. These are the parent cells of the mature bone cells called osteocytes which are unable to divide. The osteoclast is the third type of bone cell. It has a phagocytic action, i.e. it removes bone.

In addition to these cells, bone consists of collagen fibres embedded in a ground substance. This is impregnated with calcium salts giving the bone its rigidity.

A bone, although retaining its overall shape, is constantly being laid down and resorbed.

Interference with the structure of bone by a disease process will prevent it fulfilling its function to the full. For example, it may be more prone to fracture.

INFECTIONS

These may be divided into acute and chronic infections.

Acute osteomyelitis

This term refers to acute infection in bone. It literally means inflammation of bone and bone marrow. It is the soft tissue components which are involved, i.e. the contents of the medullary cavity, the Haversian systems and the periosteum.

Acute osteomyelitis is caused by a bacterium. This is most frequently *Staphylococcus aureus*. It occurs most commonly in young children between the ages of two and ten years. In nearly all cases at this age the infecting organism is blood-borne from a distant focus of infection, e.g. a boil, or even a minor skin abrasion. Other portals of entry include the throat, the teeth and the tonsils.

There is often a history of trauma, and it is possible that this might cause minor damage to the bone involved, presenting an area more susceptible to invasion by any circulating bacteria.

It is the more vascular part of the bone which is frequently involved. This is the metaphysis which is that part of a long bone between the shaft and the growth plate. The latter structure acts as a barrier to the spread of infection. However, in young infants, where the growth plate is not fully developed, infection may invade the epiphysis. This in turn may lead to joint infection and growth disturbance (Fig. 5/2).

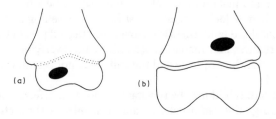

Fig. 5/2   Acute osteomyelitis. (a) In young infants the infection may settle in the epiphysis. (b) In children the infection is usually in the metaphysis; the growth plate now fully developed acts as a barrier to spread to the epiphysis

In adults, blood-borne infection is rare. Usually the bacteria are introduced through an overlying wound as, for example, in an open fracture. Such an injury may be associated with road traffic or other accidents. When it does occur, the infection tends to be less acute and is commonly found in the mid-shaft region of the bone.

Osteomyelitis commonly involves long bones, particularly the femur and tibia adjacent to the knee. However, no bone is immune;

for example, the mandible may be involved by direct spread from an infected tooth, or the mastoid process from a middle-ear infection. Occasionally there may be more than one bone involved.

In untreated acute osteomyelitis there are three phases to the pathological process:

1. *Suppuration*: Pus forms within the cancellous bone. This is a form of abscess. As it is in a confined space and therefore under tension, it is forced along the medullary canal or outward through the Volkmann's canals in the cortical bone to emerge under the periosteum. From there the spread is subperiosteal, lifting this membrane away from the bone. Pus may re-enter the bone at another level or burst through the periosteum into the soft tissues.

2. *Necrosis*: When its blood supply is cut off, bone dies. Here it may be due to infective thrombosis, rising pressure within the bone cavity, or by stripping of the periosteum. Pieces of dead bone become separated by the action of osteoclasts and form sequestra. These act as foreign body irritants and lead to a discharge through sinuses until they escape or are removed.

3. *New bone formation*: This occurs in the deep layer of the periosteum. If it is extensive it forms a new case of bone called an *involucrum* which may contain holes called *cloacae*, through which pus emerges.

The patient, who is usually a child, presents with severe localised pain, fever and malaise. He looks ill and toxic. The affected limb is held still. It may look normal at first but later swelling and redness appear. Localised tenderness is felt over the affected part of the bone. There is redness and increased warmth of the overlying skin. The tenderness may be exquisite and the child may not permit the part to be touched.

Although the child may be reluctant to move the affected limb, the neighbouring joint can usually be moved painlessly through a small range, whereas in acute septic arthritis any movement is prevented by intense pain.

TREATMENT

Before antibiotics were discovered, osteomyelitis tended to run the course outlined above. Nowadays prompt intensive use of antibiotics may be sufficient to bring the situation under control. The affected part should be rested in a splint and the patient put to bed. The antibiotics are continued for a minimum of three weeks. Drainage may not be required if antibiotics are given early.

However, if a subperiosteal abscess can be detected, or if the fever and local tenderness persist to the same degree after 24 hours of adequate antibiotic treatment, the pus should be drained by incision. Frequently the medullary cavity is also drained by drilling, although opinions vary about the need for doing this.

As the infection comes under control, the physiotherapist is required to supervise mobilisation of adjacent joints, and instruct the patient in crutch walking, initially non-weight-bearing, then progressing through partial to full weight-bearing.

COMPLICATIONS
1. *Septicaemia*: This may occasionally be fatal.
2. *Metastatic infection*: This is the spread of infection to other parts, including bones or joints.
3. *Septic arthritis*: This may occur: (a) in very young children where the growth plate has not formed a barrier to spread of infection from the metaphysis to the epiphysis; (b) where the metaphysis is intracapsular as in the femoral neck; or (c) by metastatic spread.
4. *Altered bone growth*: This may arise if the epiphysis is involved and damaged in an infant. It usually leads to shortening and may be severe. In older children there may be stimulation of the growth plate by the metaphyseal hyperaemia, leading to lengthening of the bone.
5. *Chronic osteomyelitis*.

Chronic osteomyelitis

Although much less common now because of effective antibiotic treatment, it may occur as a sequel to acute osteomyelitis.

An area of bone which has been destroyed by acute infection will contain cavities surrounded by dense bone. Pieces of dead bone are usually present and are surrounded by fibrous tissue and sclerosed bone. Although thus surrounded, they may act as foreign body irritants which will provoke the living tissue to produce sero-pus which escapes through sinuses. This tends to persist because the pieces of dead bone cannot escape.

Bacteria may also be imprisoned in the fibrous tissue. They often lie dormant for many years but may at any time give rise to an acute flare-up of the infection.

TREATMENT
This is usually conservative as the discharge may be no more than a nuisance. Antibiotics are probably not very effective as they do not penetrate the fibrous tissue barrier and sclerotic bone. However, some of the more recent antibiotics show some ability to do this.

Flares of the infection may occur at any time, giving a picture of acute osteomyelitis. They usually settle in a few days with rest. Occasionally an abscess may form which requires drainage if it remains painful and does not discharge itself.

Sometimes, if there are repeated flares or if there is a constant unpleasant discharge, the condition may become an intolerable nuisance necessitating amputation of the part.

Infection may occur as a complication of the implantation of artificial joints. This constitutes a form of chronic osteomyelitis which is being seen with increasing frequency as more and more joints are replaced.

Another form of chronic osteomyelitis is seen as a Brodie's abscess. This commonly occurs in the tibia. It may remain silent for years or present as recurrent episodes of pain. It constitutes a cavity surrounded by a sclerotic zone of bone. It usually contains clear fluid but sometimes contains pus from which the causative bacteria may be isolated. It is treated by drainage and curettage. Sometimes the cavity is then packed with cancellous bone graft to promote more rapid healing.

Tuberculous osteomyelitis

This is a form of chronic osteomyelitis. It is caused by the tubercle bacillus. It spreads via the bloodstream from a primary area of infection which may be in the lung, pharynx or gut. It causes excessive bone destruction over bone formation. It begins in cancellous bone, most commonly in a vertebral body, the small bones of the hands and feet and the ends of long bones. In the latter site it involves both the metaphysis and epiphysis.

It generally presents as a locally destructive lesion with normal tissue being replaced by caseous material. This process leads to increasing destruction of adjacent bone. Caseous material and tuberculous pus may be squeezed out of the bone forming a cold abscess. If this becomes subcutaneous a sinus may be formed.

The patient presents with a general illness of gradual onset and a long history. He may feel unwell and may complain of lassitude, poor appetite, weight loss and night sweats. There may be an evening pyrexia.

Tuberculous dactylitis

This affects the metacarpals or phalanges. A fusiform swelling develops and the shaft appears expanded as new bone is laid down on the surface.

Tuberculosis of the spine

This is sometimes referred to as Pott's disease of the spine. The vertebrae are the bones most commonly affected by tuberculosis. The centre of the vertebral body becomes caseous and the process spreads to destroy the intervertebral disc. This leads to vertebral collapse with an angular kyphus at that level. The angulation together with pressure of caseous material may lead to spinal cord compression and paraplegia.

A paraspinal abscess often develops. This may be a psoas abscess which tends to point just below the inguinal ligament. In the neck it may present as a retropharyngeal abscess.

TREATMENT

Treatment of tuberculosis is primarily by drugs. However, with drug cover, surgery may be more safely carried out. This may involve the evacuation of abscesses, and excision of diseased areas and dead bone. This may be particularly necessary to decompress the spinal cord.

Bone grafts are put into the defect left following removal of affected bone. Prolonged recumbency may be necessary. This will produce decreased muscular activity. General physiotherapeutic measures will be necessary to prevent wasting of muscles, chest and circulatory problems.

Acute septic arthritis

This is an acute infection of a joint. As in acute osteomyelitis, the causal organism is usually *Staphylococcus aureus*, but other organisms may be responsible.

The joint may be infected by the following routes:
1. Through a penetrating wound
2. By eruption of a bone abscess into it
3. By blood-borne spread from a distant site.

Untreated, the infection spreads throughout the joint. The articular cartilage may be destroyed, particularly in staphylococcal infection. The ligaments are softened and may give way so that the joint becomes completely disorganised and even dislocated. Occasionally the capsule may rupture allowing spread of pus to the peri-articular tissues, forming an abscess or a sinus. Where there has been destruction of tissues, fibrous or bony ankylosis may occur.

The patient becomes rapidly ill, with severe pain and swelling in the affected joint. He will have a high, swinging temperature. All movements of the joint are very painful. The pain is so intense that they are often totally abolished.

To prevent permanent joint damage treatment is urgent. The joint should be aspirated or opened and washed out thoroughly, followed by instillation of antibiotics. Intravenous or intramuscular antibiotics are given initially. They are continued orally as the infection begins to settle.

The joint is rested in a splint. The hip is always treated on traction to prevent disruption and dislocation.

As the patient's condition improves and the joint pain subsides, further damage to the joint is unlikely. At this stage the physiotherapist will commence careful active movements of the joint. The movements should *not* be passive, and should *never* be forced. As pain-free movement increases the patient will be allowed up non-weight-bearing on crutches. When the pain has completely settled, weight-bearing will gradually be increased. A careful watch should be kept for any sign of a flare-up of the infection. This will usually be heralded by the recurrence of pain.

If there is evidence of significant destruction of articular cartilage, ankylosis is to be expected. The joint is splinted in an optimum position until the ankylosis is sound.

Tuberculous arthritis

This is a chronic infective arthritis. As in tuberculous osteomyelitis, it is a local manifestation of a generalised disease. It commonly affects one joint, usually a large one. There is marked muscle wasting and the patient is sometimes unwell.

It is one of three main varieties of chronic arthritis, the other two being rheumatoid arthritis and osteoarthritis. In the former, although there is considerable muscle wasting and the patient is usually unwell, more than one joint is usually affected, in particular the small joints of the hands and feet. In osteoarthritis usually only one or two joints are involved, muscle wasting is only slight and the patient is well. This condition differs in that it is not primarily inflammatory. The associated synovitis is secondary to changes in the articular cartilage.

In the active phase of joint tuberculosis there is evidence of inflammation, namely warmth, swelling and associated muscle wasting. This disease starts in the synovium or interior of the bone adjacent to the joint. Initially the articular cartilage is normal. If the disease is arrested at this stage a return to normal in the joint is still possible. However, if the disease advances, the articular cartilage is attacked from both sides. The tuberculous granulation tissue involving the synovial membrane creeps across its surface destroying it. Similar granulations within the subchondral bone invade its deep surface. Once cartilage damage has occurred healing will take place by fibrous ankylosis of the joint.

If this occurs the joint is unsound as the fibrous tissue tends to shrink with time leading to increasing deformity. Also tubercle bacilli may be locked up in this tissue. If this is the case, later flare-up may occur. It is likely that tearing of the fibrous tissue by stress may liberate these organisms.

TREATMENT

As well as general treatment of the patient by rest and antibiotic therapy, local management of the active phase of the disease is:
1. *Rest*: The joint involved is splinted. In the upper limb the joint may simply be rested in a sling.
2. *Traction*: This overcomes spasm and prevents collapse of soft bone. As in acute septic arthritis it is particularly used if the hip is involved. It may be in the form of skin or skeletal traction.
3. *Operation*: After rest and antibiotic treatment have been in progress for a few weeks, if the disease is not settling rapidly, operation may be considered. Excision of the diseased synovium, together with other tuberculous debris, facilitates the action of the antibiotics and promotes more rapid healing. This may allow a more useful range of movement to be regained.

As in tuberculous osteomyelitis an abscess may form in the surrounding soft tissue if the joint capsule is perforated. If this becomes subcutaneous, it is liable to erupt through the skin giving rise to a sinus. This sinus track communicates with the joint and may allow secondary infection of the joint to occur. If this should be the case, ankylosis of the joint may become bony.

An abscess may be treated by aspiration or incision followed by closure of the overlying skin under antibiotic cover. Instillation of streptomycin into a sinus track may effect its cure.

As the disease heals, local treatment depends upon the stage at which its arrest occurred. If articular cartilage damage is minimal, good return of function can be expected. Stress of the joint is gradually reintroduced. In the case of the lower limb, splints are removed but the patient remains in bed on traction. The traction is then removed for increasing periods of time and then altogether. Mobilisation non-weight-bearing is commenced followed by partial, then full, weight-bearing. This allows for gradual reconstitution of the joint and adjacent bones. The patient is carefully observed and at any sign of recurrence of his signs or symptoms he is dropped back a stage in his rehabilitation programme.

In the upper limb treatment is simpler. The splint or sling is gradually removed for increasing periods and is dispensed with as use increases.

If the disease is arrested late, i.e. after articular cartilage has been destroyed, fibrous ankylosis is to be expected. Therefore the joint is splinted in its optimum position while this occurs. Movement is prevented but stress allowed, e.g. weight-bearing in the lower limb. Some form of splint may be required permanently.

In the upper limb the fibrous ankylosis will be longer as gravity exerts a constant traction force. In the shoulder mobilisation is graduated until support is dispensed with. If pain continues the joint is arthrodesed. In the elbow a permanent splint may be used, although a sling may be sufficient and even this may be dispensed with.

In the longer term, in the absence of a flare-up, the only local treatment required may be a removable splint in the upper limb and a raised shoe in the lower limb. If deformity is a major problem particularly in the hip, corrective osteotomy may be of great help.

If a joint should continue painful arthrodesis may be carried out.

TUMOURS

The word tumour means swelling. In pathological terms it refers to a swelling within the tissues and is a manifestation of neoplasia – the term neoplasia meaning new growth. Tumours are either benign or malignant.

Benign tumours show an excessive proliferation of cells but the tumour remains localised, is non-invasive and does not metastasise, i.e. does not spread to distant tissues.

Malignant tumours are characterised by:
1. Invasion of surrounding tissue.
2. Recurrence after removal or radiotherapy
3. Metastases, i.e. spread to local lymph nodes or distant tissues
4. Rapidity of growth
5. Abnormal changes in the cell nucleus
6. Anaplasia: A malignant tumour fails to reproduce the structure of the tissue from which it grows whereas a benign tumour may reproduce it perfectly. This lack of differentiation is called anaplasia. The more anaplastic the tumour, the more malignant it is likely to be.
7. Fatal outcome: A malignant tumour as the name implies tends to kill the patient.

Benign bone tumours nearly all occur in adolescents or young adults. On a radiograph their benign character is demonstrated by the clearly defined edges.

Malignant tumours are either primary, i.e. they arise from bone itself, or secondary, i.e. they are metastatic deposits from tumours of other tissues. Primary malignant tumours of bone are generally highly malignant and fatal. They tend to occur in young people, are painful and do not show a definite edge on the radiograph.

All primary bone tumours whether benign or malignant are rare.

Secondary malignant tumours are, on the other hand, relatively common and occur mainly over the age of 50. Tumours which most commonly metastasise to bone are carcinoma of breast, kidney, lung, prostate and thyroid.

The principal tumours, benign and malignant, will be summarised and then a more detailed description of osteosarcoma and secondary tumours of bone will be given. The general basis for any classification of bone tumour is based upon the tissue of origin of the tumour. Recollection of the tissues involved in the formation and structure of bone, briefly outlined at the beginning of the chapter, will serve as a general guide to the possible tumours that may arise.

VASCULAR (ANGIOID) TISSUE TUMOURS
Benign: (a) Angioma
     (b) Aneurysmal bone cyst
Malignant: Angiosarcoma

BONE-FORMING TISSUE TUMOURS
Benign: (a) Osteoma (exostosis)
     (b) Osteoblastoma
     (c) Osteoid osteoma
Malignant: (a) Osteosarcoma
     (b) Juxta cortical osteogenic osteosarcoma

CARTILAGE TUMOURS
Benign: (a) Osteochondroma (similar to exostosis but includes cartilage)
     (b) Chondroma: Within bone=*enchondroma*. If protruding beyond confines of bone=*ecchondroma*
     (c) Chondroblastoma
Malignant: Chondrosarcoma

EMBRYONIC VESTIGIAL TISSUE TUMOUR
Chordoma (locally malignant, i.e. invades local tissue)

FIBROBLASTIC TISSUE TUMOURS
Benign: Fibroma (variants non-ossifying fibroma, chondromyxoid
        fibroma)
Malignant: Fibrosarcoma

TUMOURS FROM NON-OSSEOUS CONNECTIVE TISSUE FOUND IN BONE
Benign: (a) Lipoma
              (b) Neurofibroma
              (c) Neurolemmoma
Malignant: (a) Liposarcoma
              (b) Reticulosarcoma
              (c) Myeloma
              (d) Ewing's tumour (Fig. 5/3)

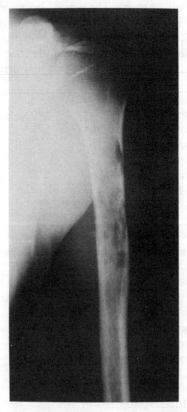

Fig. 5/3   Radiograph showing a Ewing's tumour of the shaft of humerus

UNDIFFERENTIATED CONNECTIVE TISSUE TUMOUR
Giant cell tumour

The treatment of a benign tumour is either by excision or curettage
and bone grafting.

The reasons for carrying out such treatment are:

1. If the tumour is painful, e.g. osteoid osteoma
2. If the tumour interferes with function of a tendon, or causes a
   prominent lump which is either disfiguring or prone to being
   knocked, e.g. exostosis
3. If by weakening the bone the tumour gives rise to a pathological
   fracture, e.g. enchondroma
4. If the tumour becomes larger, painful and the outline on the
   radiograph becomes less distinct. This may indicate malignant
   change and is occasionally seen in an osteochondroma
5. Where there is significant inherent risk of malignant change, e.g.
   giant cell tumour.

Osteosarcoma (osteogenic sarcoma) (Fig. 5/4)

The term sarcoma is given to malignant tumours of connective
tissue. An *osteogenic* sarcoma is, therefore, a malignant, specialised
connective tissue tumour arising in bone.

There are three varieties of the tumour which are based upon the
principal tissue seen on histological examination. They have in
common the fact that they all form osteoid (uncalcified bone matrix)
and bone.

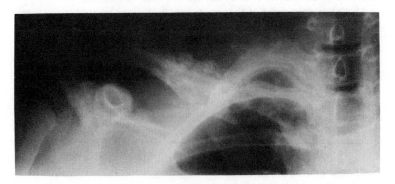

Fig. 5/4   Radiograph showing an osteosarcoma of the clavicle
(this is a rare site)

Where chondroblasts (cartilage cells) predominate it is called a *chondroblastic osteogenic sarcoma*. If fibroblasts predominate it is called a *fibroblastic osteogenic sarcoma*. If bone formation predominates it is called an *osteoblastic osteogenic sarcoma*.

They most commonly occur in the metaphysis of a long bone, mostly in the lower end of the femur or upper end of the tibia. They are twice as common in males and the highest incidence is between the ages of 10 and 25 years.

Pain is usually the first symptom. Local swelling will quickly occur as these tumours are rapidly growing. The temperature of the overlying skin may be increased and commonly there are dilated veins in the area. The swelling becomes tender. The tumour commonly metastasises to the lungs.

Diagnosis is confirmed by a biopsy before treatment commences.

TREATMENT

Treatment may be one or a combination of the following: amputation; radiotherapy; chemotherapy.

If there is no evidence of metastases amputation is usually carried out. This must involve removal of the whole bone as so-called skip lesions may occur, i.e. the bone may be involved at levels other than the main tumour mass. For this reason if the lower end of the femur is involved a hip disarticulation amputation is carried out.

If there is metastatic spread, treatment is usually by radiotherapy. However, amputation may be carried out to remove the local tumour which may become very painful and swollen.

A combination of radiotherapy followed by amputation is sometimes used even if there are no obvious metastases.

More recently some of these tumours have been treated, with some success, by cytotoxic drugs.

If a solitary lung metastasis is formed its excision is now considered worthwhile.

If amputation is carried out the physiotherapist will be closely involved in the rehabilitation programme. This will involve stump bandaging, education in walking with crutches and management of the prosthesis.

Secondary tumours in bone

These are the most common tumours in bone. They occur mainly after middle age.

TREATMENT
1. *Drugs*: Analgesics, and, sometimes, hormones as in the case of breast and prostatic carcinoma.
2. *Radiotherapy*: Pain is often improved. The tumour mass may shrink and therefore paraplegia due to spinal deposits may sometimes improve.
3. *Operation*: If the tumour should fungate it is probably best excised although radiotherapy may be useful. Surgical treatment of intractable pain from these tumours may sometimes involve division of sensory nerves, nerve roots or nerve tracts in the spinal cord. Secondary deposits in the vertebral column may cause pressure on the spinal cord requiring decompression by laminectomy.
4. *Fixation of pathological fractures*: Such a fracture may be the presenting feature of a secondary deposit in bone. Internal fixation of a long bone fractured in such a way is the usual method of management.

METABOLIC BONE DISORDERS

While the mechanical functions of bone may be obvious, the fact that they are physiologically very active can easily be overlooked. They play an integral part in calcium and phosphate metabolism, forming a reservoir which contains 99 per cent of the calcium and 90 per cent of the phosphate in the body.

Calcium in its free ionised form is necessary for a number of important body functions, namely:
1. Blood coagulation
2. Normal cardiac and skeletal muscle contraction
3. Normal nerve function.
Maintenance of a blood calcium level between very narrow limits is essential to avoid disturbance of these functions. To maintain this level there is a delicate balance between calcium absorption from the gastro-intestinal tract, its excretion by the kidney and its uptake and mobilisation from bone. Calcium metabolism comes under the influence of many factors the chief of which are parathyroid hormone and vitamin D.

Parathyroid hormone acts at three sites to increase the plasma calcium level. First, it facilitates calcium absorption from the intestine. Secondly, it causes mobilisation of calcium from bone. Thirdly, it acts on the kidney causing an increased excretion of phosphate, which in turn leads to a fall in the plasma phosphate level which causes a rise in plasma calcium.

Vitamin D is the term used to refer to a group of closely related substances. Some are found in the diet (fish-liver oil is particularly rich in this) and some are produced by the action of ultraviolet light on certain substances found in the skin of mammals. Vitamin D is required for the absorption of calcium from the intestine. It also causes mobilisation of calcium from bone. In vitamin D deficiency, poor absorption of calcium leads to hypocalcaemia and failure of mineralisation of the protein of newly-formed bone.

An understanding of the normal physiology of bone as it relates to calcium metabolism will provide a good basis for understanding the metabolic diseases of bone, some of which will now be outlined.

Infantile rickets and osteomalacia

A lack of vitamin D, due either to dietary deficiency, insufficient exposure to sunlight or both, results in these conditions.

Infantile rickets as its name implies occurs in children. The disturbance in calcium metabolism is the same as in osteomalacia which is the adult expression of the disorder. The manifestations of both these disorders only differ in so much that in the child the bones are in a growing phase.

In both conditions there is an abundance of osteoid, that is, uncalcified bone matrix. In children there are added changes involving the growth plate cartilage. These zones become wider but the abundant cartilage is not converted into bone.

Lack of vitamin D leads to a decreased absorption of calcium and phosphate. This in turn leads to a fall in the blood calcium level which stimulates secretion of parathyroid hormone. This hormone cannot increase calcium absorption from the bowel in the absence of vitamin D, but it does cause calcium resorption from bone. The result, therefore, of this sequence of events is that calcium, rather than being laid down, is resorbed from bone in order to maintain the blood and tissue fluid calcium at the correct levels.

In the child, the effect on the growth plates leads to retarded ossification and growth. The bones are generally softened and prone to bend. This is especially noticeable in the weight-bearing bones.

In the adult, the bones become decalcified giving rise to a ground-glass appearance on the radiograph. Another radiographic characteristic is bands of radio-lucency. These are called Looser's zones or Milkman's fractures after the people who described them. They represent pseudo-fractures and occur most commonly in the upper humerus, scapula, ribs, pubis and femoral neck. The softened bones are more prone to fracture with minimal trauma (pathological fractures). A group of subcapital fractures of the femur occur in osteomalacic patients. These people are older and often housebound. They have a poor diet and little exposure to sunlight. Patients with osteomalacia often feel unwell and complain of generalised pains and muscle weakness.

TREATMENT
The primary treatment of these conditions is by administration of vitamin D with calcium supplements.

Secondary treatment may involve later correction of deformities by osteotomy. Fractures will require appropriate treatment.

Secondary rickets

This may occur in a number of rarer situations. In these, vitamin D deficiency is not the primary cause.

1. *Vitamin D resistant rickets*: This is due to hypophosphataemia (low blood phosphate). Individuals with this require massive doses of vitamin D for normal bone formation to occur. Because of this it is known as vitamin D resistant rickets.
2. *Hypophosphatasia*: This is an inherited disease where the enzyme alkaline phosphatase is lacking. Because of this, although the supply of vitamin D and calcium is normal, the calcium is not deposited in bone.
3. *Renal rickets*: This is due to malfunction of the kidneys. There is a fall in phosphate levels due to failure of its resorption by the kidneys. This gives rise to increased secretion of parathyroid hormone which mobilises calcium from bone. In a child this will produce the picture of rickets, but in an adult osteomalacia will result.

Hyperparathyroidism

In this condition too much parathyroid hormone is secreted. This may be due to a tumour (adenoma) of a parathyroid gland or, occasionally, to hyperplasia of all the glands. The result of this is excessive excretion of phosphate from the kidney giving a low blood phosphate level. There is normally a constant relationship between the calcium and phosphorus levels in blood. If one falls the other rises. In this situation, because there is a fall in blood phosphate levels, calcium is withdrawn from bone with a consequent rise in the blood calcium level. As a result of this there is a rise in urinary calcium excretion with an increased incidence of calcium containing kidney stones.

Disturbances in bone structure may also occur. There is resorption of bone leading to osteoporosis. Many cysts may be formed and there may be an abundance of fibrous tissue. These changes have given rise to the descriptive term, *osteitis fibrosa cystica*. The bones are weakened and are prone to bending and fracture.

Hypoparathyroidism

This is most commonly due to inadvertent removal of the parathyroid glands during thyroid surgery. There is a consequent fall in blood calcium level. This gives rise to neuromuscular excitability which in its full-blown manifestation produces muscular spasms referred to as tetany.

Osteoporosis

In contrast to osteomalacia where there is a lack of calcium deposition in a normal matrix, in osteoporosis there is poor formation of the protein matrix but normal calcium deposition and bone resorption.

It may occur in a variety of conditions, three of which will be considered.

DISUSE OSTEOPOROSIS

This is seen in paralysis or immobilisation of a limb. Osteoblasts lack the normal stimulus of stresses and strains on the bone, so that bone formation is decreased. There is an increase in calcium excretion with a tendency to form renal stones. General exercises are therefore important for patients who are recumbent for long periods.

POST-MENOPAUSAL OSTEOPOROSIS

Bone formation is influenced by the gonadal hormones (oestrogens and androgens). Lack of these hormones leads to osteoporosis. This is most commonly seen with the fall in oestrogen levels which occurs at the female menopause. Senile osteoporosis is for the most part based upon lack of these hormones.

HYPERCORTICOSTEROIDISM (CUSHING'S SYNDROME)

Here osteoporosis is due to hypersecretion of adrenocortical hormones, in particular the glucocorticosteroids. It is due to excessive protein breakdown which inhibits new bone formation and causes breakdown of existing bone matrix, an anti-vitamin D action and an increased urinary calcium excretion which is secondary to an increased glomerular filtration rate.

A similar effect may be seen with the administration of steroids therapeutically over a long period of time.

With osteoporosis there is an increased tendency for bones to fracture. This is demonstrated by the common occurrence of fractures of the neck of the femur in elderly female patients. There is also a tendency to compression fractures of vertebral bodies leading to spinal deformity (usually kyphosis) and loss of height. Fractures are treated appropriately. There is some evidence that calcium supplements in certain forms with vitamin D may give some improvement in this condition. These patients, unlike those with osteomalacia, are not ill and are not affected by generalised pain and muscle weakness. However, sometimes the two conditions may co-exist.

BIBLIOGRAPHY

Woods, C.G. (1972). *Diagnostic Orthopaedic Pathology*. Blackwell Scientific Publications Limited, Oxford.

Chapter 6

Principles of Orthopaedic Traction Systems

by G.K. ROSE, OBE, FRCS *and* E.R.S. ROSS, FRCS, FRACS

THE TRACTION SYSTEM

Traction means the *act of exerting a pulling force* and the example of a tractor pulling a plough is easy to understand. When traction is used clinically it must be understood as part of a system of forces. Only if the physiotherapist has an understanding of *all* the forces which comprise this system can she appreciate the way in which it acts and, importantly, the parts of the system it is permissible to move temporarily for necessary therapy. This means that the system should be as effective when it is left as it was when approached.

The essential components of such a system are:

1. A traction force which is a vector quantity having both magnitude and direction.
2. Counter-traction. This is a second reactive force used to localise the effect of the first to a desired area.

In order to pull out the cork a bottle can be held by its most convenient part, the shoulders. Suffice that the counter-force acts beyond the point at which the corkscrew acts (Fig. 6/1). Personal experience shows that the resultant has been localised to the chosen area, the cork, and that this begins to move when the friction between the cork and bottle is exceeded.

Traction force

In relationship to the part being treated, force may be generated internally or externally:

1. *Internally* from muscle activity, either spasm or voluntary contractions (Fig. 6/2).
2. *Externally* from gravity, i.e. the use of a weight; a part of the body

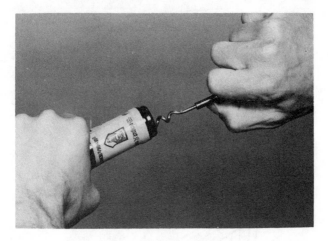

Fig. 6/1   Traction and counter-traction

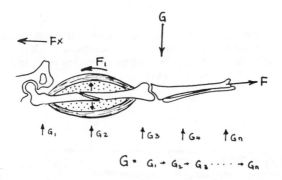

Fig. 6/2   The force F_1 generated by muscle spasm will tend to cause the femoral shaft fracture to overlap and therefore shorten. The force to maintain the length is localised at the fracture site by traction force F and counter traction Fx. *Note* that angulation of the fracture is caused by force G (gravity) and this is resisted by $G_1 + G_2 \ldots G_n$, from appropriately placed slings

(Fig. 6/3); or a bag of water or sand (Fig. 6/4). Because, initially, this weight pulls downwards, the force engendered may be changed in direction by a fixed pulley. A movable pulley or pulleys may be used to gain mechanical advantage (see Fig. 6/6).

Additionally, gravity will have a direct action on the part being treated (Fig. 6/2).

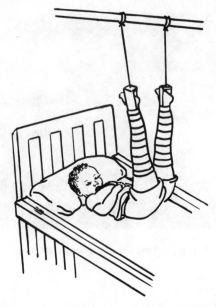

Fig. 6/3 Gallows traction. Traction is provided by part of the child's weight. Care must be taken to see that the buttocks are therefore clear of the bed. Counter-traction is provided by the rigid stand attached to the bed, which in turn pushes against the floor

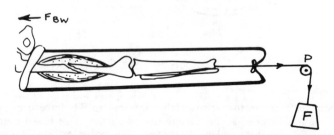

Fig. 6/4 Weight F pulling downwards is translated via pulley (P) into a transverse force. Counter-traction is Fbw deriving partly from body-weight as this slides down the sloping bed, moderated by friction

Counter-traction

This may also use gravity, or it may be provided by two fixed points joined together against which these forces react; the classic example is the Thomas' bed knee splint (Fig. 6/5).

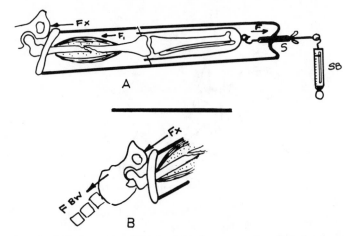

Fig. 6/5 Fixed traction. (A) The force is generated entirely by the muscle spasm around the fracture; this pulls against the splint end (F), and the counter-traction is at Fx with pressure against the ischial tuberosity. (B) Pressure against the ischial tuberosity can be alleviated initially by using Fbw from sliding traction of the body-weight – this must not exceed the force F or distraction will occur

Clinical uses of traction systems

1. The reduction and maintenance of the fracture position (Fig. 6/2).
2. The reduction of muscle spasm, and therefore pain, in inflammatory joint disease or fractures.
3. The correction of fixed deformities.
   (a) The use of external gravitational forces as in the Agnes Hunt system for the reduction of a flexion deformity of the knee in rheumatoid arthritis, with simultaneous correction of the posterior tibial subluxation (Fig. 6/6).
   (b) The use of internally generated muscle force, e.g. in the Milwaukee spinal orthosis (see Fig. 15/12, p. 286). Active extension of the cervical spine, pressing the occiput downwards against the posterior support produces longitudinal traction.

TRACTION FOR FRACTURES

In the treatment of fractures two forms of traction (often in combination) are used.

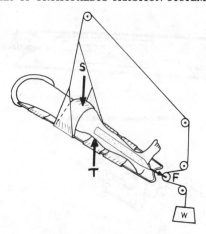

Fig. 6/6 Agnes Hunt traction for a knee-flexion contracture. By using a system similar to the Hamilton Russell the longitudinal straightening force (F) is applied and this equals 2W. A force (S) pressing down on the knee derives from the extension of the cord through a sling transverse over the knee; this in turn tends to press the knee straight, but at the same time a reactive force (T) from a sling presses upward against the head of the tibia tending to reduce the subluxation

Sliding traction (Fig. 6/4)

In this illustration traction is applied to a fractured femur in a Thomas' splint. The weight F opposes the action of the muscles around the fracture which would cause it to overlap while counter-traction localising the force to this site is FBW=body-weight. The problem with this form of traction is that as the muscles providing the internal force waste, and, therefore, weaken, the force F is greater than this and the fracture will distract, i.e. separate, and non-union is more likely. It needs careful regulating with progressive reduction of F.

Fixed traction (Fig. 6/5A)

This is a self-contained system with only one initial force, i.e. that generated by the muscles which pull against the end of the splint at F. Counter-traction is provided by the ring against the ischial tuberosity (Fx). S is a screw to pull the fracture just to length, and the force in the system can be measured by using a spring balance SB to pull on the attachment. When this just separates from the splint the force can be read off the spring balance. In the early stages, i.e. the first week, this will be very high and commonly the foot of the bed is raised. An element of sliding traction is now introduced from body-weight (Fig. 6/5B) (moderated by friction on the bed) if the splint is fixed to the end of the bed to provide counter-traction. Always providing that this sliding traction is less than that in the splint, pressure on the ischial tuberosity will be reduced without distracting the fracture. For this reason the force in the splint is measured daily and as it drops, and it does this quite sharply in 7 to 14 days, the sliding traction element is removed by levelling the bed.

In both systems gravity acting directly tends to bow the fracture downwards and must be resisted by carefully adjusted slings (Fig. 6/2).

A more directly applied form of fixed traction is an *external fixator* using skeletal traction and counter-traction (Fig. 6/7).

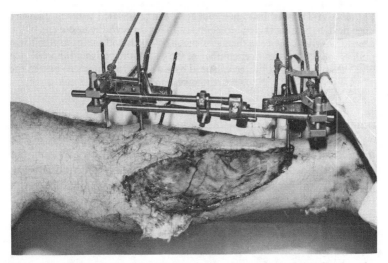

Fig. 6/7 External fixation. Traction can be produced locally by the threaded bars

This covers the elements of traction but confusion sometimes occurs because of the presence of many cords and pulleys used for a different reason.

In Figure 6/8 two cords run from the top of the Thomas' splint to the bottom. These are suspension cords. Likewise are the two cords

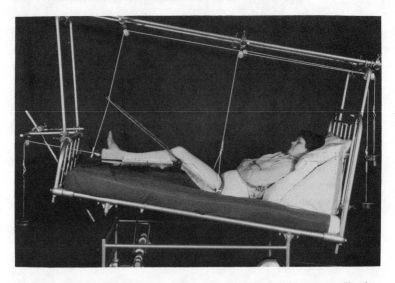

Fig. 6/8 A Thomas' bed knee splint with an articulated segment allowing knee flexion. Sliding skeletal traction is applied through the upper end of the tibia. The whole device is then suspended by cords and pulleys; from these pulleys the cord passes over a pulley at the end of the bed and the whole leg plus the apparatus is counter-balanced by a weight – this plays *no* part in the traction system

running from the bottom of the main splint to the Pearson knee-piece on which the leg lies. These cords are not an essential part of the traction system. However, by suspending the injured part plus the splint in the air the patient can move more freely. This reduces the possibility of pressure sores, aids nursing care and allows the physiotherapist to perform her task more easily.

FIXATION METHODS

Apart from 3b, page 111, all forms of traction require a satisfactory attachment to the part to be treated: two forms are used, skin or skeletal.

Skin traction

This is obtained by using friction between the skin and a material bandaged to it to transmit the force to a part (Fig. 6/3). The traction force must be spread over a large area of skin. This reduces the force per unit area or the load on the skin which reduces the danger of damaging the skin. The material used is adhesive or non-adhesive. Adhesive strapping, e.g. Elastoplast, gives a better grip than non-adhesive strapping such as Ventfoam. However, patients may be allergic to adhesive strapping, and a severe allergic response precludes its use. In general, non-adhesive strapping tends to be non-allergic. Although 6.5kg (15lb) can be applied through skin traction, in practice it is used only where much smaller weights are required. Care must be taken not to extend strapping above the fracture site. This will reduce or abolish the effect.

CONTRA-INDICATIONS
Skin traction should not be used:
(a) where there are abrasions or lacerations;
(b) where there is circulatory impairment, e.g. varicose ulcers;
(c) where there is atrophic skin, e.g. patients on prolonged steroid therapy.

COMPLICATIONS OF SKIN TRACTION
1. Allergy to components in the strapping.
2. Skin excoriation.
3. Pressure sores. These occur at prominent bony points, e.g. the malleoli and attachment of the tendo calcaneus.
4. Common peroneal palsy. This may occur if the bandaging holding the longitudinal strapping rolls up and forms a tight ring around the upper fibula.

Skeletal traction

A rigid metal pin or tensioned wire is driven into or through bone. The traction force is applied directly to the skeleton (Fig. 6/9). Some commonly used devices are shown in Figure 23/13, page 463. A Steinmann pin is a sturdy 4–6mm diameter stainless-steel rod with a trocar point to allow easier penetration of bone. The Denham pin has an additional thread which grasps the cortex as the pin is screwed in. In porotic bone commonly found in the elderly, the thread provides a better grip. A Kirschner wire is quite weak and can easily be bent. However, if it is stretched by a tightener as shown in Figure 6/10 tension is developed in the wire which will then support considerable loads.

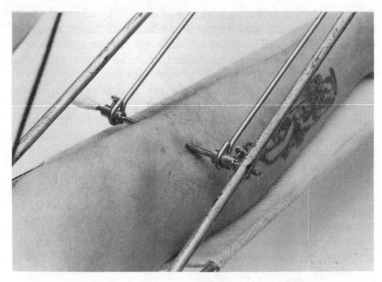

Fig. 6/9 Skeletal traction (Steinmann pin) through the upper tibia

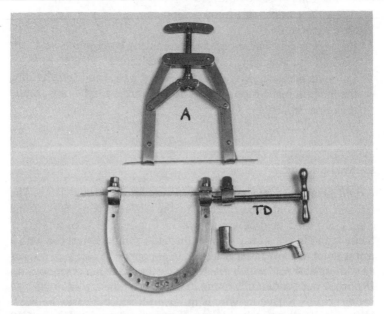

Fig. 6/10 Tension wire used in skeletal traction. (A) The screw-caliper device; (TD) a tensioning device. Either can be used to put the wire under tension

Loosening of the pin and subsequent pin-track infection are the only problems. A neglected pin-track infection could lead to osteomyelitis.

Common peroneal nerve palsy can also occur if the leg is allowed to lie in external rotation, the nerve may then be squeezed by the weight of the limb on a metal splint.

All complications can be minimised or indeed avoided if at least one member of the treatment team examines the traction device at least daily.

PULLEYS

The traction in Figure 6/11(1) shows four pulleys. Whereas the weight (water bag) hangs directly down over the end of the bed the line of action of the force which it produces is changed to produce two forces A and B acting on the body at point X. One force seems to pull the leg along the bed while the other pulls the thigh up in the air, in fact they resolve into a force C which pulls in the long axis of the femur (Fig. 6/11(2)).

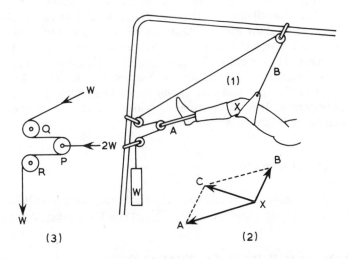

Fig. 6/11 Hamilton Russell traction to show two principles of traction. The hanging weight (W) is by a system of pulleys transformed into 2 forces A and B. A has twice the value of B and together are resolved by a parallelogram of forces into C which is in line with the fractured femur (2). It is the pulleys' system PQR (3) which produces this difference in force in A and B. Because Q and R are fixed at the end of the bed and P is movable, this causes a mechanical advantage via P which makes the force in this direction 2W

Look again at Figure 6/11(1): the pulleys at the foot of the bed form a system shown diagrammatically in Figure 6/11(3). The function of such a pulley system is to increase the mechanical advantage of this part of the system and double the force W at X. In practice if the cord jams against the pulley-casing all function is lost. As this can easily occur, it should be included on the daily inspection.

WEIGHTS
There are limits set on the weight used, by the size of the patient, e.g. child or adult; the type of fixation used, e.g. skin or skeletal; by the part under treatment, e.g. cervical spine or lumbar spine; and by the condition under treatment, e.g. a femoral neck fracture or a femoral shaft fracture. It is better to think about the requirement in each case than to concoct a recipe book for every eventuality.

OTHER TYPES OF TRACTION

There are numerous variations of traction that the physiotherapist may meet in her work. They include gallows traction (Fig. 6/3); Hamilton-Russell traction (Fig. 6/11), Perkins' traction (Perkins, 1974) (these allow early mobilisation of the knee joint) and Fisk traction. Traction may be used also in the correction of contractures, e.g. Agnes Hunt method (Rose, 1977) (Fig. 6/6); in the correction of spinal deformities, e.g. halo-pelvic traction (see Chapter 16). Full details of all these, and others, will be found in books listed in the Bibliography. It is also possible that local variants of the standard methods will be met in practice.

PHYSIOTHERAPY

This is discussed in the relevant chapters; for hip conditions (Chapter 8); for spinal deformities (Chapter 15); and for fractures (Chapter 24).

DOS AND DON'TS OF TRACTION

Do learn how the particular traction works before treating the patient.
Do check that the weights are hanging free before and after treating the patient.
Do check that cords run freely in pulleys, and that pulleys rotate freely.

Do check the skin for any signs of pressure or inflammation.

Do check that movement of the free joints is actively possible; this is important particularly for dorsiflexion of the ankle joint for the early detection of nerve injuries or compressions.

Do report any adverse findings to the nurse in charge of the ward and to the medical officer concerned.

Do not meddle with the traction unless you have been specifically trained to do so.

Do not release the traction unless the surgeon has given instructions to do so.

Do not loosen, or tighten, tapes, cords, screw extensions or slings of the traction apparatus.

REFERENCES

Perkins, G. (1974). The George-Perkins Traction. *World Medicine*, January 30.

Rose, G.K. (1977). Total functional assessment of orthoses. *Physiotherapy*, **63**, 3, 78–83.

BIBLIOGRAPHY

Adams, J.C. (1983). *An Outline of Fractures, Including Joint Injuries*, 8th edition. Churchill Livingstone, Edinburgh.

Apley, A.G. and Soloman, L. (1982). *Apley's System of Orthopaedics and Fractures*, 6th edition. Butterworths, London.

Charnley, J. (1970). *The Closed Treatment of Common Fractures*, 3rd edition. Churchill Livingstone, Edinburgh.

Owen, R., Goodfellow, J.W. and Bullough, P. (eds) (1980). *Scientific Foundations of Orthopaedics and Traumatology*. William Heinemann Medical Books Limited, London.

Stewart, J.D.M. (1975). *Traction and Orthopaedic Appliances*. Churchill Livingstone, Edinburgh.

Chapter 7

Foot and Knee Conditions

by G.K. ROSE, OBE, FRCS *and* J.A. BENTLEY, MCSP, ONC

A realistic understanding of knee and foot problems requires that these areas be considered in the context of gait and not simply during standing. Furthermore as these structures are three-dimensional, simple planal consideration severely inhibits understanding and therapeutic progress. This type of failure is well illustrated in the orthodox approach to the foot in the past.

FOOT CONDITIONS

Comparisons of the foot with a static structure such as a bridge is not only valueless but detracts from the concept of the highly mobile structure with a wide range of adaptability to allow for variations in the shape of the ground. Important concepts of functional anatomy are:

1. **Articulations** (the word articulations includes joints but is not limited to these). These are:

    (a) *Intrinsic*: Cartilage covered low-friction joints rotating about a single axis and therefore track-bound, i.e. rotating only clockwise or anticlockwise. This axis is a product of a joint shape held in contact by ligaments (Fig. 7/1) and all the joints together form a track-bound linkage which moves with a set pattern no matter at what point the force is applied, e.g. external rotation of the leg produces supination of the foot (Fig. 7/2). Conversely, supination of the foot causes external rotation of the leg. The position of these axes in space is important. That of the subtalar axis (Fig. 7/3) transmits the side to side movement of the foot to rotational movements of the leg (Fig. 7/4). Similarly there will be a distal rotation of the metatarsophalangeal joint of the great toe relative to

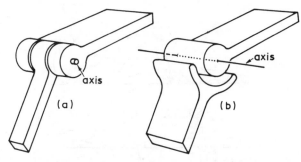

Fig. 7/1 (a) A mechanical hinge with a pin as an axis. (b) An anatomical hinge joint; the axis is a resultant of the joint shape

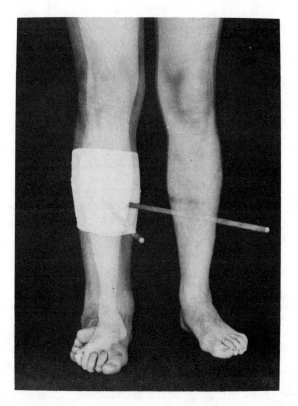

Fig. 7/2 By means of a pointer fixed to the subcutaneous border of the tibia (a patella hammer does well) rotation of the tibia compared with movements of the foot can be easily seen

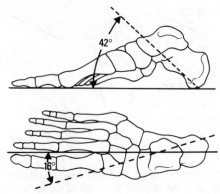

Fig. 7/3   The average position of the subtalar axis. *Note* the obliquity in space

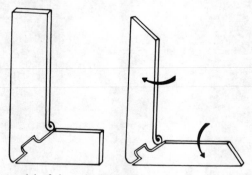

Fig. 7/4   A model of the subtalar joint showing the translation of motion through a right angle

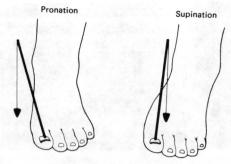

Fig. 7/5   A pointer fastened to the great toe nail indicates the rotation of the axis of the metatarsophalangeal joint depending on the posture of the hind foot

the ground (Fig. 7/5), and where this is considerable there will be an adverse ground reaction tending to push the toe into the valgus position (Fig. 7/6) and this accounts for the higher incidence of hallux valgus which occurs with abnormally pronated feet.

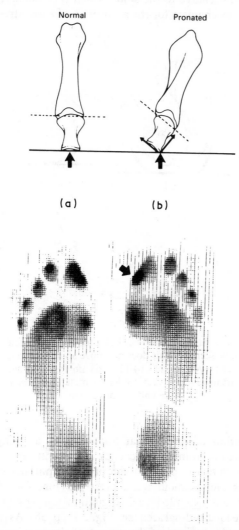

Fig. 7/6   (a) Normal alignment of the axis of the metatarsophalangeal joint in relation to the ground. (b) Where the axis is oblique due to pronation there is a resolution of the ground reaction causing valgus stress, and this can be seen on the differential pressure footprints

(b) *Extrinsic*: These are not joints but are high-friction rolling articulations beneath the under-surface of the calcaneus and the metatarsal heads with the fibro-fatty tissue beneath these (Fig. 7/7). The axis here moves in space like that of a bicycle wheel over the ground – relative to the skin – which is stationary. This is an important mechanism for the absorption of shear stress.

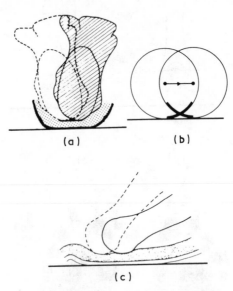

(a)   (b)

(c)

Fig. 7/7 Extrinsic articulations. (a) Calcaneo-contact articulation moving laterally. It will be seen that this does not move about a single stationary axis but rolls as does a bicycle wheel. (b) The axis moving sideways. This form of movement occurs in all planes and, under the metatarsal heads (c), shows as a fore and aft movement

2. **The function of the plantar aponeurosis,** a strong structure which extends from the calcaneus and is inserted through five digitations into the bases of the proximal phalanx of each toe, embracing the sesamoid at the great toe (Fig. 7/8). When these phalanges are extended each digitation tightens and shortens raising the longitudinal arch (see Fig. 2/17, p. 58). As the degree of shortening is maximal at the great toe, the foot inverts and the tibia externally rotates. This occurs twice during each stance phase: first just before and on the heel impact, which is consequent upon the action of the extensors of the toes; as the foot goes down to

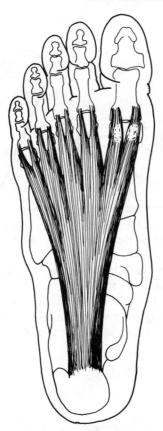

Fig. 7/8   Anatomy of the plantar fascia. Extension of proximal phalanges causes shortening of this, maximal at the great toe and arch rise occurs at the point indicated and it is this which defines metatarsal rays, the medial three being the metatarsal plus cuneiform and the outer two, the metatarsal alone

full contact position the arch is lowered and the foot pronated absorbing the internal rotation of the longitudinal rotation of the limb segments; and secondly at the end of stance when passive extension repeats the process, initiates external rotation of the limb segments and converts the foot into a rigid structure which plays its part in the rise and fall in the centre of mass of the body (Fig. 7/9).

Using these components one can now construct, as it were, a model of the foot which can be subdivided into two functional portions:

(a) That above the subtalar joint which is the talus only (although

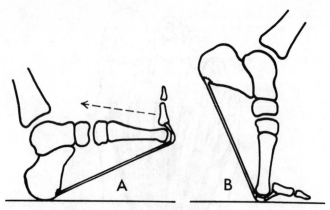

Fig. 7/9   A. The first arch rise at heel contact actively initiated by long extensors of the toes. B. Passive arch rise at the end of stance phase

because it is rotationally locked in the mortice of the ankle joint, the tibia will rotate with it).

(b) The bones distal to the talus which can be regarded as a specialised six-legged stool with a fixed posterior leg of the calcaneus with five articulated legs anteriorly, the metatarsal rays (Fig. 7/10).

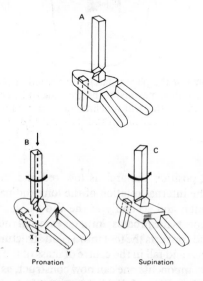

Fig. 7/10   For the sake of simplicity only two anterior rays are represented, and the talus and tibia represented as a single rotating segment

Ignoring the dynamic changes of walking, the very terminology 'flat foot' implies that some arbitrary height of the internal longitudinal arch, measured in one plane is either normal or pathological, which is not the case. The position was slightly improved by the use of the term *valgus* applied either to the heel or to the ankle as this indicated that changes in the transverse plane could also occur. However, it was assumed that this was directly related to the flatness of the foot but an investigation showed this view to be unsupported by fact. Some 177 school children between the ages of five and seven, the entire contents of two infant schools, had their feet measured and a 'valgus index' (VI) derived. The purpose of the index was to relate the proportional shift of the intermalleolar diameter of the ankle medially in respect of the heel area, in such a way that allowance could be made for the different sizes of feet and the results compared (Fig. 7/11 and 7/12). It will be seen that all feet lean inwards to some extent and the average index is in the region of 11. High arched feet can lean very considerably although those with extreme VI

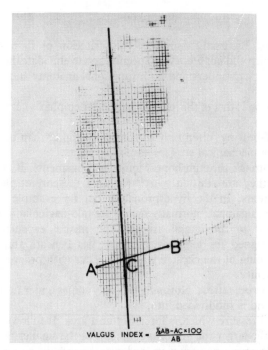

VALGUS INDEX = $\dfrac{\frac{1}{2}AB-AC \times 100}{AB}$

Fig. 7/11   A method of deriving valgus index to allow for different sizes of foot. Points A and B are the malleoli projected downwards, and C the point where the central axis of the foot crosses the line

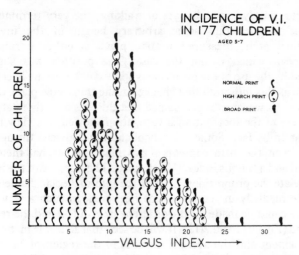

Fig. 7/12 Distribution of valgus index in 177 unselected children

were flat. By itself, therefore, this criterion of flatness or even abnormality did not seem very specific, and to elucidate the problem it is necessary to understand both functional anatomy and function of the feet.

Function is that of the legs but particular emphasis has to be placed on:

1. Load-bearing, often very considerably higher than body-weight. These mechanical stresses have two effects:

   (a) *Intrinsic* through bones, joints and ligaments. It is important that they are resisted, particularly by the correct placement of ligaments. In the hyperpronated foot for example, the strong spring ligament, normally below the talo-navicular joint, will be rotated to the lateral aspect. The medial capsule, which is ill-designed for load-bearing, now lies beneath this joint and stretching of the capsule will then occur with progression of the deformity.

   (b) *Extrinsic* stress. Normally this only comes under the soles of the feet and is subdivided into:

   (i) Pressure which is force per unit area. It follows, therefore, that the larger the uniform contact area the smaller the pressure, and from this point of view the lower the arch the better. The word uniform is important, for if within this area, the load is maldistributed either by a bony prominence which projects downwards or because it is nearer one edge than the others (as will be seen later) then the situation changes.

(ii) Shear stress. This is the application of load in a plane horizontal to the contact area and there are mechanisms in the foot designed to minimise this (see Fig. 2/18, p. 59).

2. Shock-absorbing mechanisms within the foot and leg to minimise peak loading (see Fig. 2/14, p. 53 and Fig. 2/17, p. 58).
3. Absorb internal rotation of limb segments and initiate external rotations.
4. During level walking the foot plays little part in propulsion but the matter is different in pathological situations as, for example, a patient with both hips stiff or in activities such as climbing.
5. Prehensile usage which can occur to an extraordinary degree as, for example, in patients born without arms.

Functionally each of the three inner rays comprises a cuneiform bone with its associated metatarsal, and the outer two are the metatarsals only, and are so defined because it is at the basal joint of these rays that elevation of the longitudinal arch occurs in consequence of the function of the plantar aponeurosis. These, like all other intrinsic joints, are hinge in type and in the static standing position are locked in full extension giving a foot with a support area like a three-legged stool, normally stable. The foot requires no muscular activity to maintain this because the talo-tibial load-line falls within the triangular support area (Fig. 7/13). Should this line fall

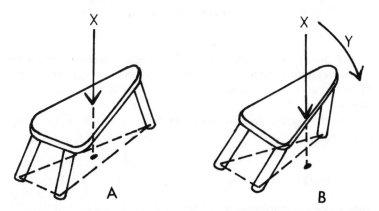

Fig. 7/13   A. Stable position of a subtalar stool where X represents the tibial force. B. Where the force falls medial to the support area the stool becomes unstable and the amount of subsequent movement will depend on the degree of mobility in the subtalar joint. If small this will cause intrinsic strain, if large the stool will rotate to lie sideways on the ground

outside the support area, whether medially or laterally, the consequences depend on the range of movements in the subtalar joint. Normally this allows very considerable inversion of the foot and in these circumstances the stress is not put on the intrinsic joints of the foot but occurs in the ankle as a rotation of the talus. Should this stress occur vigorously then a series of classical rotational ligamentous and bony injuries occurs in the ankle. The pronation range is short and does not allow a corresponding situation to occur, and in these circumstances excessive stress on the intrinsic joints of the foot occurs. However, where the foot is hypermobile the foot will then pass to the classical hypermobile flat-foot position (Fig. 7/14).

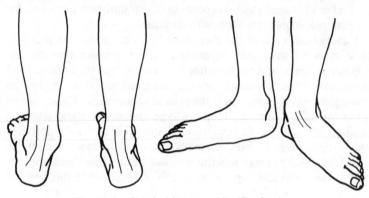

Fig. 7/14   Classical hypermobile 'flat foot'

In reality the position is not quite as simple as this and some degree of independent movement can occur in the mid-tarsal region and while it frequently corresponds to that of the subtalar, does not always do so.

With this biomechanical background we can now turn to foot pathology.

FLAT FOOT

This term as commonly used is a nebulous mixture of normal anatomical variants with a very small core of pathological conditions. The normal variants will be determined by somatotype, ethnic derivation and by age (Asher, 1975) (Fig. 7/15). Just what happens to the vast number of children seen with flat foot in orthopaedic clinics

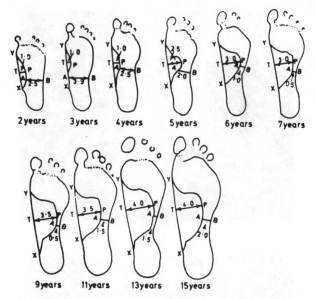

Fig. 7/15 Variation in footprint shape with age in an untreated foot

and given varieties of treatments is speculative. Certainly adult clinics are not filled with a proportionate number of patients suffering from the fact that some 40 or 50 years ago they had no treatment. The only useful, albeit limited, follow-up has been that of Harris and Beath (1947) who examined over 3500 recruits to the Canadian Army. Of these 6 per cent had hypermobile flat foot with short tendo calcaneus and 2 per cent spasmodic valgus (Harris, 1948). Only these foot conditions caused significant disability and must therefore be diagnosed as early as possible and treated efficiently.

The hypermobile foot presents as a painless condition at about the age of two. Because of the loss of stable foot support it is often associated with delay in walking and signs are (Rose, 1982):

1. A high valgus index. This is not specifically diagnostic.
2. Abnormal great toe extension test. With the child standing evenly on both feet and looking forward, the great toe is pushed upwards by the examiner and the plantar aponeurosis tightened. In the normal foot the medial arch will rise and the tibia externally rotate (Fig. 7/16). Absence of these is highly significant.
3. Inward rotation of the great toe-nail relative to the ground. This is invalid in the presence of toe deformities.
4. The shape of the footprint preferably on a Harris and Beath mat.

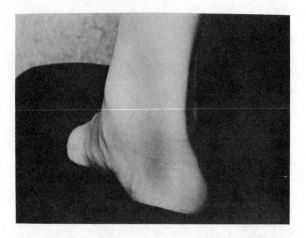

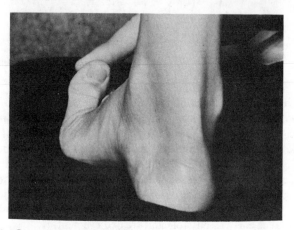

Fig. 7/16 Great toe extension test. *Note* that the arch rises and, as will be seen from the external malleolus, the tibia externally rotates

Lowness of the arch is not significant. Only reversal of the curve of the footprint, associated with an inward rotation of the heel oval and increased pressure under the medial columns of the foot is of importance (Fig. 7/17).

5. Associated hypermobility in other joints, at the elbow, the metacarpophalangeal joints of the fingers, the knee and the ease with which the thumb can be brought into alignment with the forearm (Fig. 7/18). At this stage the tendo calcaneus is long, but secondary shortening subsequently occurs. The importance of this

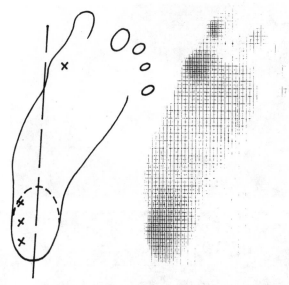

Fig. 7/17   Characteristics of the hypermobile flat foot on a Harris and Beath differential pressure mat

is that stretching of the tendo calcaneus or surgical elongation does not improve the posture of the foot.

Because of this hypermobility and the associated tibial bowing these feet fall into a position with the load-line medial to the support area.

As such feet are mobile, if held within the corrected position efficiently for an appropriate length of time, i.e. six years or so, an excellent prognosis can be expected with the spontaneous recovery of the underlying hypermobile condition. If left untreated the condition progressively worsens because of the stretching of joint capsules as already indicated. A very small number of cases, particularly those associated with well-defined syndromes such as those of Down, Marfan or Ehlers-Danlos, will not recover with this regime and may, rarely, require surgical intervention.

The emphasis is, however, on efficient conservative treatment and this can be monitored, even with the foot in the shoe, by observing the external rotation of the tibia. Using this method the efficiency of wedges applied to the outside of the shoe was investigated (Rose, 1958: 1962) and this indicated that the commonly prescribed crooked and extended heels produced no correction. Wedges on the inside border of the sole and the heel did so, but did not promote growth

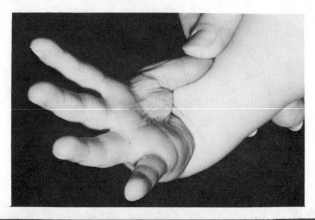

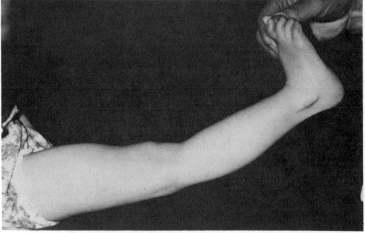

Fig. 7/18   Hypermobility of joints. *Note* that the thumb can be brought to the forearm

changes to improve foot posture. Additionally, there is the objection to such methods that they require the shoes to be taken away for varying periods (and this now imposes a considerable financial load on the parents) and furthermore will quite rapidly wear down and become ineffective. It seemed important therefore to look at other methods of rolling the foot from the hyperpronated position to the normal and it was shown that this was most efficiently done by applying a transverse horizontal force in the mid-tarsal region.

In the very small child this is best done by either (1) a specialised outside iron and an inside Y-strap (*note* Y not T) (Fig. 7/19); or (2) a polypropylene extended heel cup (Fig. 7/20).

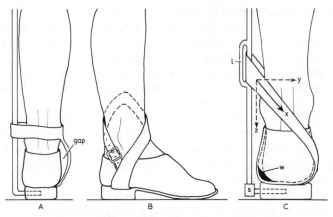

Fig. 7/19 (A) Classical T-strap which exerts no force on the foot but only on the lower tibia. (B) Y-strap. (C) Mechanical complement necessary for correction. The force in the Y-strap (x) which resolves into (y) and (z) will cause the Y-strap to travel downwards and lose effect unless loop (1) is provided. The reacting wedge (w) is necessary to complete the moment and stress-relieving articulation (s) to prevent breakage at this weak point

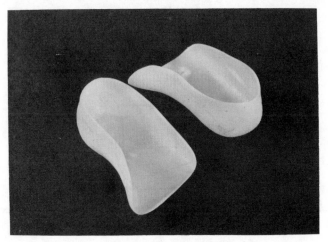

Fig. 7/20   Polypropylene extended heel cups

OUTSIDE IRON AND INSIDE Y-STRAP

To produce the desired effect mechanically four components are required:

1. A Y-shaped strap not a T which applies force only to the lower end of the tibia.

2. A restraining loop on the iron to accommodate the strap which is thus prevented from sliding distally instead of correcting the foot.

3. A wedge lateral to the heel to provide a counter-reaction and it is convenient to use a Rose-Schwartz insole.

4. Some form of stress-relieving articulation at the spur-iron junction to avoid recurrent fractures of this area due to the mechanical efficiency now introduced.

It will be noted that in situations like this where the foot is correctable, the forces to be applied to the foot in order to hold it in the corrected position are small because the load is taken through the foot itself and not through the apparatus which is only required to hold the foot in the stable position.

This is the optimum device for children from one to five years whose feet are chubby and difficult to hold by other means.

POLYPROPYLENE EXTENDED HEEL CUP

The polypropylene extended heel cup transfers body-weight through a right angle to provide a horizontal force (Fig. 7/21). It should be made from a plaster cast of the foot in the fully corrected position.

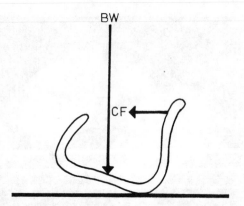

Fig. 7/21 BW (body-weight) translated into a horizontal CF (corrective force)

Casting is assisted by externally rotating the tibia of the standing patient and then locking the foot in the corrected position by dorsiflexion of the great toe, care being taken to press the first metatarsal head on to the floor. The heel cup requires to be extended to the first and fifth metatarsal heads. The normal torque of the foot causes marked discomfort over the neck of the fifth metatarsal in the shorter heel cups if these have any function.

It is used as a follow-on device for the iron and being custom-built is reserved for the most marked cases. Commonly it produces a little skin thickening over the inner border of the foot, but this is well tolerated and disappears when the treatment is discontinued.

A third method of correction works on a different principle, namely the wedge placed behind a wheel to prevent it turning and rolling (Fig. 7/22). A plastic meniscus provides both an internal wedge at the

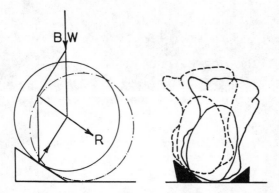

Fig. 7/22 A theoretical analysis of the function of the wedge in action where BW represents body-weight and R represents the resultant corrective force

calcaneo-contact articulation, therefore limiting pronation, and also an external counter-wedge to prevent the foot sliding laterally from the correction. The divergence of the two arms is prevented by a membrane between them (Fig. 7/23). It comes in stock sizes, is self-adhesive but needs to be reinforced by two penetrating nails to prevent torque displacement. It can, therefore, be provided immediately in outpatients. It is very suitable for a majority of cases of 'flat feet' treated in orthopaedic clinics and can be used in cases of foot strain later in life.

As has been indicated in Figure 4/7, page 87 it is important that the orthosis should itself be supported if it is to function.

There appears to be no beneficial function for the internal longitudinal arch support apart from the fact that some, made in rather firm material, do have a similar function to the heel meniscus posteriorly.

Operative intervention essentially moves the support area so that it contains the load line and this is best done by a calcaneal osteotomy which moves the posterior leg of the 'stool' medially.

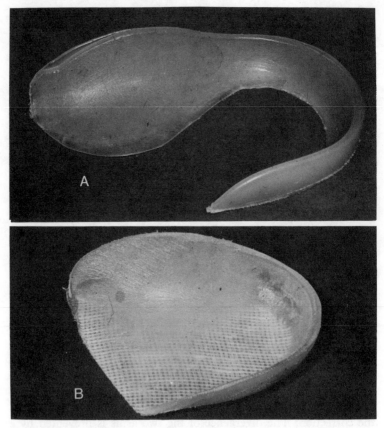

Fig. 7/23 Rose-Schwartz meniscus. (A) The essential medial wedge with lower outer rim to prevent foot sliding away from the wedge. (B) The completed orthosis

SPASMODIC VALGUS

This condition is painful and usually becomes apparent in early adolescence. It derives its name from the fact that in some cases the peroneal muscles are in spasm. This does not necessarily occur and is a secondary feature. The characteristic of the foot is that it is held in fixed eversion which quite commonly occurs in high arched feet. The essential pathology is an impingement of the calcaneus and the tarsal-navicular joint which is only revealed by special oblique radiographs. Providing the patient is under 14, treatment of choice now seems to be excision of the impingement or bar, always providing there are no other changes to be seen in the foot. In these circumstances 90 per cent of the patients can be relieved and can return to full sporting activities. For those who have relatively minor symptoms, but do not come into this category, the use of an iron or Y-strap or an extended heel cup may well prove sufficient, and after a few years the symptoms appear to settle leaving no significant disability, although there may be restricted mobility. Only rarely is it necessary to fuse the subtalar joint.

RHEUMATOID VALGUS

This condition develops because of hypermobility of the foot joints consequent upon the disease and comes to resemble closely that of the hypermobile flat foot of childhood. It may, however, come on quite acutely because initially the early stages of deformity are resisted by overaction of tibialis posterior. At some time in the progression of the disease this will quite suddenly rupture and the foot roll into the full hyperpronated position. Commonly this is not correctable and in these circumstances the use of the iron and Y-strap or extended heel cup are less efficient than in childhood. If any attempt is made to achieve correction the interface pressure is commonly intolerable because the device becomes supportive and not stabilising and the treatment of choice is a calcaneal osteotomy.

CAVUS FOOT

As in all foot conditions some distinction has to be made between the natural variation in foot shape and the pathological. Pes cavus is not simply a non-progressive high arched foot but is now regarded as being neurological in origin although it is not always possible to identify this positively. It is, however, important that in all suspected cases a thorough neurological and radiological examination be undertaken which may reveal lesions of:
1. Muscle, such as muscular dystrophy.
2. Peripheral nerves or lumbo-sacral spinal nerve roots, e.g. Charcot-Marie-Tooth disease, polyneuritis, trauma or various forms of congenital lesions such as diastematomyelia.
3. The anterior horn cells of the spinal cord, e.g. poliomyelitis, cord tumours.
4. Spinocerebellar tracks, e.g. Friedreich's ataxia.

5. Pyramidal or extrapyramidal systems of the brain, e.g. cerebral palsy.
6. Psychiatric disorders such as hysteria.

Such feet are characterised by the progressive development of a high arch, associated with tightening of the tendo calcaneus, inversion of the heel and clawing of the toes, and these deformities commonly become fixed. Particularly in lesions category 2 (above) there may be associated sensory loss and vascular disturbance which may be demonstrated as severe chilblains, combined with sensory loss and the development of trophic ulceration.

The problems of such feet derive from both abnormal extrinsic and intrinsic stress. The extrinsic derives from the small support area which is characteristic of the higher arch combined with the inversion of the foot which reduces this further to the outer border only. The clawing of the toes makes the metatarsal heads prominent in the sole because of the tightened plantar fascia and because of the supination so produced contributes to the inversion. Both this and the tightening of the tendo calcaneus largely negates the shock-absorbing mechanisms of the foot.

The condition becomes apparent at various ages ranging from the myelomeningocele type apparent at birth, the rapid appearance of a unilateral foot at about the age of three in diastematomyelia, that of Friedreich's ataxia and muscle dystrophy from six onwards while others, particularly of a mild degree, become symptom-producing during the third decade.

Early diagnosis is therefore valuable particularly if this leads to the recognition of a treatable condition such as diastematomyelia. In some cases this is not possible and the distinction between the normal high arch and the mild degree of cavus can only be made after the foot has been followed-up for a number of years, careful measurements and Harris-Beath footprints being taken at regular intervals.

Because the underlying condition is neurological and often associated with muscle imbalance, particularly of the intrinsic muscles of the foot, there is little reason to suppose that physical therapy or shoe alterations have a significant effect on the natural history of the disease, and attention has to be directed toward alleviation of the results of distorted mechanics. Conservative treatment for early cases includes re-distribution of pressure beneath the foot by the use of thermoplastic foam insoles and, where there is sensory loss, reduction in shear stress by combining these with appropriately shaped rigid soles. Insoles with metatarsal bars are best avoided, for while they may initially give some relief of pressure they will soon give rise to pressure atrophy of the already jeopardised tissues of the sole.

Operative intervention has been designed to:
1. Delay progression. This has included detachment of the sole muscles and overlying aponeurosis from the calcaneus to defunction the plantar aponeurosis, and/or by the transfer of the long toe-extensors to the necks of the metatarsals or transposition of the long flexors to the extensors in order to moderate the intrinsic muscle imbalance.
2. Correct the foot posture by bony operations. This has included calcaneal osteotomy to overcome inversion of the heel and thereby improve the support area, various mid-tarsal resections to reduce the height of the arch of the foot and at the same time realign if necessary supinated metatarsal rays. This increases the area of support and it again tends to place the load line more centrally within it.

HALLUX VALGUS

Hallux valgus is the deviation of the great toe at the metatarsophalangeal joint away from the mid-line commonly associated with a varus of the first metatarsal. Secondarily there develops a protective adventitious bursa at the medial aspect of the joint (the 'bunion'), hypertrophy of the medial side of the first metatarsal head and the development of osteoarthritic changes which eventually may involve the whole of this joint. As the deformity increases and the bunion enlarges, rubbing on the shoe may damage the skin covering and the bunion becomes septic.

A facile explanation of this condition is that it is consequent upon the wearing of shoes or socks which are too tight. Certainly pressure can deform the foot as was seen in the Chinese and to a lesser extent as caused by women's fashion footwear. Similarly women with 20 degrees or less of angulation when put into sandals with a single strap over the metatarsal heads show in the course of a few months considerable improvement. While hallux valgus does occur in unshod races it is noticeably less. Nigerian women for example had a mean value of nil with a maximum up to 7 degrees angulation, while British women of a similar age-group had a mean value of 17 degrees with a maximum up to 25. While it is therefore clear that considerable improvement in the general situation could be obtained by the scrupulous avoidance of such external pressures both during childhood and adult life, there are problems in accepting this as the basic cause. It is 10 times more common in women than men yet there is little evidence that a significant difference in shoe fit occurs during the early years of life. The great toe angle increases in both equally up to the age of five, and it is only at the age of nine that any significant divergence occurs, the average in girls going up to 13 degrees at 21 compared with 10 degrees in boys. Additionally a significant relationship has been established between pronation of the foot and a higher incidence of hallux valgus. The practical implications of these considerations lie in the main with a selection of patients for operative intervention. If best results are to be obtained this should be made in relationship to the general assessment of the foot.

Surgical intervention

In general the following types of procedure are adopted.:
1. Simple trimming of the head of the first metatarsal which is generally unsatisfactory as it ignores the fact that this prominence is a secondary phenomenon.
2. Trimming associated with an arthroplasty of the metatarsophalangeal joint. Removal of the proximal end of the proximal phalanx: the Keller-type of operation has the inherent disadvantage of retraction of the sesamoid proximally because of the division of the plantar fascia. Trials are now being made of the insertion of a silicone spacer to try and avoid this but it seems extremely unlikely that such inserts will survive the mechanical stresses of walking over a number of years. The alternative approach has been to remove the first metatarsal head (Mayo's procedure), but this has the disadvantage of shortening the first metatarsal and removing some support from the inner side of the foot.
3. These objections have led to arthrodesis of the metatarsophalangeal joint which can be an eminently satisfactory and robust operation provided there is adequate hyperextension in the interphalangeal joint, and providing arthrodesis is done in the correct position for that particular foot.
4. Because it is recognised that if any operation is done in the immature foot recurrences are almost inevitable with growth, operations have been proposed to try and modify the attachment of the small transverse muscles of the foot to provide some active correction. This is only partially successful and, indeed, because of the variations in attachment, can be disastrous producing an even more troublesome varus of the toe. The lesson here is to delay operation as long as possible in the young, and then, if at all possible, to do an arthrodesis of the metatarsophalangeal joint.

Various types of orthosis have been proposed to keep the toe straight or correct it but there is no evidence that these are successful in either objective.

HALLUX RIGIDUS

In this case the metatarsophalangeal joint of the great toe becomes progressively stiffer and more painful. It is generally caused by repeated minor injury during adolescence; it is more preponderant in females and is often a familial affliction, when it is sometimes associated with corresponding stiffness in the metacarpophalangeal joints of the thumb. The articular cartilage of the joint becomes progressively thin and may disappear and this is associated with the formation of osteophytes around the rim. Many patients may have a short period of painfulness which can be relieved by the use of an appropriately stiffened sole of the shoe with a rocker contour which avoids the recurrent extension stress on the stiffened joint. The joint may then continue to stiffen and, depending on the general foot posture, become painless. In other cases where this does not occur arthrodesis of the joint provides the best chance of success although occasionally it is necessary to do an arthroplasty because the great toe is long and the interphalangeal joint stiff.

METATARSALGIA

Metatarsalgia is a name given to pain experienced under the metatarsal heads and there are two types:

1. Where the normal level alignment of the metatarsal heads has become disturbed and one or more heads become prominent in the sole and symptom-producing because of the excessive localised pressure. This is associated with some stretching of the inter-metatarsal ligaments. Occasionally relief can be obtained by appropriate exercise therapy with the intrinsic muscles where the clawing is mobile. Commonly, however, this is associated with fixed clawing of one or more toes (Fig. 7/24), as in this condition the relevant digitation of the plantar aponeurosis is tightened and the metatarsal head pulled downwards into the sole relative to those which are not. The cure lies in the surgical correction of the deformed toes. A severe degree occurs with rheumatoid arthritis, and this can be treated by removal of all metatarsal heads and parts of the shafts to achieve a level tread and allow the toes, now largely defunctioned, to lie in a position of minimal pressure.

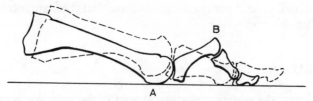

Fig. 7/24   Interrupted line is first metatarsal ray. Fixed clawing of second toe (continuous line) causes metatarsal head to become prominent in sole and cause pressure (A). Shoe presses at (B)

2. The other quite different type is Morton's metatarsalgia where there is a sharp pain often associated with a burning sensation occurring usually between the third and fourth toes and which can on occasions be relieved dramatically by manipulation of the foot. This is because there is a thickening of a digital nerve, often referred to as a neuroma, which is now thought to be secondary to an entrapment of the nerve associated with thickening of the intermetatarsal bursa. This condition can be most satisfactorily relieved by excision of the neuroma but many patients tend to manipulate their foot themselves to gain relief and after a period the condition may resolve spontaneously.

PHYSIOTHERAPY FOR FOOT CONDITIONS

Physiotherapy for the foot conditions described is common to them all but the emphasis will vary with the condition to be treated or the type of operation performed.

The following is a brief guide to the treatment of painful feet, whether due to foot strain or following surgery.

1. Contrast baths to improve the circulation. This is a simple method of treatment which the patient can continue at home. Fill one foot bath or similar receptacle with hot water (45°C (115°F)) and another with cold water. Immerse the foot and lower limb up to the knee first in the hot water for three minutes and then in the cold water for half a minute and repeat the procedure three to four times.

2. When swelling is present, elevation of the limb, oil massage to the foot followed by ice packs and vigorous foot and ankle exercises to reduce swelling, improve the circulation and assist venous return. Intermittent positive pressure or faradism under pressure with the limb in elevation can also be used.

3. Traction and passive stretchings and gentle mobilising when applicable to maintain joint range and length of surrounding tissues.
4. Passive mobilising techniques to the small joints of the foot.
5. Faradic foot baths for the intrinsic muscles of the foot to improve muscle tone and circulation.
6. Specific active exercises for the intrinsic muscles of the foot.
7. Non-weight-bearing active and resisted foot and ankle exercises to improve strength and stability and maintain mobility – progressing to weight-bearing exercises.
8. General correction of posture taking into consideration the relationship of the trunk, hips, knees and feet.
9. Rhythmical stabilisations of the trunk in standing to develop balance reactions and co-ordination.
10. Re-education of walking to encourage the patient to use the whole foot as a stable but mobile structure and to develop a normal pattern of gait.

The exercises should be simple and well taught. The patient should continue the treatment at home and practise the exercises conscientiously. Supervision should continue for a short time until the patient is walking well and confidently, and knows the exercises.

KNEE CONDITIONS

GENU VALGUM/VARUM

These terms imply deviation of the knee either away from the mid-line or towards it respectively. In children it must be appreciated that both these conditions can be entirely physiological and that there is normally a change from varum to valgus with growth as indicated in Figure 7/25. Much treatment, varying from shoe alterations to physiotherapy, has been declared successful by doctors and patients because of this spontaneous change, and even very extreme appearances can change dramatically and spontaneously (Fig. 7/26).

In both conditions it is necessary to eliminate the rare but important pathological conditions and these include:
1. Rickets. Simple vitamin D deficiency rickets has reappeared in this country, particularly among immigrants, and it is associated with the continuance of cultural dietary habits in a country where the synthesis of vitamin D from sunshine is inadequate. Similar changes may occur in consequence of renal tubular insufficiency

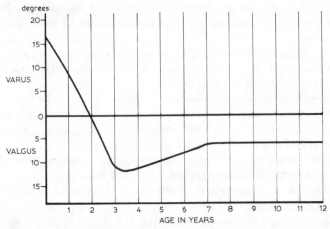

Fig. 7/25   Graph showing rate of normal change from varus to valgus

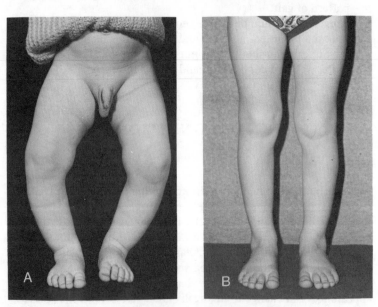

Fig. 7/26   Change in untreated patient in three years

which can be relieved by carefully controlled administration of vitamin D and phosphates. Such control is of vital importance because vitamin D in large doses can cause irreversible renal damage and possibly death. An even more serious condition is the rickets of generalised kidney failure, for while the rickets can be easily corrected, the renal problem then requires either dialysis or preferably transplantation.

2. Tibia vara (Blount's disease) is a localised development abnormality occurring at the medial aspect of the proximal tibial epiphysis. There are two types, one occurring in the infant and the other in adolescence. It is progressive and requires operative correction.

3. A wide range of rare skeletal disorders. General involvement of the skeleton including the skull combined with radiography often make the diagnosis clear. In the milder cases a disproportion between the skeletal segments and the trunk will excite suspicion and in this respect it is useful to bear in mind that the child is not simply a scaled-down adult (Fig. 7/27). Raised hairy pigmented patches on the skin point to a possible neurofibromatosis which is often associated with a rather marked angular varus deformity of the lower tibia and may be unilateral.

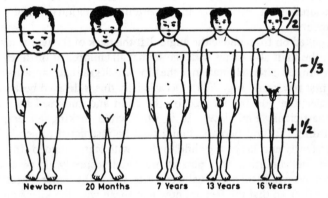

Fig. 7/27   Change in body proportions with age

4. Localised disturbances of epiphyseal growth may occur in consequence of trauma to the epiphysis or infection. In the past it was customary to correct the deformity by osteotomy once progression had ceased, but it is now appreciated that by early intervention progression can be prevented in cases of localised premature epiphyseal fusion by removal of the fused portion and replacement by fat.

The vast majority of cases will therefore be physiological and the major problem is one of therapeutic restraint in those cases which are not obviously improving. This is greatly assisted by appropriate recorded measurement but there will remain a small number of cases where pressure from patients and parents for cosmetic reasons demand correction. For a time the insertion of staples across one side of the epiphysis in the knee region to limit growth there was practised; while this *could* be successful a significant number of complications, worse than the original condition, has resulted in a considerable diminution in enthusiasm. It is better and safer to wait until almost full skeletal maturity has occurred and then to correct the condition by an appropriate osteotomy either in the lower femur or proximal tibia and fibula.

Splintage has *no* place in treating these cases apart from the early, marked deformity where in the first year or two of life moulding of the bones under general anaesthetic and application of plaster casts done on two or three occasions at three-weekly intervals does seem to stimulate natural correction.

It is appropriate once again to say that these conditions cannot and should not be considered in a planal manner as they are often associated with variations in longitudinal rotation of the limb segments.

Looked on from above the angle that the neck of the femur makes with the shaft also varies with age so that all children at birth tend to have limited external rotation of the hips which gradually appears over the first few years (Fig. 7/28). Occasionally this is delayed because of the sleeping posture adopted by the child and endorsed by many paediatricians (Fig. 7/29). It is worthwhile making an enquiry regarding this and parents should then be instructed to gently but persistently encourage the child to sleep with legs extended. In some cases the condition will persist into adolescence with persistent in-toeing, which then gradually corrects, not at the femoral neck but in the tibia so that the feet are now line ahead with the knees turned inwards. This condition may be worrying from the point of view of cosmesis but appears to be the cause of little or no disability. Similarly, varying degrees of torsion in the tibia can develop independently. Again formidable operations have been proposed but at this time there is no evidence that they significantly improve function nor delay the onset of degenerative changes in the neighbouring joint but certainly carry some element of risk.

In adults valgum/varum can occur as a result of either the lateral or medial compartment of the joint being affected following meniscectomy or osteoarthritis. In rheumatoid arthritis this may be accompanied by collapse of a tibial plateau, and laxity of ligaments so that the deformity may become extreme. In small degrees of deformity the

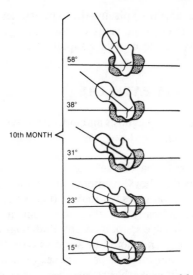

Fig. 7/28   Normal variation of neck/angle of femur with age

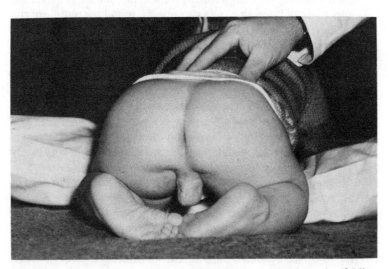

Fig. 7/29   Common sleeping posture which tends to delay normal unfolding of internal torsion/bowing of legs

compartment can be restored to width by insertion of a metal plateau (Mackintosh's prosthesis), and in more severe cases corrective osteotomy of the tibia (and less often with the lower femur or both) may be undertaken, the aim being to stabilise the joint by realignment, at the same time placing the joint parallel to the ground. Many types of complete knee replacement (endo prostheses) have been used with varying success (see Chapter 21).

CHONDROMALACIA PATELLAE

This term is not a precise diagnosis and indeed is often used simply to describe pain behind the knee cap. Two main types can be distinguished:

1. That occurring between the ages of 8 to 17, three times more common in girls than boys, commonly bilaterally and frequently persistent over several years without getting better or worse. It is rarely accompanied by any limitation of movement or effusion into the joint and can resolve spontaneously. Radiologically there is no abnormality. Treatment should be as far as possible conservative and this ranges from quadriceps exercises (which hardly seems logical as this is to increase the pressure between the patella and the femur); resting the compartment for several months in a long-leg caliper; steroid injection; or a garter worn round the middle of the patellar ligament. All can be successful, and all failures. Exploration of the knee joint (now replaced by arthroscopy combined with palpation of the articular cartilage with a blunt probe) can for a similar, and often severe, symptom picture reveal a variety of conditions varying from complete normality through to large areas of osteochondritis dessicans (this is the separation of articular cartilage from the underlying bone), either hinging as a flap or completely eroded leaving an ulcer. Removal of this area is commonly undertaken and symptoms tend to abate but very rarely patellectomy is undertaken.

   It should be emphasised that routine examination of children in this age-group by moving the patella over the underlying femoral condyles while the knee is extended will commonly reveal quite painless patella grating and this sign is of very little value in diagnosis therefore. There is no evidence that such grating gives rise to adverse effects later in life or indeed that even when chondromalacia is established that this does so.

   Furthermore microscopic examination shows that a surface degenerative lesion is frequently found in youth and regularly in maturity and its presence cannot be held responsible for this form of patello-femoral pain. Basal degeneration of the cartilage however can occur which goes on to blistering and the separation described.

2. In the sixth decade patello-femoral pain due to the development of typical degenerative arthritis of the knee occurs and this type is accompanied by effusion and limitation of joint movement. Radiological signs are present, with the symptoms tending to increase gradually. Coarse painful crepitus is present. As before the conservative treatment range is wide. Operatively, patellectomy is occasionally undertaken depending on the condition of the other compartments of the knee. Where knee-joint replacement has been undertaken it has been customary to leave the patella and in these circumstances it can become troublesome so attention is now being paid to the resurfacing of this.

RECURRENT DISLOCATION OF THE PATELLA

This condition, almost always lateral displacement of the patella usually occurring spontaneously without history of injury, has a definite familial tendency and occurs most commonly in females with ratios of three to one or even higher being reported. Predisposing causes include:
1. Generalised ligamentous laxity in just over one-third of all patients.
2. Abnormal attachment of the ilio-tibial band to the upper pole or lateral border of the patella, which can pull the patella laterally when the knee is flexed.
3. Genu valgum which displaces laterally the insertion of the patellar ligament.
4. A high-lying patella often secondary to Osgood-Schlatter's disease (osteochondritis of the tibial tubercle) which can cause elongation of the patellar tendon. When the knee is flexed the normal buttressing effect of the lateral femoral condyle is lost.
5. Congenital hypoplasia and flattening of the lateral femoral condyle. A rare form of this is the *nail-patella syndrome* associated with abnormalities of the nails and projections of bone from the posterior pelvis known as iliac horns.
6. Injury.

The diagnosis of this condition must always be borne in mind when considering knee problems; oblique radiographs of the patello-femoral compartment taken with the knee flexed at 40 degrees are likely to reveal malpositioning of the patella (even when undislocated) and hypoplasia of the lateral femoral condyle or early degenerative changes.

In the early stages, particularly after injury, conservative treatment is indicated with strengthening of the vastus medialis muscle. Once it becomes apparent that a condition is not improving early surgical treatment is indicated to avoid degenerative changes. In children only soft tissue operations are considered, the commonest being excision of any contracted ilio-tibial band and mobilisation of the attachment of vastus lateralis. The attachment of vastus medialis is then separated and re-implanted into the lateral border of the patellar ligament and distal border of the patella. After skeletal maturity the tibial tubercle can be transplanted medially and somewhat distally in the tibia with appropriate lateral capsular release, thereby realigning the patella in the femoral groove.

In both cases the patient is in a plaster cast for four weeks and during this time partial weight-bearing is permitted. The cast is then bivalved and gradual remotion and muscle strength are promoted by appropriate physiotherapy.

PHYSIOTHERAPY FOR KNEE CONDITIONS

Physiotherapy for the conditions of the knee joint discussed in this chapter is common to all; but the emphasis will vary with the condition to be treated, the degree of pain and disability, and the surgery performed. Treatment aims to relieve pain, develop muscle power and strength, and maintain full range of movement.

Physiotherapy following total knee replacement and osteotomy around the knee joint is described in Chapter 22.

Pain may be relieved by:
1. The application of heat or cold in whatever form is appropriate or available.
2. Hydrotherapy; the warmth and support of the water relieving pain and facilitating movement.

The development of muscle power and mobility throughout the limb and particularly around the joint may be achieved by:
1. Isometric exercises and passive mobilisation techniques.
2. Proprioceptive neuromuscular facilitation techniques (PNF) and techniques to elicit normal postural reactions.
3. Weight-resisted exercises and, where applicable, heavy weight-resisted exercises as described by de Lorme (1945).
4. Hydrotherapy.
5. Knee class.

The physiotherapist must observe and assess the effects of treatment and change, adapt or discontinue it as necessary.

Patients who require corrective surgery, for example recurrent dislocation of the patella, are usually young people who have had intermittent bouts of pain and discomfort over a period of time and who, after operation, tend to be very apprehensive and reluctant to move the limb and need reassurance and encouragement.

POSTOPERATIVE PHYSIOTHERAPY

Following surgery the limb is supported in a plaster of Paris cast or by a pressure bandage and back splint. Gluteal exercises, isometric quadriceps exercises and foot movements are encouraged immediately but a satisfactory quadriceps contraction may not be achieved until pain and discomfort have diminished, and straight leg raising is not usually attempted for the first few days. Weight-bearing is determined by the type of operation and at the discretion of the surgeon.

When the splintage is removed knee mobilising and strengthening exercises are given but care must be taken to avoid excessive leverage over the knee until sound healing has occurred.

Hydrotherapy is an effective form of treatment in the initial stages of mobilisation, the warmth and support of the water helping to overcome apprehension and facilitate active movement. The back splint is retained for walking until the patient has achieved full active extension of the knee, 70–90 degrees of flexion and good control of movement through the range. Once confidence has been restored rehabilitation progresses quickly and the patient gradually resumes normal activities.

REFERENCES

Asher, C. (1975). *Postural Variations in Childhood*. (Apley, J. overall editor.) Butterworths, London.

de Lorme, T.L. (1945). Restoration of muscle power by heavy resistance exercises. *Journal of Bone and Joint Surgery*, 27, 645–67.

Harris, R.I. and Beath, T. (1947). *Army Foot Survey – An Investigation of Foot Ailments in Canadian Soldiers*. National Research Council of Canada, Ottawa.

Harris, R.I. (1948). Hypermobile flat foot with short tendo Achilles. *Journal of Bone and Joint Surgery*, **30A**, 116.

Rose, G.K. (1958). Correction of the pronated foot. *Journal of Bone and Joint Surgery*, **40B**, 674.

Rose, G.K. (1962). Correction of the pronated foot. *Journal of Bone and Joint Surgery*, **44B**, 642.

Rose, G.K. (1982). *Pes Planus*. In *Disorders of the Foot* (Jahss, M.H. (ed)). W.B. Saunders Co, Philadelphia.

BIBLIOGRAPHY

Hollis, M. (1981). *Practical Exercise Therapy*, 2nd edition. Blackwell Scientific Publications Limited, Oxford.

Maitland, G.D. (1977). *Peripheral Manipulation*, 2nd edition. Butterworths, London.

ACKNOWLEDGEMENT

Figures 7/15 and 7/27 reproduced by permission of Butterworths, London, and Figure 7/16 by permission of W.B. Saunders Co, Philadelphia.

Chapter 8

Disorders of the Hip and Inequality of Leg Length

by G.A. EVANS, MB, BS, FRCS, FRCS(orth)
and V. DRAYCOTT, MCSP, ONC

CONGENITAL DISLOCATION OF THE HIP

Epidemiology

Congenital dislocation of the hip occurs more frequently in females than males with a ratio of 3:1 at neonatal diagnosis. The reported incidence at birth is between 3 and 5 cases per thousand live births. The left hip is affected more frequently than the right, and it is bilateral in 20 per cent of cases (Fig. 8/1). Familial and environmental factors predispose to this condition. It is probable that the most

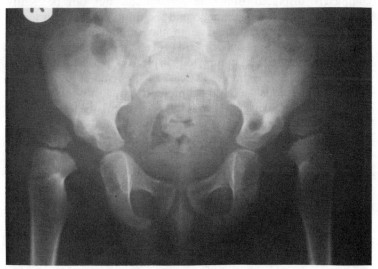

Fig. 8/1 Bilateral dislocation of the hips in a three-year-old child. It is associated with acetabular dysplasia and a straight femoral neck-shaft angle due to excessive anteversion

important familial factor is excessive generalised joint laxity, and if one parent has suffered from congenital dislocation the risk of presentation in a child is 12 per cent (sons 6 per cent, and daughters 17 per cent) (Wynne-Davies, 1973). Antenatal environmental factors associated with an increased incidence of a dislocation are first-born child, breech presentation, and oligohydramnios.

It is possible that intra-uterine compression, fetal position, or a combination of the two, results in a dislocation in those babies with a genetic predisposition. The joint laxity may be further increased in the perinatal period by maternal hormones responsible for relaxing the ligaments of the birth canal crossing the placenta and affecting the baby. In the post-natal period it is known that the majority of unstable hips undergo spontaneous resolution (Barlow, 1962). On the other hand if the hips are maintained in an unfavourable extended and adducted position spontaneous resolution does not occur, with the result that the incidence of dislocation appears much higher in societies in which it is customary to 'swaddle' infants.

Pathology

Neonatal hip instability varies in severity and has three different presentations. The first is frank dislocation, when the femoral head is completely displaced from the acetabulum, but can be gently relocated by the examiner. The second presentation is the dislocatable hip, when the femoral head is in the acetabulum but, with a provocative manoeuvre of backward pressure on the adducted thigh, the femoral head can be completely displaced from the acetabulum (Barlow, 1962). Once the leg is released the femoral head usually reduces spontaneously. The third presentation, a subluxable hip, is the most difficult to diagnose, and is associated with the least capsular laxity. Subluxation occurs when the femoral head can be moved significantly, but not completely out of the acetabulum.

The shape of the femoral head and acetabulum is normal in the neonatal period, but persistance of the instability results in secondary anatomic abnormality. The acetabular labrum (limbus) becomes deformed, and may become inverted between the head and acetabulum. When a dislocation has been present for a prolonged period, the inferior capsule and psoas tendon develop contractures, which prevent relocation of the femoral head. The femoral head begins to lose its spherical shape and the anteversion of the femoral neck tends to increase, rather than decrease as in the normally located joint. The acetabulum becomes shallow through lack of growth of its lateral and anterior margins (Fig. 8/1). These features are progressive with the persistence of the dislocation. It is therefore important to diagnose and treat the condition at birth in order to prevent the development of the soft tissue and bony changes described, and to reduce the magnitude and morbidity of the treatment. Rarely the dislocation may be present *in utero* and is usually associated with other joint problems such as arthrogryposis. In these circumstances the secondary changes will be present at birth.

Clinical presentation

All new-born children should be examined to try to identify dislocation or abnormal laxity of the hip. Frank dislocation is associated with shortening of the leg, a high-riding prominent trochanter, a relative emptiness of the femoral triangle, and telescoping on proximal pressure. The head can be felt to relocate on performing Ortolani's manoeuvre, which involves abducting and raising the flexed thigh forwards gently. Occasionally on performing this manoeuvre the sensation of a click can be elicited from the joint. In the absence of displacement of the femoral head this is of no serious significance. With such neonatal screening, Barlow (1962) claimed that he was able to diagnose all cases in the new-born period and eradicate the late presentation of hip dislocation. However, in most centres worldwide, we have not been able to reproduce this success, and a minority of cases continue to present later in life. Apart from failure to recognise a neonatal dislocation, a further possible explanation is that the occasional neonatal subluxation, which is difficult to detect clinically, may result in progressive acetabular dysplasia and displacement of the femoral head (Kepley and Weiner, 1981).

In the older child the classical clinical signs of dislocation include limited abduction, a high greater trochanter, and relative femoral shortening. The dislocation is no longer reducible by the Ortolani manoeuvre. After the age of walking, there is a noticeable limp with a positive Trendelenburg test. Bilateral cases present with a symmetrical waddling gait, which may not be recognised as being abnormal until the child has grown out of the toddler age.

Treatment

The objective of treatment is to reduce the femoral head into the acetabulum without producing damage to it or its blood supply by forceful manoeuvres. The specific treatment depends on the age of the child at diagnosis. It is advantageous to start treatment in the neonatal period, before the onset of secondary soft tissue and bony changes. For this reason all children are screened for congenital dislocation as part of the neonatal examination, and at the developmental screening usually undertaken by the community physician at approximately six weeks and six months of age.

When the diagnosis is made in the *newborn* the principle of treatment is to retain the hip in flexion and abduction, so that the femoral head is reduced in the acetabulum. The initial capsular laxity regresses, and after approximately three months' treatment the joint is stable, requires no further treatment, and the prognosis for a normal joint is excellent. Treatment usually starts once the diagnosis has been made, although in some centres it is deferred for two to three weeks because, as mentioned above, a large number resolve spontaneously and only the minority of hips with residual instability are then treated. There are many different devices available to maintain the flexed and abducted posture of the hips, and these include the Craig nappy splint, the Von Rosen splint, and the Pavlik harness. The former two splints tend to hold the hips in one position, whereas the Pavlik harness allows motion, but within a constrained range (Fig.8/2) (Lovell and Winter, 1978).

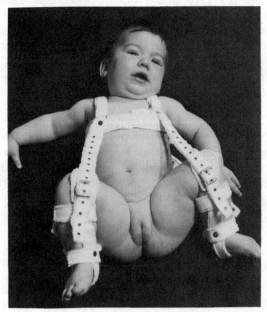

Fig. 8/2   Pavlik harness applied

When treatment is started later, *up to six months of age*, the Pavlik harness achieves reduction in the majority of cases. When the harness is first applied the hip is still dislocated, but the active movement and kicking of the child within the constraints of the harness achieve a spontaneous reduction. The complications of this treatment in terms of damage to the femoral head are negligible. When successful, the reduction is achieved within three weeks, but the harness is usually retained for up to a further six months depending on the appearance of the bony growth and remodelling on radiographic examination. The treatment described so far can be undertaken as an outpatient.

If diagnosed after *six months of age*, or if any of the above mentioned treatment has failed to achieve reduction, the child requires in-patient treatment. At this stage there is relative shortening of the soft tissues adjacent to the hip joint. Skin traction is therefore an important preliminary treatment to manipulative or operative reduction. This prevents excessive pressure on the head and damage to it following reduction. There are several different techniques of applying traction to the legs some of which, such as the Wingfield frame (Scott, 1953) and Alvik traction, attempt to obtain reduction during the period of traction. Other forms, such as overhead divarication traction (Fig. 8/3) are primarily used to stretch the soft tissues, followed by a gentle

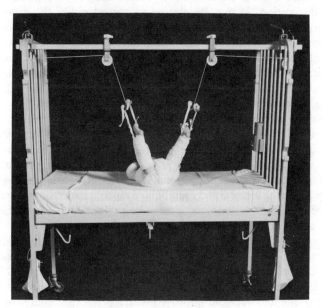

Fig. 8/3   Gallows traction

manipulative reduction under general anaesthesia. This is called a 'closed reduction'. An arthrogram of the hip joint may be performed at the same time to demonstrate absence of soft tissue interposition between the femoral head and acetabulum. In a small child the majority of the femoral head and acetabulum are made of cartilage and do not show on a plain radiograph. If a closed reduction cannot be achieved (Fig.8/1), an operation is necessary to remove the obstructive factors and this is called an 'open reduction'. The most common obstructive factors are persistent contracture of the inferior capsule, a tight psoas tendon, and an inverted limbus. Once the reduction has been achieved, by either manipulation or operation, it is maintained by application of a plaster of Paris spica. The regime thereafter depends on the individual preference of the treating surgeon. In general terms hip abduction is maintained either by a plaster cast or splint until there is evidence of satisfactory bony remodelling of the joint on the radiograph. Plaster casts are changed at intervals depending on the rate of growth of the child, with short periods of physiotherapy at the time of admission for plaster change. Stiffness is more likely to be a problem after open rather than closed reduction.

Additional operative procedures may be required in an older child, when there is less potential for bony remodelling following reduction of a dislocation. It may be elected to correct either the excessive femoral anteversion, or the dysplasia of the acetabulum in order to improve the stability of the reduction while the leg is in the weight-bearing functional position. This reduces the need for prolonged splintage in abduction and flexion. The anteversion is corrected by derotation osteotomy of the proximal femur (Figs. 8/4a and b), and the acetabular dysplasia by a pelvic osteotomy, described by Salter, which tilts the acetabulum downwards, forwards, and laterally (Figs. 8/5a and b) (Salter, 1961). Following such surgery, the child is immobilised in a plaster spica for six weeks until the osteotomy has united, and then requires physiotherapy to assist progressive mobilisation. In the very occasional case presenting after three years of age, both the femoral and acetabular dysplasia may require surgical correction. The whole correction can be performed at one operation but there is an increased risk of postoperative joint stiffness.

Very occasionally a child may present for the first time during adolescence with a limp or discomfort in the hip due to subluxation and acetabular dysplasia (Fig. 8/6). If the subluxation is irreducible, as is frequently the case at this age, the position is accepted and the cover of the femoral head improved with a pelvic osteotomy. At this age a Chiari osteotomy is appropriate, dividing the ilium immediately

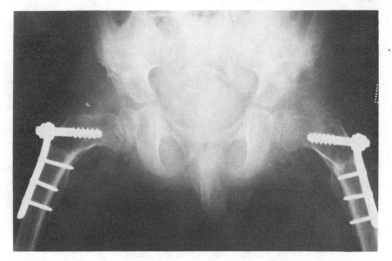

Fig. 8/4a Open reduction and femoral derotation osteotomy to correct the anteversion (same patient as Fig. 8/1)

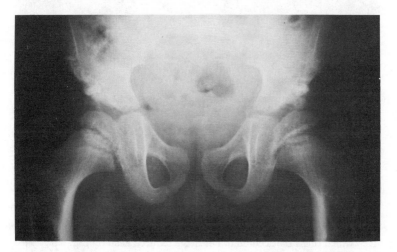

Fig. 8/4b The surgical plate and screws have been removed, and the acetabulae are slowly remodelling as the child grows (*cf* Figs. 8/1 and 8/4a)

above the level of the head and displacing the lower fragment with the head medially under the cover of the upper fragment. The superior joint capsule remains between the articular surface of the femoral head and the exposed bone of the osteotomy surface (Chiari, 1974). Unlike

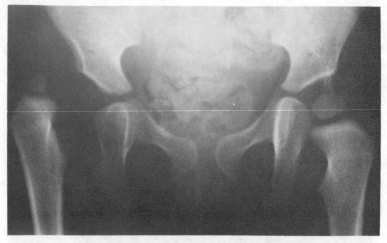

Fig. 8/5a Unilateral dislocation in a 22-month-old child

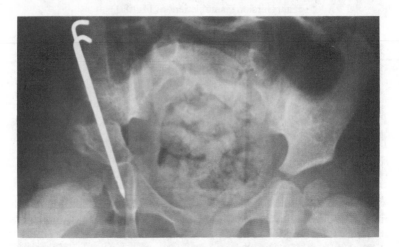

Fig. 8/5b Following combined open reduction and a Salter pelvic osteotomy which turns the acetabulum over the reduced head (*cf* Fig. 8/5a)

the Salter osteotomy performed at a younger age, this does not place normal articular cartilage over the head, and is therefore regarded as a salvage rather than a reconstructive operation. Sometimes a bony shelf is constructed over the femoral head rather than performing the Chiari osteotomy (Wainwright, 1976). Following a period of immobilisation in plaster to allow the osteotomy to unite, the patient

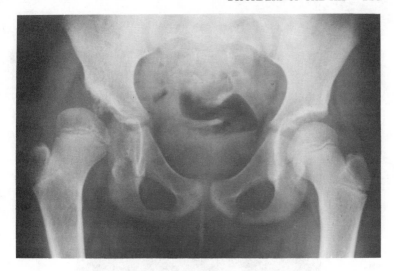

Fig. 8/6   Adolescent child with subluxation of the femoral head and
acetabular dysplasia

requires physiotherapy to mobilise the joint and to strengthen the
abductor and extensor muscles.

Physiotherapy

Dislocation of the hip is the most common of the congenital disorders
and the physiotherapist has only a small part to play in the early stages
of the treatment. Initially the child should be carefully and gently
assessed for clinical signs such as limited range of abduction,
asymmetrical thigh and buttock creases, apparent limb length
inequality and, in the child who has already begun to walk, assessment
of the gait, looking for 'dipping' or 'toe walking'.

The majority of children are treated initially on gallows (Bryant's)
traction or Alvik traction, the choice being dependent upon the age
and size of the child. Young babies up to the age of approximately 18
months are put on gallows traction (Fig. 8/3); this allows bonding to
continue between mother and child, and still maintain a gentle pull
(Fig. 8/7). The Alvik traction is a more permanent arrangement and
the child should not be removed from the bed. The purpose of the
traction is to stretch the soft tissues around the hip joint prior to
reduction which may be either open or closed. During this time, if it is
possible to get co-operation from the child, the physiotherapist should

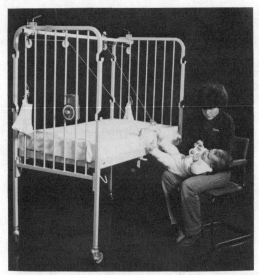

Fig. 8/7   Baby on gallows traction allowing bonding with the mother

encourage active movements of the feet, and static (isometric) contractions of the quadriceps and gluteal muscles. It may mean that treatment takes the form of play, and parents and nurses should be encouraged to attempt to achieve this aim during their stay with the child. Once reduction of the hip has been achieved the child is usually immobilised in a plaster of Paris double-hip spica for a minimum period of six weeks, which may extend to 10 weeks, depending upon the procedure involved.

Once the plaster is removed then physiotherapy is of value. Exercises to regain mobility of the hips and knees, combined with strengthening of the muscles, especially the gluteals, are of vital importance. The timing and progression of treatment is determined by the individual consultant. Wherever possible mobilisation should include hydrotherapy. This serves to relieve any apprehension in the child, and at the same time allows the physiotherapist to give gentle exercises in the form of play. Weight-bearing is commenced once the hips and knees are mobile and strong enough to allow a reciprocal gait, that is at least 90 degrees of hip and knee flexion, and the gluteal muscles strong enough to prevent waddling. Once walking is begun it is important to discourage any asymmetry of gait as, if left uncorrected, it may become habitual and lead to further acquired deformities.

PERTHES' DISEASE

Epidemiology

Perthes' disease is a transient ischaemic necrosis of the capital femoral epiphysis which occurs in children between the ages of 2 and 12 years, but mainly between 4 and 8 years of age. Boys are affected four times more frequently than girls and the condition is bilateral in approximately 12 per cent of affected children. It was described almost simultaneously at the beginning of the 20th century by Legg from the United States, Calvé from France and Perthes from Germany. There is no obvious pattern of inheritance. Many children appear to be undersized and skeletally immature at the time of developing Perthes' disease. There is also a slightly higher incidence of minor congenital anomalies in these children compared to a control population. It is speculated that there may be a congenital abnormality affecting skeletal development which in some ways makes the hip susceptible to Perthes' disease. However, the precise aetiology is unknown.

Pathology

The pathological process involves the death of part or the whole of the capital femoral epiphysis followed by gradual revascularisation of the area. The articular cartilage is normal or, at most, shows faint signs of degeneration in its basilar layers. At an early stage a radiograph will show flattening and increased density of the femoral head (Fig. 8/8a, p. 167). On microscopic examination there is pronounced necrosis of the bone with grossly distorted marrow trabeculae, and the bone fragments are of a soft consistency. Later the radiograph appears to show the femoral head broken up into areas that are relatively dense interspersed with areas of radiolucency. This represents the resorption of the dead bone with added areas of osteoid and new bone. The femoral head may become distorted, flattened, and extruded laterally from its normal location under the acetabulum. There is a gradual increase in the amount of living bone, and on the radiograph the femoral head usually regains its homogenous density over two to four years. In the meantime it may lose its normal spherical shape and become flattened superiorly. This is important as the final shape of the head influences the long-term prognosis of the joint. If the head remains spherical, even if it is slightly larger, the prognosis is good. Increasing loss of sphericity and congruity predisposes to a proportionate increase in the severity of secondary osteoarthritis during adult life (Lloyd Roberts and Ratliff, 1978).

Clinical presentation

The most frequently observed symptom is a limp, which may or may not be associated with pain in the groin and inner thigh. Occasionally the pain may be referred to the distal thigh and knee. Muscle spasm is usually present and limits abduction and internal rotation of the hip. The absence of pyrexia, with normal haematological investigations excludes the differential diagnosis of pyogenic arthritis or osteo-myelitis of the femoral neck.

Treatment

Perthes' is a self-limiting condition, and all affected femoral heads heal. The objective of treatment is therefore to try to minimise the deformity during the active stages of the disease in order to reduce the incidence of osteoarthritis during adult life. The age of onset of the condition, and the amount of femoral head involved appear to be the two major prognostic factors. Children under five years usually do very well, especially if the femoral head is only partly necrotic. However, onset after six years of age, has a less favourable prognosis. When the child first presents, it is generally agreed that the appropriate treatment consists of bed rest and skin traction in order to relieve the muscle spasm and regain the range of hip motion. The majority of children will have regained full abduction and internal rotation after two or three weeks' treatment. The management thereafter varies widely within Great Britain, and throughout the world. There has been a general trend to try to select the appropriate cases which would benefit from further treatment. For example, the prognosis for presentation under four years of age with partial head involvement, and without lateral displacement of the head, is excellent and does not justify the imposition of restricted activities or surgical intervention.

Although there are many different specific methods of managing Perthes' disease, there are two basic treatment principles, which may be applied individually or in combination. The first principle is *weight relief* and the second is *containment*. The latter principle refers to the fact that if the femoral head can be maintained deeply within the acetabulum during the soft vulnerable phase of the disease process, the acetabulum will function rather like a mould, and a more normal femoral head will result. Since it is the lateral and anterior portions of the capital epiphysis which become uncovered, the containment can be achieved by abduction and internal rotation of the hip (Figs. 8/8a and b).

Non-weight-bearing treatment includes bed rest with or without

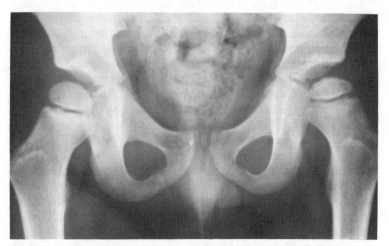

Fig. 8/8a   Early flattening and lateral displacement of the femoral head (right) due to Perthes' disease

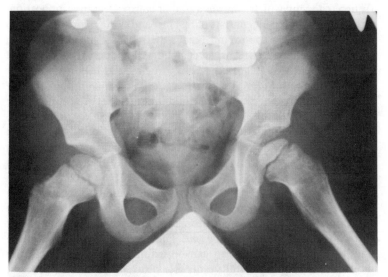

Fig. 8/8b   Femoral head 'contained' in the acetabulum by application of an abduction brace

traction, and was traditionally applied on a Robert Jones frame. Bed rest for longer than is necessary to regain motion in the hips is now no longer considered practical. Weight relief is also achieved with a Snyder sling and by the Birmingham splint. Ischial weight-bearing braces are not truly weight-relieving and on occasions may increase the pressure across the joint. The hip usually remains adducted with this brace and the results of treatment are inferior to those of containment methods. However, treatment on the Jones frame and with the Birmingham splint applies a combination of weight relief and containment. There are several methods of the treatment that rely on containment of the femoral head but allow weight-bearing. These include plaster casts to maintain the abduction, so called broomstick or Petrie plasters (Fig. 8/9); abduction splints and surgical intervention. There is probably little difference in the results of these containment methods and the choice will depend on the availability of an orthotist to undertake prompt delivery and repairs of a splint, and on the geographic and social factors which influence the indications for operative treatment. One type of abduction splint was developed at the Scottish-Rite hospital in Atlanta, USA and allows the child to walk in abduction with minimal other restriction, to attend school and sit at his normal desk, and to play out of doors (Figs. 8/10a and b). This particular splint does not maintain internal rotation of the hip, but on weight-bearing there is usually a minimum of 20 degrees flexion of the hip which achieves a similar cover of the anterior portion of the femoral head.

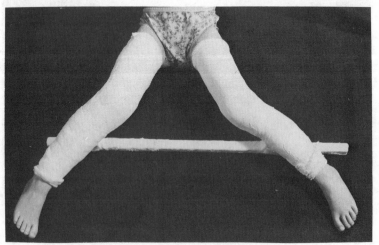

Fig. 8/9 Petrie or broomstick plasters

Surgical containment of the femoral head can be produced by either a proximal femoral varus derotation osteotomy (Fig. 8/11), or by

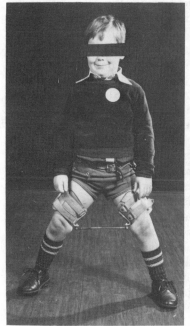 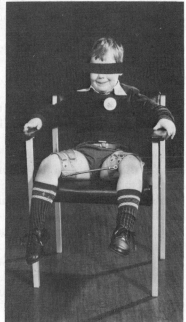

Fig. 8/10a The Scottish-Rite brace (standing)   **Fig. 8/10b** The Scottish-Rite brace (sitting)

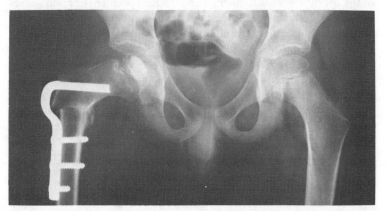

Fig. 8/11 Perthes' disease presenting with a dense infarcted capital epiphysis which has been treated by femoral osteotomy

altering the acetabulum to provide further coverage with a Salter pelvic osteotomy. Surgery is more often indicated when the prognosis indicates that the healing phase may be prolonged, as in older children. It can also be used for patients who will not tolerate a bracing programme. The range of movement must be almost normal prior to surgical treatment.

Physiotherapy

Providing the decision is made to institute active treatment, this may again be in the form of conservative or operative intervention. In both cases *containment* of the hip is the ultimate aim. Conservative measures may include both weight-bearing and non-weight-bearing means. If prolonged bed rest is advised as a method of non-weight-bearing the child must be taught all static exercises, particularly quadriceps and gluteals, together with resisted exercises to avoid muscle wasting. The Snyder sling may also be used; this allows the child to be mobile on axillary crutches and still remain non-weight-bearing on the affected side. However, other methods which allow weight-bearing with containment, appear to be more satisfactory.

Such a one is the Scottish-Rite brace which holds the legs in abduction, yet allows flexion of the hip joint. The brace is custom-made by the orthotist and the child should be taught to be completely independent within the splint, leading as near normal life as possible. Once the brace is fitted the child has to be taught to balance in the abducted position, and from then on to progress to a reciprocal gait making use of the universal joints on the abduction bar of the splint. In order to maintain an upright posture the child stands with flexed hips and knees, thus self-inducing containment. While the child is in the brace the parents should be taught how to look after the splint and be shown the exercises to be done with the child, daily, to maintain hip range and muscle power, particularly hip extensors.

A second method of weight-bearing with containment is the application of Petrie plasters, i.e. long-leg plaster of Paris cylinders with the knees flexed at approximately 15 degrees and, by attaching a broomstick at the lower end of the plaster cylinders 30 degrees of hip abduction and 20 degrees of internal rotation are maintained. This method does not allow reciprocal hip flexion because of the rigidity of the broomstick. Once again the child is taught to stand in the plasters and progress to walking, being completely independent on discharge. Such children are readmitted to hospital at three-monthly intervals when the plasters are removed and a period of hip and knee mobilising begun, strictly non-weight-bearing. Hydrotherapy has proved invaluable during this time. Once full range of movement has been regained, particularly in the knees, the plasters are re-applied and the child discharged. This procedure is repeated until, based on radiological findings, healing is complete.

Surgical means of achieving containment involve an adduction and external rotation osteotomy usually with plate fixation. Routine postoperative care for a femoral osteotomy should be followed, with weight-bearing delayed for at least six weeks. During the initial postoperative period every effort should be made to maintain the pre-operative range of movement and, where possible, to increase the same. In some instances the child may be discharged home in a plaster hip spica for a six-week period. On readmission, once the plaster is removed, vigorous physiotherapy is required to regain hip and knee joint range prior to weight-bearing.

SLIPPED UPPER FEMORAL EPIPHYSIS

The term slipped capital femoral epiphysis refers to a displacement of the femoral neck in relationship to the head, usually during adolescence. The femoral neck rotates externally and slides upwards causing the radiological appearance of a femoral head which is displaced posteriorly and inferiorly (Fig. 8/12a, p. 173).

Epidemiology

Boys are more frequently affected than girls and because of the delayed growth spurt in boys the condition occurs on average about two years later than in girls. The age range for boys is 10 to 17 years, with an average of 11 to 12 years. The black population is apparently more frequently affected than the white population. The skeletal age is usually below chronological age, and approximately half the patients have body-weight at or above the 95th percentile. The condition occurs bilaterally in approximately 1/5th of cases. There is frequently a positive family history of the condition.

Aetiology

The precise aetiology is still unknown. The plane of separation is at the bone-cartilage junction of the growth plate and it is thought that there may be increased structural weakness at this site during the adolescent growth spurt. There are some interesting mechanical factors which have been observed. The growth plate normally changes from a horizontal to an oblique position during the early adolescent period and the periosteum of the femoral neck, which is the main stabiliser of the epiphysis, atrophies at the same time. In addition there may be hormonal factors which relate to the balance of pituitary growth hormone and sex hormones. The sex hormones induce growth plate closure at skeletal maturity, and growth hormone stimulates the proliferation of the cells of the growth plate. A frequent condition associated with slipped epiphysis is the adiposo-genital syndrome, a condition characterised by obesity and deficient gonadal development, which suggests that it may be due to excessive loading of the relatively weak growth plate. Less frequently the condition occurs in a very tall, thin boy, which may indicate a relative excess of growth hormone and weakness of the rapidly proliferating growth plate. When the slip is bilateral and symmetrical, other conditions such as hypothyroidism should be excluded.

Clinical presentation

There are three classical presentations:
1. The *acute* slip is the result of significant injury with no previous history of pain. It is usually severe enough to prevent weight-bearing.
2. The *acute on chronic* slip presents with some aching in the hip or distal thigh for weeks or even months prior to an acute episode as described above (Fig. 8/12a, p. 173).
3. The *chronic* slip is the commonest presentation, the child complaining of a limp, pain, and loss of motion which may have been present for several weeks (Fig. 8/13a, p. 175). Occasionally the only symptom is pain referred to the knee.

Examination reveals restriction of internal rotation and abduction, and as the thigh is flexed it tends to roll into external rotation and abduction. There is frequent shortening of the leg, which tends to lie in external rotation. Radiographic examination will confirm the diagnosis and indicate the severity of the displacement. In chronic cases there is remodelling of the inferior and posterior aspects of the femoral neck adjacent to the growth plate, which begins to develop a slight hook. The opposite hip should be examined carefully for early involvement, which may simply be a widening of the epiphyseal line.

Treatment

Once the diagnosis has been made, the child should not be allowed to weight-bear and arrangements should be made to admit the child

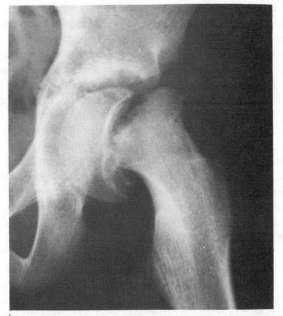

Fig. 8/12a   Displacement of the capital femoral epiphysis which occurred suddenly after a preceding history of an ache and occasional limp

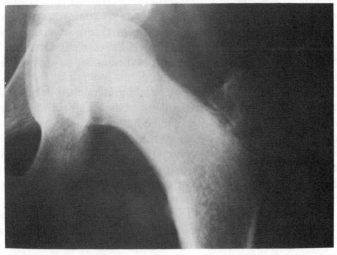

Fig. 8/12b   Improved position of the epiphysis as the result of skin traction applied with progressive abduction and internal rotation of the hip

directly to hospital for treatment. This is in order to prevent any further displacement. The child is placed in bed with skin traction on both legs in order to reduce spasm and relieve discomfort.

If the slip is acute the displacement can be corrected with skin traction, by slowly and progressively abducting and internally rotating the leg (Fig. 8/12b). Alternatively, the reduction can be achieved by gentle manipulation under general anaesthesia. If the acute slip has been present for more than two weeks, there is considerable risk of avascular necrosis from manipulation, and because of this problem there is divided opinion as to whether manipulative treatment should be used at all. If an acute slip has occurred on a pre-existing chronic slip, it is important that the repositioning only reduces the acute aspect of the slip. The greater threat to the hip is avascular necrosis, and not incomplete reduction. Further displacement is prevented by surgical insertion of pins along the femoral neck into the epiphysis.

The objective of treatment in the child with a chronic slip is to stabilise the femoral head in situ and maintain the range of motion. This is usually preceded by a period of bed rest and traction, which relieves muscle spasm and synovitis, and apparently reduces the risk of the complication of chondrolysis. Further displacement is then prevented by operative insertion of pins along the femoral neck into the epiphysis (Fig. 8/13b). In cases with severe displacement this may be technically very difficult. Operations have been devised either to correct the displacement at the level of the open growth plate (Dunn's osteotomy) (Dunn and Angel, 1978) or to compensate for the deformity with a subtrochanteric osteotomy (Southwick osteotomy) (Southwick, 1967). There appears to be an increased risk of avascular necrosis with the former procedure, and of chondrolysis with the latter procedure.

If the opposite hip shows widening of the growth plate, or early slip, it should also be pinned. There is debate as to whether prophylactic pinning of the contralateral hip should be undertaken routinely. As pinning of the hip can be associated with complications, it is probably better reserved for selected cases such as those with predisposing hormonal abnormalities, for example the adiposo-genital syndrome.

The main complications of this condition and its treatment are avascular necrosis and chondrolysis. Avascular necrosis occurs as a result of tension and occlusion of the retinacular vessels passing along the femoral neck to the capital epiphysis. This causes necrosis and collapse of the femoral head with loss of sphericity. The potential for retaining a spherical head is very much poorer at this age than in young children with Perthes' disease, and usually results in secondary

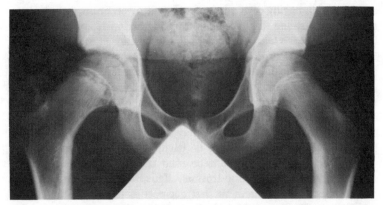

Fig. 8/13a A chronic slip of the capital epiphysis (left). There is slight widening of the growth plate, and early medial and backward displacement of the epiphysis

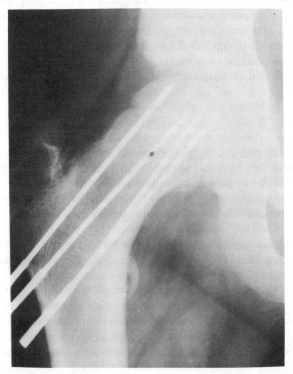

Fig. 8/13b Surgical fixation of the epiphysis by insertion of pins which pass along the femoral neck and across the growth plate

osteoarthritis during early adult life. Chondrolysis presents with acute pain and restricted motion of the hip joint. The precise cause is not known. There is a loss of articular cartilage, which is later replaced by fibrocartilage which does not have the same properties of wear, and predisposes to secondary osteoarthritis. The initial treatment is to try to reduce the joint reaction with traction and salicylates, and to retain a range of motion with physiotherapy. This is followed by a prolonged period of non-weight-bearing and motion exercises. Despite this treatment the range of motion may be very limited. The natural history of even the severe slips is that they do well into middle life before the development of osteoarthritis, if there has been no avascular necrosis or chondrolysis. This therefore suggests that simple methods of treatment that decrease or eliminate the risk of avascular necrosis or chondrolysis should be most commonly used.

Following pin fixation of the femoral epiphysis the patient is encouraged to regain active control of the hip and, in particular, the ranges of abduction and internal rotation. When this has been achieved the child is allowed to partially weight-bear with the aid of crutches, and the decision to allow full weight-bearing will vary according to the degree of displacement and security of fixation. The growth plate usually fuses prematurely, which prevents any further possibility of displacement, and it is usual to remove the pins at this stage.

Physiotherapy

Following surgery, it is important that early active assisted movements are given to the hip. Progressive exercises are given over the initial 10-day postoperative period, bearing in mind the need to maintain and, if possible, increase the muscle power of the unaffected leg, as the child will have to be non-weight-bearing for at least six weeks.

During the non-weight-bearing period it is important that the child and his parents continue with exercises to the affected hip. Isometric exercises for the gluteal and quadriceps muscles should be taught, together with maximum movement in all ranges at the hip joint. During treatment it is important to examine the sound hip at regular intervals as, occasionally, the contralateral epiphysis may slip, even during the 10-day postoperative period of bed rest. As she is handling the patient daily, it is often the physiotherapist who first detects this.

COXA VARA

Coxa vara is an abnormality of the proximal end of the femur which is characterised by a decrease in the neck shaft angle. This angle measures approximately 150 degrees at one year of age and gradually decreases to 120 degrees in the adult. A neck shaft angle of less than 120 degrees in a child is arbitrarily labelled as coxa vara.

Aetiology

There are many different causes of coxa vara. *Infantile* coxa vara is regarded as a distinct entity and is characterised by having a triangular bone defect in the inferior part of the metaphysis of the femoral neck (Fig. 8/14). It is sometimes bilateral but is not associated with any other developmental defect. Several reports of a family history suggest that the condition has a genetic transmission.

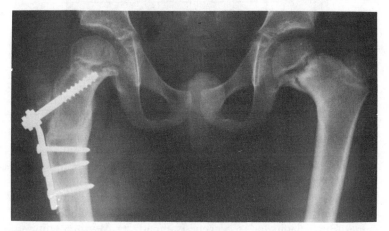

Fig. 8/14 Bilateral coxa vara which has been corrected on one side by a valgus osteotomy. On the other side the triangular bone defect persists at the inferior margin of the metaphysis

Other focal forms of coxa vara include children with a congenital short femur, which may sometimes be associated with lateral bowing of the proximal femoral shaft and sclerosis on the concave side (Fig. 8/15). In the more severe forms a pseudoarthrosis may be present between the femoral neck and shaft, and this represents the minor end of the spectrum of congenital anomalies known as proximal focal

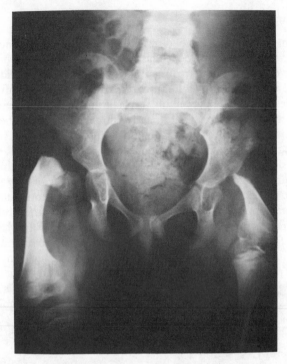

Fig. 8/15 Congenital shortening of the femur with coxa vara. On the opposite side there is congenital absence of the femoral head and proximal shaft

femoral deficiency. Other causes of coxa vara include any skeletal disorder or dysplasia which result in softening or weakening of the bones. Examples include osteogenesis imperfecta, Morquio's disease, achondroplasia, and metaphyseal dysostosis.

Clinical presentation

In infantile coxa vara the deformity is diagnosed when the child first walks, usually with a painless limp or waddling gait. Trendelenburg's sign is positive and hip abduction limited. The greater trochanter is elevated sometimes so that the tip of the trochanter impinges upon the ilium resulting in marked gluteal deficiency. In unilateral cases there is usually a leg length discrepancy.

Treatment

Treatment depends on the degree of deformity, the functional impairment, and the evidence as to whether the deformity is progressive. Conservative treatment may be employed in mild cases where the varus deformity is not progressing and the neck shaft angle approaches normal. However, in the majority of children with the infantile variety of coxa vara, early surgery provides the best opportunity to achieve a painless and fully mobile hip without further shortening of the limb. The indications for surgery are the presence of a vertical defect in the femoral neck, a neck shaft angle of less than 100 degrees, and progression of the coxa vara, which may or may not be associated with discomfort. An intertrochanteric or subtrochanteric valgus osteotomy accompanied by internal fixation is the preferred form of treatment (see Fig. 8/14). The operative goal is to place the proximal femoral growth plate in a normal alignment, perpendicular to the resultant weight-bearing force acting across the hip joint. This in turn improves the hip abductor function, and reduces the leg length discrepancy. Postoperatively a plaster spica is applied for approximately six weeks until the osteotomy has united, and then mobilising and strengthening exercises are prescribed.

Physiotherapy

Treatment is based upon the aim to preserve hip joint function and surgery is most often a femoral osteotomy. The physiotherapist becomes involved at the pre-operative stage when she will explain to the patient what will be required postoperatively. Following surgery the patient is usually immobilised in a plaster of Paris hip spica for six weeks. After this time the plaster is bivalved and gentle active assisted exercises are given to the hip and knee joints. Often the posterior half of the plaster is retained as a night splint until the child is able to control active leg movements adequately. Progressive non-weight-bearing exercises are given, combined with hydrotherapy, until a full range of movement is achieved. Weight-bearing is started as soon as union of the osteotomy is confirmed radiologically.

INEQUALITY OF LEG LENGTH

Aetiology

The problem of leg length discrepancy is common despite the fact that the aetiological factors have changed considerably during the past 20 years. Prior to the advent of poliomyelitis vaccine, shortening due to the muscle paralysis of polio was the most common. Other causes of discrepancy have now assumed greater importance, and may result in either shortening or lengthening of a limb. A short leg may be caused by a congenital abnormality (Figs. 8/16a and b), infection of bone and joint, and fractures of the long bones, especially those which result in damage and tethering of the growth plate. Neurological conditions such as spinal dysraphism and spastic hemiparesis may also sometimes cause significant shortening. Overgrowth of the limb may be associated with a haemangioma or arteriovenous malformation, neurofibromatosis, and fibrous dysplasia. Rarely, significant overgrowth may occur due to stimulation of bone growth following fracture of the femur or tibia, or the stimulus of osteotomy and subsequent plate removal.

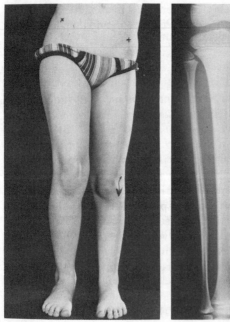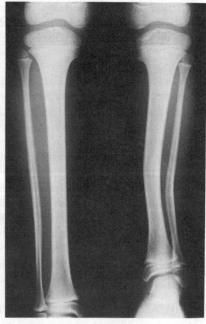

Fig. 8/16a   Inequality of leg length. The child stands with pelvic obliquity and compensatory scoliosis

Fig. 8/16b   Radiograph showing the short and slightly bowed tibia and fibula

Clinical presentation

The child may present with a limp, and other symptoms or signs which relate to the aetiology of the discrepancy. The inequality of leg length does not cause pain. When standing with both feet flat on the floor there is a pelvic obliquity and compensatory scoliosis, which the child tolerates without symptoms (Fig. 8/16a). Alternatively the child can stand with a level pelvis either by flexing the knee on the longer leg or by weight-bearing on the forefoot of the shorter leg. If the condition is not associated with weakness or derangement of the joints, the gait may appear remarkably normal. The child frequently vaults on the forefoot of the short leg in order to compensate for the discrepancy.

Treatment

The most significant factor in deciding the appropriate management is the degree of discrepancy. Differences of less than 2cm are usually accepted by the patient and can be treated by non-surgical methods, such as a shoe-raise. At the other end of the scale, any projected inequality exceeding 15cm is usually in excess of the amount that any combination of operations can be effectively or predictably employed to equalise. The only exception is when surgical conversion (amputation or disarticulation) and application of a prosthesis are employed. For the most part therefore, only discrepancies between 2 and 15cm warrant serious consideration for surgical equalisation. These are not rigid figures and they represent only practical guidelines which may be modified by the many other factors involved in the aetiology of the discrepancy. It is assumed for the purpose of the following discussion that the problem is a true discrepancy of length, rather than an apparent shortening or lengthening of the limb produced by a fixed adduction or abduction contracture respectively at the hip.

In addition to the severity of the discrepancy, the other factors which influence the nature and timing of treatment include the skeletal age, anticipated adult height, and sex. The progression of discrepancy can be measured accurately by taking serial radiographs known as grid films or scanograms. These also allow assessment of the relative discrepancy within the femur and tibia. Serial radiographs of the hand will allow an assessment of bone age and development, which may precede or lag behind chronological age by up to two years. Serial measurement of height on a percentile chart will allow prediction of the anticipated adult height. These measurements are important to help decide the most appropriate treatment, and to monitor the effect if started prior to skeletal maturity.

Surgical equalisation of limb length can be achieved either by shortening the long side, lengthening the short side, or utilising a combination of shortening and lengthening.

A limb can be shortened in one of three ways;

1. The growth plate of the distal femur, or proximal tibia and fibula can be arrested prematurely by epiphyseodesis (Phemister, 1933).
2. The same centres can be arrested temporarily or permanently by epiphyseal stapling (Blount, 1958).
3. The femur or tibia (or both) can be shortened by resection of bone.

Epiphyseodesis is performed on the longer leg at an appropriate time prior to skeletal maturity and, if successful, the short limb continues to grow and will exactly correct the discrepancy by the completion of growth. It is critical to time the operation correctly and this depends on the information gained from serial pre-operative grid films and bone-age assessment. Epiphyseodesis is usually reserved for discrepancies not exceeding 5cm. It is a relatively simple operation, without significant complications, and the rate of acceptable correction is high. Stapling of the epiphysis has a similar effect and convalescence is more rapid. Theoretically the principle advantage that this operation offers over epiphyseodesis is that the operation can be reversed by removal of the staples if overcorrection is occurring. However, practical experience has shown that the response of the growth plate to staple removal is not predictable and the reliability of this procedure is not really proven. The operation is also technically demanding and if the staples are not inserted in precisely the correct site there is a risk of producing asymmetrical growth arrest and deformity. Unlike the former two procedures, bone-shortening operations can be used during or after completion of growth. Up to 6cm of subtrochanteric bone can be resected from the femur without permanent weakening of the thigh or hip, and even more bone can be resected at a midshaft shortening. Shortening below the knee requires resection of a portion of tibia and fibula. These operations are usually associated with internal fixation of the bone fragments.

Correction of inequality can also be achieved by lengthening of bone, and interest has focused recently on the possible benefits of electromagnetic stimulation of the growth plate. Its benefit and indications are as yet undetermined, whereas mechanical lengthening of the femur and tibia is well established (Wagner, 1977). The method which has remained most consistently acceptable is osteotomy followed by gradual distraction. The technical steps include an osteotomy, application of a mechanical distraction device, and

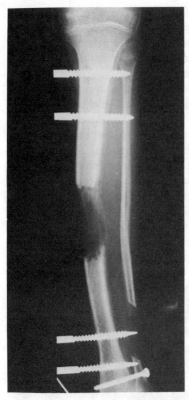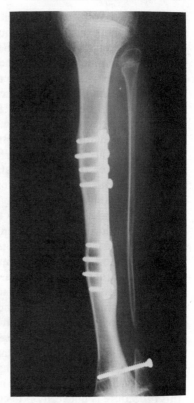

Fig. 8/16c Treatment by osteotomy and lengthening. The screws of the Wagner external fixator have been inserted into the tibia and a separate screw inserted distally to maintain correct alignment of the malleoli

Fig. 8/16d Consolidation of the lengthened tibia after removal of the external fixator and application of a plate

gradual distraction of approximately 1–2mm per day (Fig. 8/16c). Electromyographic study of the lengthened muscles indicates that a 10 per cent lengthening of the bone's initial length is a safe limit, with 15 per cent being the absolute maximum. Slow lengthening protects the soft tissues, in particular the peripheral nerves, and during distraction daily clinical assessment should be performed to exclude early or minor neuropraxia. If present, further distraction is temporarily discontinued until nerve function has recovered, and then further gradual lengthening is usually possible until the desired lengthening is achieved. Clinical guidelines which are helpful in governing the rate of distraction are the degree of pain, the development of sensory or motor neurologic deficit, alterations in local circulation, and any significant elevation of the diastolic blood pressure. Once the desired length is achieved the bone is usually fixed internally with a plate and the external distraction device removed (Fig. 8/16d). Bone grafting of the defect is sometimes required, especially after skeletal maturity. The lengthening operations are more extensive surgical interventions, and are accompanied with greater morbidity, than the shortening operations. Lengthening is therefore reserved for patients who either have a short stature and would be unsuitable for shortening, or have a discrepancy which cannot reasonably be corrected by shortening procedures alone.

There is one situation where the *cause* of discrepancy may be remedied. Following a fracture across the germinal layer of the growth plate a bony tether sometimes forms between the epiphysis and metaphysis. This retards growth, and if the tether is not central it causes angular deformity. An operation may be performed to resect the bony bridge or tether and this was first described by Langenskiold (1981). The surgical defect created is then filled with inert material, such as a fat plug or bone cement, in order to prevent the bone from growing into the defect and retethering the growth plate (Fig. 8/17a).

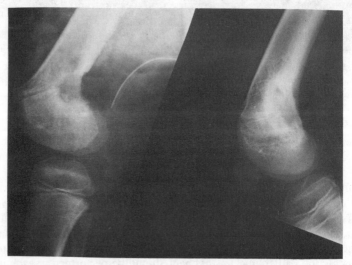

Fig. 8/17 (*Left*) Postoperative appearance following resection of a bony tether. (*Right*) The appearance nine months later showing continued growth of the femur and realignment of the growth plate to a more normal transverse position

Minor angular deformities will correct spontaneously with further growth (Fig. 8/17b) and the operation may be of benefit for tethers which affect up to 40 per cent of the growth plate. Following this procedure the leg is initially protected in a plaster, and subsequently physiotherapy is required to mobilise and strengthen the limb. A brace is sometimes applied to protect the leg until the weakened area of bone has remodelled.

Physiotherapy

LEG SHORTENING

Following epiphyseodesis the patient is encouraged postoperatively to perform isometric quadriceps exercises as soon as possible, progressing to straight leg raising. As soon as the patient is comfortable, usually 48-hours postoperatively, full weight-bearing in a plaster of Paris cylinder may begin. This regime continues for a further six weeks after which the plaster is removed and knee mobilisation commenced. Initially the knee is often very stiff, and a great deal of encouragement is needed. It often helps to involve the child by measuring the joint range and charting it daily – the child being responsible for filling in the chart. Hydrotherapy should be used wherever possible. Full weight-bearing without the plaster is commenced once the quadriceps are strong enough and the knee has a joint range of at least 90 degrees.

It is important to point out to the child and his parents that at the end of the procedure the limb length will appear exactly the same as pre-operatively and a shoe-raise will still be necessary. This often leads to disappointment, but when the explanation is such, namely the attempt to compensate by reducing the growth on the sound side as the short limb catches up, the patient and his parents will accept the necessity for a shoe-raise, reducing in size as growth becomes complete.

LEG LENGTHENING

This is carried out by means of a distraction device. Close observation of the limb is of vital importance postoperatively, and the physiotherapist should be aware of the complications such as interference with blood and nerve supply to the limb. During the period of active lengthening, intensive physiotherapy is necessary to stretch the soft tissues around the site and maintain the length of muscle, parallel with the bone length. In *lengthening of the tibia*, the posterior tibial group of muscles must be stretched frequently to prevent equinus deformity of the foot, and in *lengthening of the femur* the quadriceps must be stretched by maintaining full knee joint range thus preventing a stiff, extended knee.

The patient is encouraged to be mobile, non-weight-bearing, using axillary crutches for six weeks. After this period the distraction device is removed, the lengthened bone is plated and, where necessary, a bone graft given. The leg is then immobilised in a plaster cast until radiological union is confirmed. This is a minimum period of three months. Once the plaster is removed, intensive physiotherapy should be given to mobilise the joints involved. Care should be taken, however, when exercising the affected limb, to avoid any stress upon the lengthened area.

REFERENCES

Barlow, T.G. (1962). Early diagnosis and treatment of congenital dislocation of the hip. *Journal of Bone and Joint Surgery*, **44B**, 292–301.

Blount, W.P. (1958). Unequal leg length in children. *Surgical Clinics of North America*, **38**, 1107.

Chiari, K. (1974). Medial displacement osteotomy of the pelvis. *Clinical Orthopaedics and Related Research*, **98**, 55–71.

Dunn, D.M. and Angel, J.C. (1978). Replacement of the femoral head by open operation in severe adolescent slipping of the upper femoral epiphysis. *Journal of Bone and Joint Surgery*, **60B**, 394–403.

Kepley, R.F. and Weiner, D.S. (1981). Treatment of congenital dysplasia–subluxation of the hip in children under one year of age. *Journal of Paediatric Orthopaedics*, **1**, 413.

Langenskiold, A. (1981). Surgical treatment of partial closure of the growth plate. *Journal of Paediatric Orthopaedics*, **1**, 3.

Lloyd-Roberts, G.C. and Ratliff, A.H.C. (1978). *Hip Disorders in Children*. Butterworths, London.

Lovell, W.W. and Winter, R.B. (1978). *Paediatric Orthopedics*. J.B. Lippincott Co, Philadelphia.

Phemister, D.B. (1933). Operative arrestment of longitudinal growth of bones in the treatment of deformities. *Journal of Bone and Joint Surgery*, **15**, 1.

Salter, R.B. (1961). Innominate osteotomy in the treatment of congenital dislocation and subluxation of the hip. *Journal of Bone and Joint Surgery*, **43B**, 518.

Scott, J.C. (1953). Frame reduction in congenital dislocation of the hip. *Journal of Bone and Joint Surgery*, **35B**, 372.

Southwick, W.O. (1967). Osteotomy through the lesser trochanter for slipped capital femoral epiphysis. *Journal of Bone and Joint Surgery*, **49A**, 807.

Wagner, H. (1977). *Progress in Orthopaedic Surgery. 1: Leg Length Discrepancy.* Springer-Verlag, New York.

Wainwright, D. (1976). The shelf operation for hip dysplasia in adolescence. *Journal of Bone and Joint Surgery*, **58B**, 159.

Wynne-Davies, R. (1973). *Heritable Disorders in Orthopaedic Practice.* Blackwell Scientific Publications Limited, Oxford.

BIBLIOGRAPHY

Adams, J.C. (1981). *Outline of Orthopaedics*, 9th edition. Churchill Livingstone, Edinburgh.

Anderson, W.V. (1967). *Lengthening of the Lower Limb: Its Place in the Problems of Limb Length Discrepancy.* Included in *Modern Trends in Orthopaedics* – 5. Butterworths, London.

Catterall, A. (1971). The natural history of Perthes' disease. *Journal of Bone and Joint Surgery*, **53B**, 37.

Catterall, A. (1975). The management of congenital dislocation of the hip. *Nursing Mirror*, March 6th.

Lovell, W.W. and Winter, R.B. (1978). *Pediatric Orthopedics.* J.B. Lippincott Co, Philadelphia.

Petrie, J.G. and Bitenc, I. (1971). The abduction weight-bearing treatment in Legg-Perthes' disease. *Journal of Bone and Joint Surgery*, **53B**, 54.

Powell, M. (1981). *Orthopaedic Nursing and Rehabilitation*, 8th edition. Churchill Livingstone, Edinburgh.

Wagner, H. (1977). *Progress in Orthopaedic Surgery. 1: Leg Length Discrepancy.* Springer-Verlag, New York.

Chapter 9

Examination and Assessment of the Spine and Peripheral Joints

by P.M. WOOD, MCSP, DipTP

When a physiotherapist is requested to treat a patient suffering from a spinal disorder, or a peripheral joint disability, the sequence of events is similar. There is a need to examine the patient to assess how the signs and symptoms of which he complains actually affect his activities, which structures are involved, and how therapeutic techniques may be used to relieve pain and restore normal function.

Sometimes restoration to full function is not possible due to irreversible changes in joints or soft tissues. In this case the physiotherapist must assess how much functional improvement may be expected, and then teach the patient to manage within his capabilities. Liaison with the occupational therapist, general practitioner and social services may be required if the provision of aids or home structural changes are needed.

In this chapter examination and assessment of the spine, hip, knee and shoulder will be discussed. Chapter 10 will discuss principles of treatment. The aim is to give a logical sequence of questioning and testing which will lead to an adequate understanding of the patient and his disability. Physical treatment can then be used to its best advantage.

SPINAL DISORDERS

The physiotherapist treating patients suffering from spinal disorders needs a clear knowledge and understanding of the anatomy and biomechanics of the vertebral column. Particular attention should be paid to the functional aspects of the abdominal muscles during movements involving a load as in heavy lifting.

The complexity of the joints, muscles and other structures involved in vertebral movement means that when dysfunction occurs the actual diagnosis of the disability may be difficult to pinpoint. It is common for a patient to be 'labelled' *low back pain* rather than a definite diagnosis being given. The physiotherapist must be sure that the referring doctor has discarded diagnoses which rule out physical treatment, although this would not prevent her from carrying out a full 'indications' examination and assessment prior to treatment.

The purpose of the examination by the physiotherapist is to obtain a complete picture of the disability of the patient. This, together with appropriate consideration of the anatomical structures involved, will indicate where and how physical treatment is directed. During both the subjective and objective examinations, the physiotherapist is looking for contra-indications to physical treatment of the vertebral column. These depend to some extent on the type of treatment to be considered, but the following would be contra-indications to most forms of treatment.

Contra-indications

MALIGNANCY INVOLVING THE VERTEBRAL COLUMN
This is usually metastatic since primary tumours of the vertebral column are rare. The patient complains of severe, unremitting pain, often of root distribution and perhaps affecting more than one root. There is obvious weight loss. There may be a history of a primary tumour which has been treated – look for a surgical scar or evidence of telangiectasia following radiotherapy. Metastatic deposits in the vertebral column are frequently noted when the primary tumour is in the breast, thyroid or prostate gland.

SPINAL CORD INVOLVEMENT
This is indicated by bilateral paraesthesia in the hands and feet. Loss of co-ordination in the legs may lead to gait disturbance.

CAUDA EQUINA LESIONS
If there is any question of a cauda equina lesion the patient should be asked specifically about bladder and bowel function.

RHEUMATOID ARTHRITIS
If there is an acute inflammatory stage of the disease anywhere in the body, active or passive movement of the vertebral joints is contra-indicated. This is because of ligamentous and bony changes, softening and erosion, occurring in the joints of the vertebral column

as elsewhere in the body. These changes, particularly in the cervical spine, can lead to the danger of subluxation or even dislocation at the atlanto-axial joint.

ACTIVE INFLAMMATORY OR INFECTIVE ARTHRITIS OF THE VERTEBRAL COLUMN

The patient will look ill, be pyrexial and complain of severe pain.

BONE DISEASE OF THE SPINE

Such conditions as Paget's disease or ankylosing spondylitis may be contra-indications to physical measures, although palliative treatment may help relieve pain.

Pain sensitivity of the spine

The following vertebral structures are highly pain-sensitive. Injury or disease processes will lead to the production of pain which often has a specific pattern of localisation/referral and nature.

Structure	Pain pattern
Bone	The periosteum is highly sensitive, and gives rise to deep pain which may radiate
Facet joints (apophyseal joints)	Synovial joints which have nerve endings in both capsule and ligaments. They may refer pain a considerable distance, but it is a dull, diffuse type which may show specific radiation patterns
Ligaments	The long ligaments of the vertebral column are innervated to a greater or lesser degree. The posterior longitudinal ligament is richly innervated and gives rise to local deep pain
Muscle	All muscles show pain sensitivity, and give rise to a dull aching pain. This is usually localised. Pain may also arise due to ischaemia of muscle in spasm

Disc	Controversy arises when pain sensitivity of intervertebral discs is discussed. Many authorities advocate that pain from a disc occurs only when rupture disrupts the surrounding pain-sensitive tissues, e.g. the posterior longitudinal ligament giving rise to lumbago; or pressure on the nerve root as in sciatica
Spinal dura	This has a rich innervation anteriorly but not posteriorly
Nerve roots and cauda equina	These are richly innervated and give rise to pain of marked dermatomal distribution. In inflammatory conditions pain may arise throughout the length of the affected nerves
Blood vessels	The blood vessels in the vertebral canal, particularly the vertebral venous plexuses, are richly innervated and can give rise to deep pain. Venous congestion will also cause pressure on other pain-sensitive structures

This knowledge of pain-sensitive areas/structures may help to pin-point structures which could be involved and therefore aid the choice of therapeutic techniques.

Although the above facts relate to the spinal structures, the corresponding tissues of peripheral joints show similar reactions. One is aware of how pain from an arthritic hip can be referred down the thigh to the knee. Problems involving peripheral joints are usually more circumscribed and consequently less difficult to pin-point in terms of tissue involvement.

EXAMINATION OF THE PATIENT

The great majority of patients present with *pain* as their main complaint. The loss of function is usually secondary. Pain is a subjective symptom of disorder, and despite a great deal of research is still not fully understood. It has been described as an 'affective state' which implies the psychological element which must always be present (Wyke, 1976). The physiotherapist needs to understand the nature of the patient's pain in the context of his personal circumstances, before she can assess the effect of his suffering on his daily life.

Subjective examination

After the details of age, sex, occupation, hobbies, etc, have been noted, it is logical to start the examination of the patient with a detailed description of his pain.

Before being asked to describe exactly where he *feels* the pain the patient must undress down to pants for a man, and bra and pants for a woman. What the patient feels should be recorded on a body chart (Fig. 9/1). In this way the *pain pattern* is depicted. This chart can then be annotated to give details of the nature, depth, severity, frequency and precipitating and/or relieving factors. Altered sensation, e.g. paraesthesia, can be added.

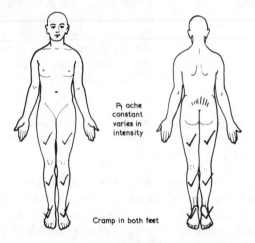

P₁ ache constant varies in intensity

Cramp in both feet

Fig. 9/1 Pain chart

The patient is then asked to describe the pain throughout a typical day. The sleeping position, and the number of pillows used may indicate a position of comfort. If the patient says that his sleep is so disturbed by pain that he has to get out of bed, this should be carefully noted and thoroughly investigated as it may indicate a more serious pathological condition.

When the pain has been fully described, associated signs and symptoms such as stiffness, swelling, feelings of weakness or even breathlessness should be queried. Also at this point in the subjective examination, the patient's lifestyle and social history, together with changes precipitated by disability, can be ascertained. A note may be made to ask more about work or home conditions at a later stage when ergonomic advice needs to be given.

When passive movement or manipulative techniques are being contemplated, special questions relating to the regions of the vertebral column will be asked to eliminate any contra-indications to treatment.

Once the patient's symptoms have been fully described, the history of the present complaint can be discussed together with past problems and any background medical history. By leaving the history to the latter part of the subjective examination, it can be listened to in the context of the complaint and is often more relevant. Supplementary questions can complete the picture.

Drugs which have been prescribed by the general practitioner, together with other relevant medication taken or used by the patient (for any reason), should be noted. During the whole of this discussion the physiotherapist will have been able to form an opinion of the patient and his attitude to his disability in the context of himself, as well as his expectation of physical treatment.

Objective examination

The essence of the objective examination is to obtain information by observation of, and testing of, the musculo-skeletal system. When necessary further testing of the cardiovascular and/or respiratory system(s) can be carried out. The physiotherapist is trying to pin-point the tissue, e.g. muscle, joint or soft tissues, involved, and measure the effect of the lesion on functional ability.

The patient is undressed as already indicated, and an experienced physiotherapist will have noted the general posture, the habitual posture and the willingness to move during the previous subjective examination. A general plan of examination of the vertebral column will include:

Observation of posture

Testing of active and passive range of movement

Testing of isotonic and isometric muscle power

Neurological testing to detect alteration of muscle power, sensation in dermatomal distribution and upper and lower limb reflexes. These will show the presence of nerve root or long tract abnormalities

Palpation
Functional tests.
(It may be considered necessary quickly to examine peripheral
joints and muscles.)
It is advisable to use acceptable methods to record joint ranges and
muscle power.

The plan is modified for each vertebral region, the examination
being carried out in a way which necessitates the least discomfort for
the patient, and avoids frequent change of position.

The equipment required will include a stool, a plinth and pillow, a
tendon hammer, tape measure, goniometer, test tubes and perhaps a
pin and cotton wool. Occasionally other testing apparatus may be
required.

CERVICAL SPINE

The patient sits in a good light. The posture is observed from behind,
in front and from the side; the following are noted: head carriage,
bony deformity, muscle wasting, asymmetry. The pain pattern is
borne in mind and the dominant hand noted.

Active movements of the cervical spine are tested. If they are full
and pain-free, over-pressure at the end of the range is applied gently.
During the movement a note is made of the range, behaviour of pain,
protective deformity and movement pattern in both upper and lower
cervical segments. While the patient is sitting, isometric and isotonic
muscle power of the upper cervical muscles are tested. Both arms are
elevated to test the glenohumeral joint and shoulder girdle function.

The patient is then asked to lie supine with his head on one pillow.
Neurological tests are carried out: reflexes, isometric muscle power in
nerve root distribution together with sensation in the dermatomal
distribution in the upper limbs are tested. Sensation is tested by light
touch. When necessary, differentiation of pin prick and cotton wool
may be used. Heat sensation is tested using hot and cold test tubes.
The upper limb muscles are tested isotonically and isometrically; the
upper limb joints are tested if necessary.

Vertebral artery insufficiency may be tested by rotating the head
passively to each side, and asking about the sensation of dizziness.

The patient is then asked to lie prone with his forehead supported
on cupped hands. Palpation examination of the cervical spine and
shoulder region begins with feeling for temperature change and
sweating. Soft tissues are palpated for tenderness, muscle spasm or
fibrous thickening. The alignment of the vertebrae is considered
before any intervertebral accessory movement testing is carried out.

Functional tests may follow to see the effect on the pain when the previous tests have not provoked the pain of which the patient is complaining.

THORACIC SPINE

The patient sits in a good light. The posture is observed from behind, in front and from the side; the following are noted: head and shoulder girdle carriage, scapular position and the general contour of the ribs and vertebral region, deformity, muscle wasting, asymmetry. The pain pattern is considered.

Active movements of the thoracic spine are tested. Flexion is a slumping movement followed by extending to the erect position including any further extension which may be possible. Care is taken to ensure that movement is restricted to the thoracic spine. Measurements are difficult to make. If movements are full and pain-free, over-pressure is gently applied at the end of the range. During movement a note is made of the range, behaviour of pain, protective deformity and movement pattern. Neck movements may be tested for upper thoracic pain. Respiration – full inspiration and expiration followed by a cough – is tested.

The patient then lies supine with the head on one pillow. Neurological tests are carried out for the lower limbs as considered necessary by the distribution of pain and the symptoms described during the subjective examination. Straight leg raising and passive neck flexion tests may indicate dural tension (for details see p. 196).

The sacro-iliac joints may be tested (see p. 196).

The patient is then asked to lie prone with the arms by the sides. General contour, the 'sky-line view', is considered with the head turned to each side. The patient is then allowed to keep the head turned to the preferred side. Isometric and isotonic muscle power of the thoracic muscles are tested, followed by sensation testing. Palpation of the thoracic spine is then carried out. Temperature change and sweating are noted, and the soft tissues palpated for tenderness, muscle spasm or fibrous thickening. An additional test in this region is the *flat-handed springing test*. The physiotherapist gently uses her body-weight through her flattened hand placed on the vertebral spines, to 'spring' the vertebral column from above downwards. Areas of spasm are easily detected. The alignment of the vertebrae and ribs are considered before intervertebral accessory movement, and costovertebral and costotransverse ranges are tested.

Functional tests may follow when previous tests have not provoked the patient's pain.

LUMBAR SPINE

The patient sits in a good light. He is then asked to stand and move away from the chair. In this way his ability to rise from sitting, move, and his gait can be seen. He then stands and his vertebral posture is noted from behind, in front and from the side. Particular attention is paid to pelvic and shoulder symmetry, muscle wasting and deformity. The pain pattern is considered.

Active movement is then tested – flexion, extension and side-flexion. Rotation does not occur to any degree in the lumbar spine because of the alignment of the apophyseal joints. Rotation may be tested in upper lumbar problems when the patient would be in a sitting position. If movements are full and pain-free, gentle over-pressure is applied at the end of the range. Functional movements may be tested with the patient in standing. He is asked to stand on each leg in turn, and rise on to tiptoe repeatedly to test calf muscle power. During movement, the range, behaviour of pain, protective deformity and movement pattern, are all noted.

The patient then lies supine with his head on one pillow. Neurological examination of the lower limbs includes reflex testing, sensation in dermatomal distribution and isometric muscle tests for root abnormalities. The patient then lies prone and isometric and isotonic muscle power in the lower limbs are tested as considered necessary. Similarly, peripheral joint movements may be tested. The abdominal muscles are tested isometrically and isotonically.

Special tests carried out in the lumbar spine examination, and perhaps in the thoracic spine examination, are those testing movement of neural structures within the spinal canal.

Passive straight leg raising may give rise to pain if tethering or restriction of movement has occurred in the lower lumbar and upper sacral roots.

Passive neck flexion will cause pain if movement of neural structures is restricted.

Passive prone knee flexion is carried out when the patient turns into prone lying, and pain indicates restriction of movement in the roots of the femoral nerve.

Sacro-iliac joint testing may be carried out quite quickly by compression and distraction of the anterior superior iliac spines. This leads to gapping and compression respectively in the sacro-iliac joints.

Pain on these tests will require further examination.

These tests are done with the patient in the supine position.

The patient then turns to the prone position with his head turned to each side while the lumbar contour is noted. He then lies with his arms at his sides and the head turned to the preferred side. The extensor muscles of the vertebral column are tested isometrically and isotonically. Any neurological testing is completed. Palpation of the lumbar spine starts with noting temperature change and sweating; the soft tissues are palpated for tenderness, muscle spasm or fibrous thickening. The alignment of the vertebrae and the position of the iliac crests are considered before intervertebral accessory movements are tested. It may be considered necessary to palpate and further test the sacro-iliac joints.

OBJECTIVE EXAMINATION OF THE HIP JOINT

The patient sits in a good light. The physiotherapist should watch him as he rises from sitting and walks a short distance, including steps if possible. She should particularly note the amount of weight the patient takes on the affected leg.

The patient then stands, and his posture together with any deformity or muscle wasting is noted. Active movement of *both* hip joints should be tested, and should include squatting, standing on one leg and hopping if capable. Balance should be checked. Active movements of the lumbar spine and other lower limb joints should be tested.

The patient is then asked to lie supine: the passive range of both hip joints should be tested, the patient turning into side lying if necessary. Both legs should be measured, and checked for any fixed deformity. *Leg length* is measured using a tape measure, from the umbilicus to the medial malleoli for the *apparent length*, and from the anterior superior iliac spines to the medial malleoli for the *true length*. *Fixed flexion deformity* is tested using *Thomas' test*: the opposite leg is fully flexed with the knee up to the chest and held by the patient. If fixed flexion is present, the leg being examined will rise off the plinth, and the degree of loss of range can be measured. Muscle power is tested isometrically and isotonically. The joints should be palpated for any temperature alteration, muscle spasm, soft tissue thickening or swelling. Sensation should be tested. Accessory movements of the hip joints should be tested, and range, pain, resistance and spasm noted. It will be necessary for the patient to turn into prone and side lying during this examination.

Functional testing may be left until last when the physiotherapist should observe the patient dressing, tying shoe laces and so on.

OBJECTIVE EXAMINATION OF THE KNEE JOINT

The patient sits in a good light. The physiotherapist should observe him as he rises from sitting and walks a short distance including steps. She should note his gait. As he stands, his lower limb posture and weight-bearing should be noted. Quadriceps and calf muscle bulk should be checked. Active movements should be tested including squatting on both legs and on each leg, standing on tiptoe, and hopping. Asymmetry is looked for, and balance tested.

The patient then lies supine and passive range of knee movement is tested including the patello-femoral movement (the latter is done by moving the patella diagonally on the femur). Quadriceps power should be tested isometrically and isotonically. The leg lengths should be measured and any fixed deformity noted (this can be done as described previously or, for the knee joint only, the measurement may be made from the greater trochanter to the medial malleolus). Measurement of muscle bulk, particularly the quadriceps, should be made: this is made by tape measure round the circumference of the thigh (for the quadriceps) at one or more given distances (e.g. 5cm and 15cm) from the superior pole (border) of the patella. The knee joints should be palpated, testing particularly for any effusion and/or temperature around the synovium and bursae. The accessory movements of the joints should be tested. During the examination the patient may need to move into sitting over the side of the plinth, prone lying and side lying. The other lower limb joints may need to be tested.

Functional testing can be left to last when the physiotherapist should observe the patient as he dresses.

OBJECTIVE EXAMINATION OF THE GLENOHUMERAL JOINT (INCLUDING THE SHOULDER GIRDLE)

The patient sits on a stool in a good light. The posture of the upper trunk, head and shoulders, together with any deformity, asymmetry or muscle wasting should be noted. The pain pattern should be borne in mind. Active movements of the glenohumeral joints should be tested: the method of measurement needs to be carefully defined and should include the movements of the shoulder girdle. Range and pain should be carefully noted and where necessary movements should be isolated. Active movements of the cervical spine need to be checked.

The patient is then asked to lie supine on the plinth. The passive range of movement at the glenohumeral joints should be tested by fixing the scapula with one hand placed under the body. The area should be palpated for altered temperature, swelling, muscle spasm and soft tissue thickening; sensation should be tested. The accessory range of movement in the sternoclavicular and acromioclavicular joints, as well as those of the glenohumeral joints, should be tested, noting the range, resistance, muscle spasm and pain. The other upper limb joints should be checked as necessary.

Functional testing can be left to last and should relate to the patient's home circumstances and/or occupation.

FOLLOWING THE EXAMINATION

At the conclusion of the full examination of the patient, the physiotherapist will have the information required prior to physical treatment. Now is the time to read the patient's case notes, look at the relevant radiographs and confirm that there are no contra-indications to treatment.

As a considerable amount of time will have been spent with the patient, it is acceptable to delay the start of treatment techniques until the next day. Indeed, when a detailed objective examination has been carried out it is often wiser to do this so that any soreness which may have been provoked has subsided. In this way such soreness cannot be attributed to treatment. It also gives the physiotherapist time to assess the findings fully and plan the treatment regime.

ASSESSMENT

This is the interpretation of the examination findings in terms of how physiotherapy can be used to relieve signs and symptoms.

An illustration of this is given in relation to how the physiotherapist may decide to relieve the pain of which the patient has complained.

Example

The patient is a middle-aged housewife who has been referred with low back pain. She is slightly overweight, has poor posture and her pain pattern, shown in Figure 9/1, indicates a diffuse aching pain. Comparison of this pain pattern with dermatome, myotome and sclerotome charts (Figs. 9/2 and 9/3) will enable the therapist to differentiate pain of deep origin from that of nerve root irritation which would show a dermatomal type of superficial radiation.

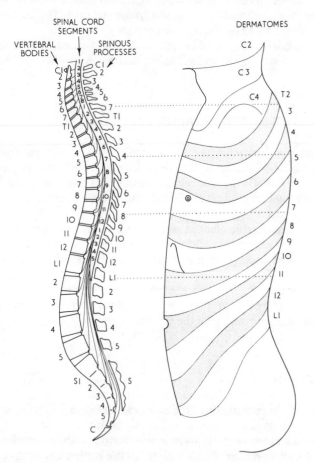

Fig. 9/2 Spinal cord segments and spinal nerves, showing the dermatomes

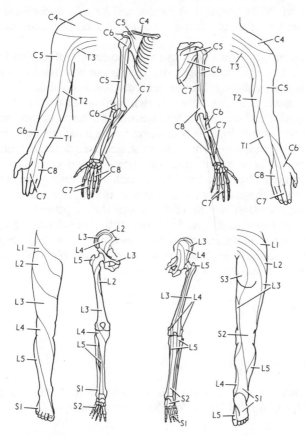

Fig. 9/3 Dermatomes and sclerotomes of the upper and lower limbs. Paraesthesia is generally referred to the dermatome and pain to the sclerotome

The patient has said that the pain is worse early in the morning when stiffness is apparent, and wears off a little during the day. Her movement is somewhat restricted in all directions; there is slight muscle wasting, but no neurological changes. On palpation there is generalised tenderness.

Having picked out the salient points from the examination the physiotherapist then considers the therapeutic techniques which may be used. In this case some form of heat, hydrotherapy, and gentle mobilising activities might be included; postural re-education and abdominal strengthening exercises would be given. Advice and supervision in back care, particularly lifting and ergonomics in the home, would be given. The patient will be told to continue home exercises which should be carried out first thing in the morning.

Assessment also means the continuing comparison of results obtained with the expected progress so that changes of treatment techniques, duration or frequency, may be made as soon as possible.

A subjective and an objective sign are chosen during the initial examination and are used as the assessment criteria. Improvement in one or both would indicate continuing a certain regime; no change, or indeed a deterioration, would show the need for a different treatment. The physiotherapist, in most instances, should expect to see an improvement, however small, after each attendance. The aim is to bring about the maximum improvement in the minimum amount of time with the least amount of discomfort for the patient.

Finally, assessment is needed to decide the overall value of a course of treatment. Does it lead to the full functional recovery of the patient or, as occasionally happens, to the decision that physical treatment will not help and should be discontinued?

REFERENCE

Wyke, B. (1976). *Neurological Aspects of Low Back Pain*. In *The Lumbar Spine and Back Pain*. (ed Jayson, M.). Sector Publishing Ltd, London.

BIBLIOGRAPHY

Melzack, R. and Wall, P.D. (1982). *The Challenge of Pain*. Penguin Books, Harmondsworth.
See also end of Chapter 10.

Principles of Treatment Following Joint Examination and Assessment

by P.M. WOOD, MCSP, DipTP

The aim of physiotherapy is to relieve pain and restore full function. After assessing the examination findings the physiotherapist selects appropriate techniques, and decides on the initial dose (if relevant) and frequency of treatment. The therapeutic means of achieving this may be considered under the following headings.

HEAT

Some form of heat may be used to relieve muscle spasm before more active techniques are used. This might be infra-red irradiation, microwave therapy or short wave diathermy. These forms of heat offer a range of depth of penetration of effects from the superficial to the deeper tissues. The patient with pain in the vertebral column may find it difficult to maintain the position for the safe application of one of these forms of heat, and this should be remembered by the physiotherapist. Testing to ensure that the patient has normal sensation of temperature is essential.

The simpler methods of applying direct heat, for example hot packs, a hot water bottle or a small electric heat pad, are often as effective as the more sophisticated methods. They have the advantage of being safe (provided the patient remembers that 'extra hot' does not mean extra effectiveness!), and can be used at home prior to doing home exercises or as a means of pain relief.

COLD

Ice packs, or towels wrung out in ice-cold water, may be used to relieve the pain of muscle spasm; they may be left on the part for approximately 10 minutes when used for relief of pain. Application of ice over the area of skin supplied by the dorsal rami may have a greater than expected sedative effect on the nervous system. Ice applied to the dermatomes supplied by the lower sacral nerves can lead to temporary alteration in bladder or bowel function.

ULTRASOUND

Ultrasound may be used for its mechanical and analgesic effects in improving circulation, and reducing oedema following soft tissue trauma. It can be useful in relieving muscle spasm. Care should be taken in applying ultrasound over the vertebral column because of the oscillatory molecular effects on sensory input to the nervous system. This is particularly relevant when it is applied over the dermatomes supplied by the dorsal rami and lower sacral nerves. Reflex neurological effects, similar to those described with ice treatments, may occur.

HYDROTHERAPY

Exercise in warm water (temperature 33°–38°C) is a valuable way of allowing pain-free movement of the vertebral and peripheral joints, either assisted, free or resisted muscle work. The warmth of the water promotes relaxation of the muscle spasm and therefore relieves pain; the buoyancy of the water gives a sense of freedom from the effects of gravity.

Other hydrotherapy techniques, e.g. whirlpool baths, may be used also.

All patients (provided they enjoy it) should be encouraged to swim regularly as part of their daily activity in the future to avoid further joint problems.

TRANSCUTANEOUS NERVE STIMULATION (TNS) (Figs. 10/1a, b, c.)

Transcutaneous nerve stimulation is being used increasingly on suitable patients for the relief of the more intractable forms of vertebral pain. It is usually applied via small electrodes which are attached to a portable stimulator. The actual stimulation sites need to be found individually by trial and error, and similarly the intensity and duration of stimulation will be judged.

TNS should not be required by the majority of patients who are referred for physical treatment.

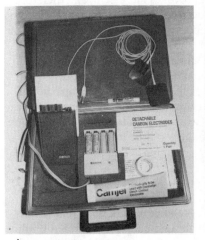
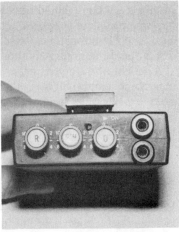

A   B

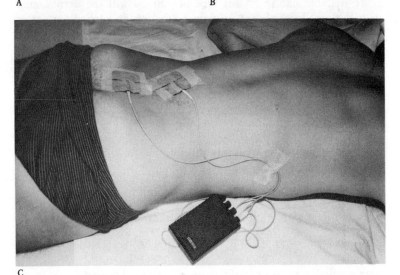

C

Fig. 10/1 A series of photographs to demonstrate a transcutaneous nerve stimulator (TNS). (a) The stimulator electrodes and jelly as supplied in a case; (b) A close-up of the top of the stimulator showing slots for insertion of electrode leads; (c) The stimulator held in position over the pain source area. The battery is of small size and is conveniently carried in a special wallet or pocket

COLLARS AND CORSETS

In acute vertebral pain movement provokes more pain, and therefore rest for a few days should be advocated. The physiotherapist should have the means of supplying temporary collars (soft foam for night wear, and Plastazote for day wear), and elasticated adjustable corsets. These should be accurately fitted and supervised.

A patient who is given a collar should be advised that the restriction in neck movement will alter other proprioception, for example he will need to take care in the dark or on entering darkened rooms when he may lose his balance. A patient wearing a collar should not drive because judgement of relative distances will be impaired.

TRACTION

Vertebral traction should be the first choice of pain relief for patients suffering nerve root pain. The initial examination will emphasise the acute irritable nature of this type of pain as will the dermatomal distribution. Intermittent sustained traction is carried out after careful positioning has localised the involved segment. In such cases treatment at least once a day is essential; prolonged pain relief will take several days to obtain.

The more chronic aching pain of osteoarthritic changes in the apophyseal joints may respond to regional intermittent traction used as a passive mobilising technique.

SOFT TISSUE MANIPULATION

Soft tissue techniques including massage, may be used to stretch tissue or relieve muscle spasm. These techniques are usually used prior to manipulative procedures or exercise therapy.

EXERCISE THERAPY IN SPINAL DISORDERS

The use of exercise regimes in the treatment of spinal disorders is valuable. The exercises are chosen carefully to suit the needs of the patient after assessment.

Re-education of vertebral posture with its emphasis on pelvic tilt and head carriage may require mobilising, stretching and strengthening exercises; these should be carried out with the patient in a recumbent position and then progressing to functional positions.

Muscle strengthening regimes should be carefully selected. The abdominal muscle group will require the most emphasis, although in some cases strengthening of the extensor muscles in their middle range may be required. Hyperextension exercises for the vertebral column are seldom necessary. A balance of activity between the abdominal muscles and the extensor muscles is required to achieve a relaxed vertebral posture.

MOBILISING EXERCISES

Vertebral mobility, including thoracic and shoulder girdle work, is necessary for full functional activity. The physiotherapist may regain mobility by using free exercises, stretching or passive mobilisation techniques.

Passive mobilising techniques

Skill in mobilisation or manipulative techniques is probably the most valuable therapeutic tool in the treatment of spinal disorders (p. 216). Passive oscillatory movement of a vertebral segmental joint through an accessory and/or physiological range can restore pain-free, full range movement very quickly. Meticulous examination and palpation plus skilful handling are required to pin-point the level of dysfunction.

Physiotherapists trained in manipulative techniques will consider the patient as a whole and give advice on ergonomics and functional activities.

STABILISING EXERCISES

On examination it may be found that the patient suffers pain from an unstable segment of the vertebral column. Often there is a 'catch' on movement particularly as the patient returns to the upright position from full flexion. Such patients need a regime of exercise to strengthen all muscle groups so that co-contraction acts as a splint to the unstable region. They may require the use of a supporting corset permanently.

SPECIAL EXERCISE REGIMES

A number of physiotherapists have specialised in the conservative management of spinal disorders. They have evolved schemes of treatment including passive movement, localised manual traction and specific exercise patterns. Kaltenborn (1970) uses traction and passive techniques followed by specific exercise; McKenzie (1972) has a specific regime of vertebral shifting for acute disc lesions.

EXERCISE THERAPY FOR PERIPHERAL JOINTS

This follows basic physiotherapeutic principles. Mobilising techniques may be applied actively or passively in a physiological or accessory range of movement at the individual joint. A suspension frame or other form of suspension may be used, or a re-education board.

Strengthening of muscle groups may be carried out by progressive resistance exercises (PRE) using dead weights, weight and pulley systems, circuit training or proprioceptive neuromuscular facilitation (PNF) techniques.

Functional activities such as dressing and undressing, housework and gardening should be included, and advice given as to the most effective way of carrying them out without aggravating the complaint.

A home exercise programme should be taught to each patient, and they should be encouraged to carry it out regularly even if they are no longer suffering any pain or loss of function.

ERGONOMIC ADVICE

Back and neck care: lifting

In recent years, back pain schools have been set up in hospitals and in industrial physiotherapy departments. The aim is to instruct patients, individually and in small groups, in the management of their back problems. Lectures are given on the vertebral column and the mechanism of pain production. Patients' own problems are analysed, and a scheme of exercises worked out (Fig. 10/2). All are taught back care, lifting and any necessary specific advice (Fig. 10/3).

The physiotherapist may be asked to teach lifting techniques to various groups of people, not only spinal pain sufferers but also normal people in particular work circumstances (e.g. nurses).

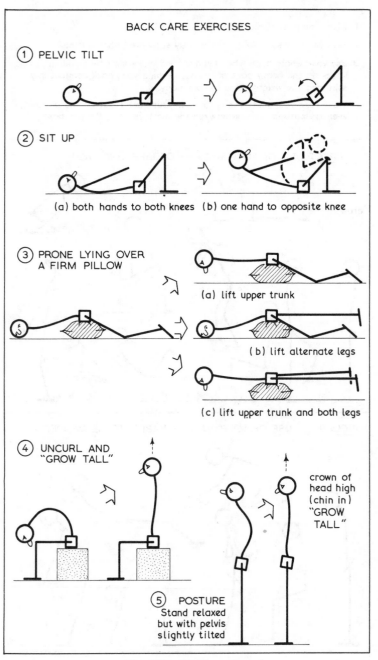

Fig. 10/2 Back exercises

1. Stand and walk tall and slim.

2. Always make sure your back is fully supported when sitting.

3. Use your whole body when bending and make sure that your hips and knees do the heavy part of lifting, keeping your back comfortably still and the weight close to your body.

4. Make sure your mattress is firm; if your back troubles you at night, even try putting boards between the mattress and the bed base.

CORRECT USE OF YOUR BACK — OF LIFELONG VALUE :-

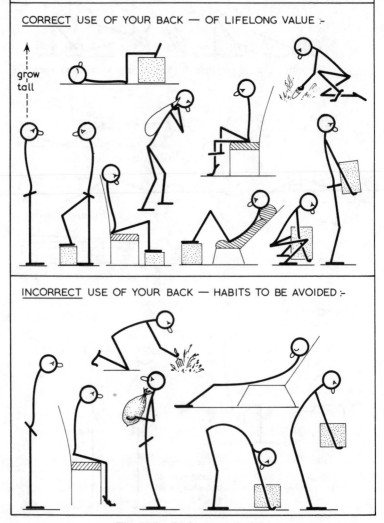

INCORRECT USE OF YOUR BACK — HABITS TO BE AVOIDED :-

Fig. 10/3 Back care and advice

Preventive advice is an important part of the physiotherapist's role in the case of back care (Fig. 10/3).

When dealing specifically with vertebral pain patients, the advice will include a discussion about sleeping positions and the use of pillows – how many, whether soft feather or foam rubber and so on. Most neck pain sufferers benefit from using one soft pillow tied in the centre to produce a 'butterfly' shape. The neck is placed in the centre so that the side wings support either side of the head.

Many low back pain patients find the Fowler's (psoas) position, i.e. hips and knees flexed and supported (Fig. 10/4), the most comfortable resting position. Indeed many back pain sufferers can stand for longer periods in greater comfort if they flex one hip and knee.

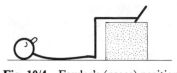

Fig. 10/4   Fowler's (psoas) position

All patients with neck or back complaints must have a firm supportive mattress.

Sitting positions should be analysed; an increase or decrease in hip and knee flexion may be used to give greater comfort. The chair must fit the patient and give vertebral support where it is needed. If the patient drives a car or some other vehicle it is advisable to discuss not only the driving position but also whether it might be wiser to stop driving until the back complaint has been treated and cured.

Suggested advice for patients with vertebral problems

The following can be adapted according to the physiotherapist's requirements, typed out, duplicated and handed to patients as reminders of what they should and should not do to avoid a recurrence of the problem.

REST POSITIONS
1. Side-lying head support, with the top leg supported.
2. Fowler's position (psoas position), see Figure 10/4.
3. Supine, with one pillow under the knees.
4. For patients who are used to lying prone, teach a three-quarter prone position – pad with pillows.

POSTURE CORRECTION

Sensible shoes – point out the distortion produced by high heels. Emphasise that if the pelvis is correct then the rest of the posture will fall into place, therefore make certain that the 'stomach' muscles are pressed toward the spine, and the 'bottom' is tucked in.

SITTING POSITION

1. If sitting irritates – ration the time spent sitting, get up before the pain comes on.
2. Have a firm chair with no wheels on it (i.e. avoid unexpected jarring of the back).
3. Hips should be well back, feet firmly on the ground with support at the small of the back.
4. Pick a chair which fits your size.
5. If you feel comfortable it means that it is mechanically right.
6. Show the patient a picture of the correct sitting position.

SITTING TO STANDING

1. For patients who note an increase in pain on this manoeuvre, explain why the pain increases as they bring the upper trunk forward flexing the lumbar spine.
2. Use of arms to take the weight of the upper trunk off the lumbar spine.
3. Use of walking on hips to reach the edge of the chair, i.e. keeping the back extended, thus enabling the patient to get up without flexing the lumbar spine.
4. Place one foot at the side of the chair to help getting up from sitting to standing.

WORK TIPS FOR THE HOUSEWIFE

1. Never lift a child from sitting, always crouch down keeping the lower back straight.
2. For standing jobs: (a) have the weight evenly on both legs (b) teach a lordotic patient the value of placing one foot on a low stool.
3. Making beds: (a) kneel at the side of the bed, smooth one half of a double bed, then repeat for the other side or (b) place one knee on the bed and repeat (a). Never stretch across the bed with straight knees.
4. Cleaning the bath: kneel at the side (use this position for washing hair if no overhead shower present).
5. Never walk up or down stairs in floppy shoes (tripping could cause a sudden stress on the back).

6. Cooking: work surfaces should fit *your* height. Discuss adaptations.
7. Keep heavy utensils on waist height shelves.
8. Keep light objects on lower shelves.
9. Shopping: use a trolley or take husband! If carrying bags, distribute weight evenly within capacity.
10. Hanging washing: use a stool if arching the back increases pain.
11. Remember the danger of slipping on wet floors, particularly kitchen/bathroom.
12. Hoovering: use two hands to spare your back.
13. Clean up spilled water or fat from the floor to avoid any danger of sudden slipping.

WORK TIPS IN THE OFFICE
1. Have the chair well up to the desk.
2. Support the small of the back.
3. Have no wheels on the chair.

WORK TIPS FOR THE FACTORY
1. Non-slip shoes. Your back cannot cope well with sudden stress.
2. Wear protective clothing where necessary.
3. Work surface should fit your height.
4. Never over-reach. Top of work surface should correspond with your arm length.
5. Lifting: always within your capacity. Remember it is better to wait five minutes for assistance with lifting, rather than be off work for five weeks or months because you have lifted beyond your capacity.

LIFTING
1. Always place one foot flat and at the side of the object to be lifted.
2. Never lift with your body-weight on the balls of your feet as it flexes the small of the back.
3. Always tuck the weight to be lifted into your stomach.
4. Lift within your capacity.
5. Have feet pointing in the direction you will be walking.
6. Use 'feet' to turn when taking the weight from one surface to another.
7. When there is two-man lifting see that one is in command, take a firm grasp and lift to a count.

DRIVING
1. Check seat.
2. Hips into the car first *then* feet in.
3. Pelvic tilting as you drive (i.e. from time to time).
4. Break up long journeys by stopping before you have tired of one position.
5. Young males (or females) on motor cycles or bicycles should check the position of the handlebars re: the position of the small of the back.

TOILET
1. Kneel at the side of the bath to wash hair/face.
2. Never use long sitting in the bath.
3. Use a non-slip mat.

CLOTHING
Slacks easier than tights for an acute back.
Shoes should be well supporting.
Avoid slippers.
Soft heels on shoes rather than leather heels.

Peripheral joint ergonomic advice

As with back problems so with peripheral joint problems, advice is of paramount importance. Work and home circumstances need to be analysed and, where necessary, alterations should be made. Co-operation with the occupational therapy department can produce much practical help for some patients who can try out appliances before accepting them for use in their homes.

REFERENCES

Kaltenborn, F. (1970). *Mobilisation of the Spinal Column*. New Zealand University Press, Wellington, New Zealand.
McKenzie, R.A. (1972). Manual correction of sciatic scoliosis. *New Zealand Medical Journal*, **76**, 484, 194–9.

BIBLIOGRAPHY

Caillet, R. (1981). *Low Back Pain Syndrome*, 3rd edition; *Neck and Arm Pain*, 2nd edition; *Shoulder Pain*, 2nd edition. F.A. Davis Co, Philadelphia.

Cyriax, J. (1978). *Textbook of Orthopaedic Medicine*, Vol I: *Diagnosis of Soft Tissue Lesions*, 7th edition. Baillière Tindall, London.

Cyriax, J. and Russell, G. (1980). *Textbook of Orthopaedic Medicine*, Vol II: *Treatment by Manipulation, Massage and Injection*, 10th edition. Baillière Tindall, London.

Grieve, G.P. (1979). *Mobilisation of the Spine*, 3rd edition. Churchill Livingstone, Edinburgh.

Grieve, G.P. (1981). *Common Vertebral Joint Problems*. Churchill Livingstone, Edinburgh.

Jayson, M. (ed) (1980). *The Lumbar Spine and Back Pain*, 2nd edition. Pitman Books Ltd, London.

Kapandji, A. *The Physiology of the Joints*. Churchill Livingstone, Edinburgh.
(1982) Vol 1: *Upper Limb*, 5th edition.
(1970) Vol 2: *Lower Limb*, 2nd edition.
(1974) Vol 3: *The Trunk and the Vertebral Column*, 2nd edition.

Maitland, G.D. (1977). *Peripheral Manipulation*, 2nd edition. Butterworths, London.

Maitland, G.D. (1977). *Vertebral Manipulation*, 4th edition. Butterworths, London.

Chapter 11

Principles of Manipulation

by J. HICKLING, MCSP

An attempt to select principles must be confined to discussion of prime constituents, a search for a general formula. The reader must study the literature of the subject for detailed information about the practice of manipulation, particularly about examination, contra-indications, and technique.

The endeavour to crystallise such a formula poses three immediate problems:

1. The definition of the word 'manipulation' is by no means agreed. To take extreme examples: it may be used to describe either the forcing of a painful and limited range of movement under anaesthesia, or a small painless movement on the conscious patient.
2. The purpose of manipulation is also by no means generally agreed; success in treatment being ascribed by different experts to the resolution of different pathologies.
3. A statement of general principles seems to require guidelines about the dangers of manipulation. To do this in the midst of confusion about definition and purpose seemed impossible.

The first concern here, therefore, is with terminology and definitions.

TERMINOLOGY AND DEFINITIONS

All manipulation is passive movement, but not all passive movement can properly be called manipulation. Somewhere along the line, as force, speed, complexity or purpose change, a passive movement becomes a manipulation but there might be disagreement about exactly when this occurs.

The use of force

The use of controlled force is essential to manipulation, but the word 'force' is alarming because it has connotations of ruthless intention, lack of control, and provocation of pain.

Terminology in which 'relaxed passive movement' is contrasted with 'forced passive movement' and 'manipulation' carries the suggestion that forced passive movement and manipulation are not relaxed. This in turn suggests that the resistance which is being encountered is that of muscle activity, and an association is often made with the provocation of pain. In fact, of course, the whole art of manipulation lies in having the patient perfectly relaxed, and the resistance that is being overcome is practically never that of muscle activity.

Some re-definition is needed here, and the terms 'free' and 'stressed passive movement' are offered, to be used in the following way:

Force in normal movement

Free passive movement is movement in which there is no encounter with tissue resistance at all, and which therefore requires no force for its performance. As soon as there is even the lightest encounter with tissue resistance, the movement is called *stressed passive movement*, necessarily demanding the use of force for its completion.

By the use of the word 'stressed' in this way it is hoped to avoid the rather dire nuances that surround the word 'forced', while emphasising that in most movements in the body, full range can only be achieved by using a degree of force to overcome normal increasing tissue resistance.

The term 'end-feel' is used by Cyriax (1978), to describe the quality of the factor limiting a passive movement, as perceived by the hand. It thus refers to the element of palpation which exists in passive movement, and is related to the term 'tissue tension sense' that is used by manipulators.

There are three 'end-feels' in the normal:

The first is *bone-to-bone*, in which active and passive ranges are equal.

The next two are *tissue approximation* and *tissue tension*, and in both of these, passive range is greater than active. Passive movement into such ranges is partly free and partly stressed, and the point at which the change occurs, i.e. the point of encounter with first tissue resistance, is earlier in the range than is usually recognised.

The term *accessory range* is here used to denote that part of stressed passive movement which lies beyond the end of active movement. The end of active movement lies somewhere beyond the end of free passive movement and before full stressed passive movement.

The relative proportions of free passive movement, active movement, and stressed passive movement vary endlessly in different movements, positions, physiques and ages, as does the resistance offered by the tissues. A general formula may be offered as illustrated in Figure 11/1.

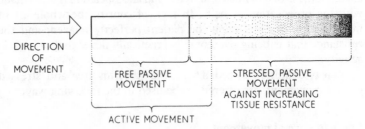

DIRECTION
OF
MOVEMENT

FREE PASSIVE
MOVEMENT

STRESSED PASSIVE
MOVEMENT
AGAINST INCREASING
TISSUE RESISTANCE

ACTIVE MOVEMENT

Fig. 11/1   Full stressed passive movement is greater than active movement and greater than free passive movement

In the normal, bone-to-bone and tissue approximation are painless. Tissue tension may also be painless, but in some physiques it may be anything from slightly uncomfortable to downright painful in the normal. This must be borne in mind when evaluating the abnormal.

With the gross primary movements which can be achieved actively there are elements of slide, roll and spin which together constitute prime movement, but which can be isolated when the joint is in an appropriate position. These isolated movements together with distraction of joint surfaces, we tend to call accessory movements. Important components of normal movement, therefore, are *accessory movement* and *accessory range*; Mennell (1964), uses the term 'joint play'. These can only be achieved by applying a degree of force, and are thus all stressed passive movements. This characteristic of accessory movement and their integrity is an important safeguard against the stresses of normal life.

Force in abnormal movement

Abnormality begins when either discomfort or resistance is greater than normal. The beginnings of the abnormal are to be noticed long before there is frank painful limitation of movement and are usually to be found in accessory movement before gross primary range is affected. For example:

1. Movement is full, but becomes uncomfortable earlier in the range than is normal
2. Movement is full, but the quality of the resistance is denser, or offered earlier in the range than in the normal
3. Movement is full, but an element of muscle spasm may be picked up by quick or careless handling.

The ability to distinguish between the resistance of tissue tension and that of muscle activity (be it active resistance or spasm) is one of the first things that the manipulator must acquire. These elements are subtle and difficult to learn, but their recognition forms the basis of informed and safe manipulation. An attempt has been made to illustrate them as Movement Diagrams (Hickling and Maitland, 1970).

It is in talking of this kind of phenomenon that manipulators are sometimes accused of mumbo-jumbo. Critics should be ready to accept that the manipulator may be attempting to convey acute perception with rather inadequate terminology. It is perhaps only fair to add that the manipulator should beware of self-deception about illusory or subjective data.

Amplitude/force/velocity

The word 'amplitude' is used to describe the size of a movement, and an important skill that the manipulator must acquire is to be able to perform a forceful, high velocity movement through a small amplitude.

The distinction between 'positioning' and 'execution' must be drawn here. Many manoeuvres are quite complex and involve considerable joint movement before the position is reached from which the manipulation is performed; insufficient care in the preliminary positioning leads to ineffective, dangerous, or unnecessarily painful manipulation.

To take a single example: the manipulator may wish to apply a high velocity thrust at the end of a generalised rotation of the trunk. During this, from position of rest to the end of the manipulation, the trunk may be seen to move through about 90 degrees represented diagrammatically in Figure 11/2. The major part of this movement is positioning, and only the last few degrees are manipulation proper.

Somewhere about point B various things occur:

1. The manipulator encounters resistance and can only continue by using increased force to enter a stressed passive range.

2. The type of resistance has to be evaluated. Muscle activity (spasm or active resistance) must be distinguished from tissue tension, and the manoeuvre then modified or abandoned.
3. If the resistance is of an expected and acceptable kind, the manipulator may use considerable force and velocity to overcome it, but must be able so to control matters that movement stops at the end of normal range at point C.
4. At the same time, the manipulator must be sure that any pain provoked is of an acceptable degree and position.

If muscle activity is not recognised, or uncontrolled force takes movement beyond normal range, either the joint is not moved effectively, or trauma occurs, or both.

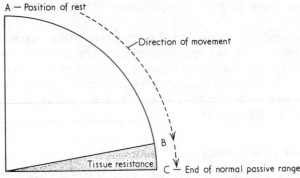

Fig. 11/2   Positioning and execution in manipulation

The skilled manipulator may choose to move from resting position to the end of the manoeuvre in one continuous, large amplitude movement, combining positioning and execution. Novices must beware of copying this, for they cannot possibly have the necessary perception and control to make such movement accurate, effective and safe. Students should separate positioning from execution, and realise that skill in the first is more difficult than, and takes precedence over, skill in the second.

Mobilisation

The word 'mobilisation' has now acquired two distinct meanings.
1. The first meaning is of long-standing use in rehabilitation. Here, 'to mobilise' means to induce and encourage mobility by whatever means are suitable. It may range from giving a recumbent patient her first gentle walk down the ward, to chasing young men round a

tough training circuit. The implication is to 'push on', to stretch the patient a bit, by whatever means seem appropriate. It thus indicates intention but does not define method.

2. In 1964 Maitland first stressed the view that the manipulator does not always need forceful techniques, but should often use more gentle methods. More gentle techniques obviously have to be carried out for longer to achieve their effect, and Maitland perfected a method of oscillatory passive movement, which he divided into Grades in order to introduce an idea of 'dosage'. Readers are referred to his books for more detail on this subject.

Maitland used the word 'mobilisation' for these techniques, and it thus acquired a second technical meaning: oscillatory passive movement, with the implication of 'holding back' from more forceful techniques. It will be seen that this is quite different from the orthopaedic use of the word described above.

Doctor and physiotherapist may well misunderstand each other here if, for example, there is a prescription to 'mobilise' a patient with back pain. If either is uncertain what the other means by the use of this word, they are strongly advised to find out.

In the ensuing text 'mobilisation' is used in the rehabilitative sense, and Maitland techniques are called 'oscillatory mobilisation'.

Manipulation/thrust techniques/Grade V

Recently the word 'manipulation' on the conscious patient has increasingly been reserved to describe a small amplitude, high velocity, forceful passive movement, usually (but not always) at the end of range. It is almost always into a stressed passive range, and the resistance being overcome may be a combination of the normal and abnormal. With few exceptions, however, it does not include forcing muscle activity, and this is an important safety factor.

This kind of manoeuvre is also called a 'thrust technique', or a 'Grade V' (linking it with the other Grades of oscillatory mobilisation described by Maitland). After positioning, the final thrust may not be in the same direction as the positioning movement. Osteopathic techniques described by Stoddard (1962), which are aimed at moving the apophyseal joints, give ample examples of this.

The above definition of manipulation is a useful one. The reader should be aware however that the word has other, slightly different meanings in the literature on the subject. For example, Mennell (1964), writes of 'examination manipulation' and 'treatment manipulation', an interesting use of the word which emphasises the interlocking relationship of examination and technique in practice.

PATHOLOGY: PURPOSE OF MANIPULATION

As already suggested, those who advocate manipulation by no means agree about what it is for. It only requires a brief acquaintance with both its literature and its exponents to make it abundantly clear that they are at odds about the disorder which responds to this treatment.

To take the simplest example – a common syndrome which presents with unilateral pain in the lumbo-sacral region and asymmetrical limitation of movement may be variously ascribed to disorder of the intervertebral disc, the apophyseal joint or the sacro-iliac joint. The manipulating physiotherapist who sits in the middle of the argument receiving similar cases with different diagnoses is perhaps peculiarly well able to appreciate this problem.

Where doctors disagree it would be unwise for the physiotherapist to have no doubt, but uncertainty need not lead to inaction. Naturally, confidence in diagnosis is a great help, but in practice no treatment is controlled by it. The diagnosis merely helps select the treatment, which is then controlled by reference to the presenting symptoms and signs, and changes which occur in them. The less certain the diagnosis, the more punctilious must re-examination become. It is this punctilious re-examination which enables the manipulator to treat, for example, the syndrome described above in a perfectly safe, methodical and effective way, while preserving a speculative approach to the nature of the underlying problem. This calls for a certain detachment of mind, which some find worrying or unsatisfactory. However, if manipulating physiotherapists can acquire this they may find that they are able to contribute evidence when the diagnosis is unsure, since the response to certain techniques can be retrospectively enlightening.

The reader is reminded that this chapter is about the principles, *not* the practice,' of manipulation. The manipulating physiotherapist is strongly advised to study all schools of thought, not only one, and to try to cultivate a dispassionate approach of the kind indicated above; an approach which may cumulatively throw light on what is now open to argument.

DISORDERS WHICH MAY RESPOND TO MANIPULATION

Disorders which may respond to manipulation are now divided very generally under two headings, mechanical derangement and contracture and adhesion.

Mechanical derangement

Here there is limitation of movement due to joint derangement or internal derangement of some kind; under this heading can be put such conditions as disc lesions, displacement of cartilage, impacted loose bodies, and possibly the impaired mobility described by osteopaths.

The purpose of manipulating is to move something: either a displacement may be reduced, returning structures to normal position and function, or it may be shifted to a 'silent position' in which it no longer causes pain. Manipulation of this kind does not involve trying to force the most painful and limited range. It is similar to the task of freeing a bit of jammed machinery – one does not usually achieve success by forcing the block, but by disengagement and perceptive jiggling in some other direction. Because of this, manipulation for mechanical derangement often includes distraction of the joint, and always involves movement into a painless or minimally affected range first. It is commonly, though not always, entirely painless.

Often it is not certain what manoeuvre will resolve the block. The manipulator must re-examine frequently to determine whether to repeat a manipulation or to use another one, and continuous information is needed about the degree and position of any pain produced. The patient's co-operation in providing this kind of clinical information is essential, and anaesthesia is therefore not used.

Contracture and adhesion

In such cases limitation of movement may be due to contracture or shortening of tissues spanning a joint; this may be due to trauma, disuse or immobilisation, or it may be secondary to some underlying pathology. In this category may also be placed the localised post-traumatic adhesion.

The purpose of manipulating here is to stretch out or rupture the constricting tissue, and the manipulator necessarily moves into a limited range to achieve this. The treatment cannot be painless, but must always remain within the tolerance of the patient and the condition itself (not always the same thing). Re-examination to determine the effects of treatment is usually carried out at the next attendance, since some treatment soreness is to be expected and may obscure immediate evaluation.

Manipulation of an adhesion is characterised by a quick, forceful, small amplitude movement. More generalised or capsular contracture requires longer, tougher handling, and 'mobilisation' is probably a better term for this than 'manipulation'.

Findings at examination

Mechanical derangement is characterised by the non-capsular pattern defined by Cyriax (1978). There may be other clues, such as sudden onset, a history of recurrence, and alterations in the position of pain and pattern of movement.

An adhesion mimics mechanical derangement in that it also presents a non-capsular pattern. The history may help to clarify, in that there will be no history of recurrence, or variation in pain and movement, and the onset will lack the typical suddenness of internal derangement. Additionally, the movements will be painful and limited in a way which suggests that they are stretching, not pinching, the source of the trouble.

Where contracture is due to arthritis or capsulitis, movement is lost in the characteristic capsular pattern for that joint (Cyriax, 1978). The value of recognising the classic capsular patterns in this context is that they will help to take the disorder clearly out of the mechanical derangement category, and thus simplify purpose in treatment.

At the spine, because of the difficulty of examining one joint at a time, these distinctions become blurred. The capsular pattern for the whole spine is a generalised, symmetrical loss of movement; asymmetrical pain and restriction can arguably be attributed to mechanical derangement, localised adhesion or capsulitis of an apophyseal joint.

Where there is doubt about the nature of the disorder, the manipulator is reminded of the attitude of mind recommended at the beginning of this section, and must rely on scrupulous re-evaluation of symptoms and signs, something which in any case is mandatory. It must be remembered that, particularly at the spine, in addition to articular symptoms and signs there may be involvement of other structures such as the nervous system, the dura mater or the arterial system. Such involvement may indicate important contra-indications, or special precautions to be taken when manipulating.

Manipulation under anaesthesia

This chapter is about manipulation of the conscious patient; mention of manipulation under anaesthesia is therefore brief.

Conditions requiring such manipulation may be either mechanical derangement (such as dislocation) or contracture. Anaesthesia is required when:

1. The manipulator is clear about the nature and the force of the manipulation needed, without relying on information that can only be provided by the conscious patient.
2. It has been decided to carry out a manoeuvre which will provoke too much pain and spasm for it to be performed kindly or effectively without anaesthesia.

DANGERS OF MANIPULATION

There are certain obvious contra-indications to manipulation, such as instability, fragility of bone or ligament, active inflammation or malignancy, where any use of force is likely to damage the structures being moved, or harmfully involve others. Examples of such conditions include rheumatoid arthritis, ankylosing spondylitis, cord or cauda equina involvement and vertebral artery involvement. This subject requires close study.

There are other situations in which the dangers of manipulation are less, but in which it is regarded with reserve, as likely to be of little help, or as more likely to exacerbate than improve. Examples in this category are the presence of distal root pain or neurological deficit. It is true that these are less responsive to manipulation, and the mechanism of spontaneous cure in disc lesions must be borne in mind. However, occasional good relief of pain can be achieved, and it is a pity to avoid all such cases. After the proper exclusion of absolute medical contra-indications, safety and effectiveness lie in a methodical re-examination by the manipulator, in acute perceptiveness in handling joints, and in observation of the rules of safety set out below. It is not prescription that can make manipulation safe, but proper application and technique.

SAFETY AND EFFECTIVENESS IN MANIPULATION

The hand

The hand must have authority, and be strong, comforting and perceptive. It receives indispensable information and is the medium for a continuous two-way process. The manipulator 'puts in' movement of precisely the kind intended, and simultaneously receives messages from the patient and the joint in the language of tissue resistance and muscle activity. This process is constant, and should be seen not only as part of technique but as continuous examination, which at any moment may modify the manipulator's intention and method.

Pain

The hand should pick up signals of pain long before the patient has any need to speak, but clear verbal communication with the patient about the degree and position of any pain provoked is essential, not only after manipulation, but during preliminary positioning.

Spasm

Never force spasm. There are exceptions to this, but the novice should beware of them.

Force and amplitude

As force is increased, reduce amplitude. Movement through one degree is unlikely to do much harm, even if the manipulation is ill-chosen.

Examination and recording

A general principle of all treatment is that re-examination is carried out at suitable intervals; on some occasions the proper intervals for such re-assessment will be longer than on others. Manipulation, especially manipulation for mechanical derangement, poses the necessity for frequent re-examination, since changes in symptoms and signs may occur immediately after a particular manoeuvre. Re-examination may be necessary several times in one treatment.

A meticulous and economical method of recording examination and technique is an integral part of the process. This cannot and must not be skipped. Only so can one keep track of rapidly changing clinical patterns in many individual cases; only so can changes in technique be remembered and future moves planned.

This is not different in kind from other forms of physiotherapy. It is just that the speed with which changes occur in manipulation may telescope the process. Grieve (1977), suggests that the allocation of time in treatment should be 'about 90 per cent thinking and 10 per cent doing'; these are fair proportions, recognising that the 90 per cent includes recording and planning future moves. It should be added that though examination must be sufficient to elicit enough information to control the treatment, there is such a thing as over-examination. In acute cases the physiotherapist must select only the critical assessment factors and so minimise examination soreness. The art of examination and recording is to achieve a balance between gathering all that is essential and eliminating what is not required.

GENERAL POINTS ON TECHNIQUE

1. Body-weight and strength must be used to advantage, and those who are lightly built must recognise that there are some physiques which they cannot handle. Those who have the advantage of strength must remember what has been said about the control of force and sensitivity in handling; otherwise their advantage may be thrown away or, worse, become harmful.

2. Explanation to the patient about what to expect, and calm reassuring directives during manipulation help tremendously in achieving the relaxation required. 'Let your foot touch the ground' said at the right moment may release tension in leg and back, and enable one to move the spinal joint effectively.

3. An ideal in manipulation is to localise movement to the affected joint alone. This may be possible at peripheral joints, but poses problems at the spine.

   (a) Even if it is felt possible to localise spinal movement in this way, it is not always clear which joint should be moved (a point already discussed). Techniques developed for moving an apophyseal joint may not be perfect for moving a disc protrusion.

   (b) The need for leverage to increase force and the desire for localisation are sometimes at odds, and a choice has to be made between them.

   A reasonable rule is to achieve as much localisation as possible, but to bear in mind the point made under (7) below.

4. A basic principle in manipulating mechanical derangement is to distract the joint surfaces during movement. In doing so one necessarily limits movement somewhat in other directions; again, a choice may have to be made here.

5. Satisfactory positioning must always be achieved before a manipulation is performed.

6. It is not forcing of movements under voluntary control that is required (if this were so most patients would cure themselves). The abnormality to be sought lies within those composite elements of joint movement which include accessory movement and accessory

range. It is within this territory that manipulation has its job to do.

7. A few techniques really mastered and done well are worth a whole bag of esoteric manoeuvres under haphazard control. The repertoire of techniques in constant use by experts is remarkably similar and remarkably small. The experienced manipulator gradually learns that what does not respond to manipulation by one person often will not respond to another; where there is success after failure it is commonly due to greater skill in performance than to a more complex manoeuvre.

DEFENDING THE LIMITATIONS OF MANIPULATION

The practice of manipulation suffers from the 'hey presto' effect, both in the eyes of the public and, sometimes, in the eyes of manipulators themselves. This phrase is used here to describe the instant, dramatic relief of pain and limitation of movement after one quick manoeuvre. This phenomenon is impressive to the patient, particularly if he has trailed round the medical and physiotherapy professions without relief, and finally found it outside the medical sphere.

The result of such an event is reputation. What the patient does not know, and what the successful manipulator sometimes seems to forget, is that this is by far from being the invariable effect of manipulation. If 10 people with back pain are selected indiscriminately and all manipulated, the chances are that one will be put right immediately; the rest will respond more slowly, not at all, or be worse for the experience.

Another factor contributes towards the prestige of manipulation, which is that there is a group of people who have a sense of well-being, of release and increased mobility, after manipulation of a normal joint (these can be matched by others who will feel stiff and sore for a while).

These two aspects of manipulation unite to produce a fellowship with a profound fidelity to its manipulators, often in the cause of prophylactic treatment. Such prophylactic effects have not been proved, and continued manipulation after the restoration of normal movement may well be harmful. If patients seek it they should be clear that it is not of proven use, and should evaluate it in terms of whether any pleasant feeling given is worth the money paid for it.

The heart of the matter, perhaps, lies in selecting a manipulator who recognises that manipulation cannot help all conditions, and who shows as much readiness to stop this treatment as to begin it in the first instance.

REFERENCES

Cyriax, J. (1978). *Textbook of Orthopaedic Medicine*, Vol 1, 7th edition. Baillière Tindall, London.

Grieve, G.P. (1977). *Mobilisation of the Spine*, 2nd edition. Henry Kimpton, London.

Hickling, J. and Maitland, G.D. (1970). Abnormalities in passive movement: diagrammatic representation. *Physiotherapy*, 56, 3.

Mennell, J.McM. (1964). *Joint Pain: Diagnosis and Treatment using Manipulative Techniques*, 2nd edition. Little, Brown and Co, Boston.

Stoddard, A. (1962). *Manual of Osteopathic Technique*. Hutchinson, London.

BIBLIOGRAPHY

Cyriax, J. and Russell, G. (1980). *Textbook of Orthopaedic Medicine*, Vol 2, 10th edition. Baillière Tindall, London.

Gray's Anatomy, 36th edition (1980). Longman, London.

Hickling, J. (1963). A defence of our limitations. *Physiotherapy*, 49, 9.

Maitland, G.D. (1977). *Vertebral Manipulation*, 4th edition. Butterworths, London.

Maitland, G.D. (1977). *Peripheral Manipulation*, 2nd edition. Butterworths, London.

McConaill, M.A. and Basmajian, J.V. (1977). *Muscle and Movements: A Basis for Human Kinesiology*. Krieger Publishing Co, New York.

See also the Bibliography at the end of Chapter 10.

ACKNOWLEDGEMENT

The author thanks Mrs B. Lindfield, DipPT, DipTeaching PT, DipPhys Anthrop, of the Department of Anatomy, St Thomas' Hospital Medical School, London, for her help in the preparation of this chapter.

Chapter 12

Degenerative Arthritis of the Spine and Intervertebral Disc Disease

by A.G. MOWAT, MB, FRCP(Ed) *and* P.M. WOOD, MCSP, DipTP

CLINICAL

ANATOMY, PATHOLOGY, INCIDENCE AND CAUSE

The spinal apophyseal joints

The spinal apophyseal joints are diarthrodial, synovial joints and are thus susceptible to be involved in the same inflammatory and degenerative processes which affect larger, peripheral joints. The apophyseal joints lie posteriorly on each side of the vertebral pedicles providing articulation with the adjacent vertebrae, and so each vertebra carries four articular surfaces (Fig. 12/1). In addition each thoracic vertebra has four small articular surfaces for the articulation of the ribs with the sides of the vertebral body and the transverse processes. The atlas and axis (the first and second cervical vertebrae) carry similar posterior apophyseal joints, but in addition there are synovial joints between the anterior arch of the atlas and the odontoid process of the axis. The third to the seventh cervical vertebral bodies differ from those elsewhere in the spine in having small synovial joints on the posterior edge of the upper and lower surfaces of the bodies – neuro-central joints.

The spinal movements which take place at each vertebra are flexion, extension, lateral flexion and rotation, the latter two being associated movements. The extent of these movements at each part of the spine depends upon the thickness of the intervertebral discs, the tension in the interspinal ligaments and the angle of contact of the intervertebral joints. In consequence, greater movements occur in the cervical and lumbar spine than in the thoracic spine and for practical purposes none occurs in the sacral region. The joints between the atlas

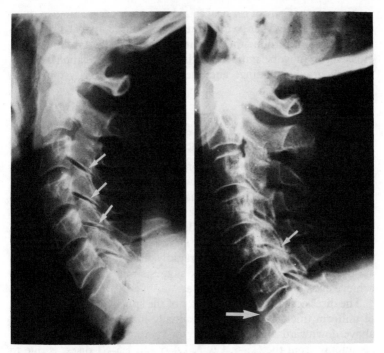

Fig. 12/1   A normal lateral radiograph of the cervical spine showing that the intervertebral discs are well preserved with little evidence of osteophyte formation on the anterior or posterior margins of the vertebral bodies. The apophyseal joints (arrowed) are normal

Fig. 12/2   A lateral radiograph of the cervical spine showing narrowing of C6–7 disc, and apophyseal arthritis

and the skull allow flexion, extension and lateral flexion of the skull while rotation of the skull upon the cervical spine is almost entirely carried out by the axis.

Degenerative arthritis in these joints, with loss of cartilage, eburnation of underlying bone and the development of marginal osteophytes, accompanied by a very variable amount of pain and decreased function, is a very common feature of advancing age (Fig. 12/2). Surveys based upon radiographic findings show that some 70 per cent of the population have such changes by the age of 60 years and that the incidence steadily increases with age. Occupational factors tend to affect the incidence, since degenerative changes are commoner in men, particularly those engaged in manual work. Further, the incidence, especially of cervical spinal lesions, is exaggerated in those patients, mostly women, with primary generalised osteoarthritis with Heberden nodes around the distal interphalangeal joints of the hands. However, it must be emphasised that there is no correlation between the radiographic findings and the presence or severity of clinical symptoms and signs.

The intervertebral discs

The intervertebral discs, lying between successive vertebral bodies from the second cervical vertebra downwards, are composed of fibrocartilage, the outer portion of which consists chiefly of concentric rings of fibrous tissue, the annulus fibrosus, while the centre of the disc, the nucleus pulposus, is softer and gelatinous. The normal disc is capable of withstanding heavy loads with relatively little deformation and serves as an efficient 'shock absorber'. It can adapt to spinal movements and should distribute rapidly changing stresses evenly up and down the spine. Recent work suggests that many spines fail to achieve even distribution of stresses.

The discs account for one-quarter of the spinal length, and are not of uniform thickness, being of gradually increasing thickness from above downwards. The frequency of symptoms, which arise most commonly from the C5–6, C6–7, L4–5 and L5–S1 discs, is due to greater stresses being present at the junctions of very mobile and relatively immobile spinal segments. By early adult life the discs are avascular and degenerative changes set in accompanied by a progressive reduction in water content. Such degenerative changes are accompanied by a tendency for the contents of the nucleus pulposus to be extruded through weakened portions of the annulus fibrosus. Such extrusion may occur through the vertebral plate into adjacent vertebrae. These Schmorl's nodes are usually symptomless, but if multiple may be associated with degenerative arthritis and a loss of height.

Extrusion of the disc in other directions is influenced by the attachment of the disc to the vertebral ligaments. The disc is loosely attached to the anterior longitudinal ligament which in turn is firmly attached to the vertebral bodies, but the disc is more firmly attached to the posterior longitudinal ligament which in its turn is only loosely attached to the posterior aspect of the vertebral bodies. Extrusion of the disc anteriorly or laterally causes anterior or lateral osteophyte growth which may be so marked as occasionally to unite and so fuse two vertebrae with consequent loss of movement of the apophyseal joints (Fig. 12/3). Extrusion of the disc contents posteriorly causes greater problems. Fixation to the posterior ligament usually means that disc extrusion occurs postero-laterally, at which site symptoms will depend upon whether the extrusion is acute or whether it occurs slowly and is accompanied by osteophyte formation. In either event the disc contents and/or the osteophytes may press upon the spinal cord, the nerve roots either as they travel downwards or through the intervertebral foramina, or upon the vertebral artery in the cervical spine.

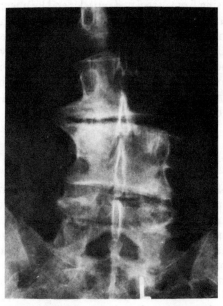

Fig. 12/3 Radiograph of lumbar spine showing how antero-lateral osteophytes from adjacent vertebrae have united. *Note* the associated disc degeneration and narrowing

The phenomenon of disc degeneration, with or without osteophyte formation and extrusion of disc contents is very common, with 60 per cent of the population having significant radiological changes in all spinal segments by the age of 60 years. The incidence in all spinal segments is higher in men. Degeneration of discs is often associated with degeneration in the apophyseal joints and once again the radiographic and clinical presentations cannot be correlated (Fig. 12/2).

The incidence of acute disc prolapse, commonest in the lumbar spine and which tends to occur in patients aged between 30 and 50 years, is difficult to determine, since the diagnosis of 'slipped disc' is a fashionable one, particularly by patients. Although acute disc prolapse produces a characteristic clinical picture, the diagnosis is medically proven relatively rarely.

Ligaments and muscles

As with joint disease elsewhere, there may be related or independent symptoms arising from associated muscles and ligaments. In addition to the anterior and posterior longitudinal ligaments, there are a variety of other spinal ligaments, the most important of which are the ligamentum flava connecting the laminae of adjacent vertebrae, and the interspinous ligaments joining the vertebral spines. A large number of muscles are attached to the spinal column, and these attachments may be the site of chronic inflammation secondary to trauma and abnormal or unbalanced loading.

THE CAUSES OF DEGENERATION IN THE SPINE

The causes of degenerative changes in the spine, sometimes called spondylosis, as with degenerative arthritis in other joints, are not clearly determined. In some patients the association with trauma, either as a single severe episode or related to repeated minor episodes over many years, usually determined by the nature of or the posture adopted at work, will be clear. In others obesity may be a major factor. However, in many patients the cause is unclear although developmental abnormalities and endocrine and metabolic factors may be involved. In the group of patients with widespread generalised osteoarthritis genetic factors are dominant, the inheritance among female members of the family often being clearly seen. It is obvious, therefore, that only some of the potential causes can be influenced during management of the patient.

CERVICAL SPINE

Clinical features

Three main groups of symptoms are produced by degenerative arthritis and intervertebral disc disease in the cervical spine. (a) Symptoms due to pressure of osteophytes or postero-lateral disc protrusion on the spinal nerves. These are by far the commonest symptoms. (b) Symptoms due to pressure of osteophytes or central disc protrusion on the spinal cord. (c) Symptoms due to pressure of osteophytes or lateral disc protrusion on the vertebral artery (Figs. 12/4 and 12/5).

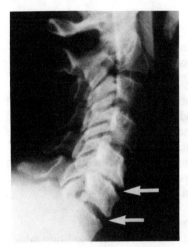 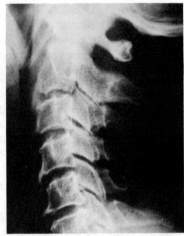

Fig. 12/4 A lateral radiograph of the cervical spine showing narrowing of the C5–6 and C6–7 discs with anterior and posterior osteophyte formation (arrowed). The apophyseal joints are well preserved

Fig. 12/5 A lateral radiograph of the cervical spine showing marked osteophyte formation

Degeneration in the neuro-central joints of the third to seventh vertebrae may contribute to both spinal cord and nerve compression.

Symptoms may be produced by acute or chronic disc changes. Acute disc prolapse usually follows trauma in younger patients and produces sudden severe pain with a further increase in intensity over a few days. Changes associated with chronic disc disease are more gradual and frequently episodic in their production of symptoms.

SPINAL NERVE ROOT COMPRESSION
Spinal nerve root compression produces pain in the distribution area of the root, but it is important to remember that the pain may be wider spread than imagined, with C4 root pain being felt in the scapular region and C7 root pain in the anterior chest. Typically, acute spasms of pain are added to a background of dull aching. The pain may

produce muscle spasm with a reduction in spinal movement or a complete loss of movement associated with a torticollis. Involvement of the motor root results in muscle weakness and diminution or absence of arm reflexes. The muscles supplied by the most commonly involved roots are listed below:

Deltoid	C5, (6)
Biceps	C(5), 6
Triceps	C(6), 7, (8)
Wrist and fingers extensors and flexors	C7, 8
Thumb abductors and extensors	C(7), 8
Intrinsic hand muscles	C8, T1

Involvement of the sensory root may produce paraesthesiae and subsequently impairment of all modalities of sensation in the affected dermatome. In the early stages, nerve root irritation may produce increased and unpleasant sensation – hyperaesthesia. Skin dermatomes are shown in Figure 12/6 but caution must be exercised in attributing symptoms to a specific root on the basis of such diagrams, as there is marked individual variation.

CERVICAL SPINAL CORD COMPRESSION
Cervical spinal cord compression is a very serious condition which occurs most commonly at the C5–6 level. Although there is a variety of presentations, the most usual involves upper motor neurone lesion

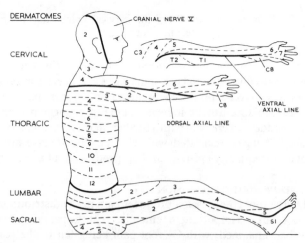

Fig. 12/6 The dermatomes of the body and the segmented cutaneous distribution of the upper limb

findings in one or both legs with lower motor neurone lesion findings in the upper limbs. In addition there will be a variety of sensory abnormalities in both arms and legs.

VERTEBRAL ARTERY COMPRESSION

Vertebral artery compression can lead, particularly in the elderly, to brainstem ischaemia and the production of vertigo, tinnitus, visual disturbances, difficulty with speech and swallowing, and ataxia and other signs of cerebellar dysfunction.

Involvement of individual spinal joints or muscle and ligamentous damage in the neck, may produce both local and referred pain often associated with secondary muscle spasm, reduced movement and torticollis. Such symptoms are the usual result of 'whiplash' injuries incurred in road traffic accidents.

DIFFERENTIAL DIAGNOSIS OF CERVICAL SPINAL DISEASE

Acute disc lesions, particularly if due to trauma, may be confused with vertebral fracture or compression. The symptoms of chronic disc protrusion associated with cord compression must be distinguished from multiple sclerosis, cord tumours, motor neurone disease, syringomyelia and subacute degeneration of the cord due to vitamin B_{12} deficiency.

The spinal apophyseal joints may be involved in a variety of inflammatory diseases which will require anti-inflammatory drugs (Chapter 16). Such diseases include rheumatoid arthritis, ankylosing spondylitis, psoriatic arthritis and Reiter's disease (Chapters 16 and 17). A variety of cardiovascular diseases may impair vertebral artery blood flow including atherosclerosis, cardiac valvular disease, thrombosis and embolism.

Spinal tumour or infective lesions (tuberculosis, staphylococcus, etc) may cause nerve root symptoms. Herpes zoster (shingles) may cause similar nerve root symptoms and diagnostic confusion until the typical vesicular rash appears. Involvement of more than one or two nerve roots suggests damage to the brachial plexus, as with viral radiculitis, thoracic outlet syndromes and drooping of the shoulders with marked downward movement of the outer end of the clavicle, often found in middle-aged women.

DORSAL SPINE

Although dorsal spinal abnormalities are found commonly in radiographic studies of the general population, the incidence of symptoms is low. Nerve root symptoms are the commonest with pain radiating to the front of the chest or abdomen. The pain may simulate that arising from thoracic or abdominal viscera.

Treatment may include use of analgesics, a firm bed, extension and rotation exercises, weight reduction, the use of a firm brassière for those with heavy or pendulous breasts, a full posterior spinal support, and occasionally nerve root blocks.

LUMBAR SPINE

Clinical features

There are some differences between the type and causes of symptoms in the lumbar spine compared with the cervical spine. In particular, there are no vascular symptoms. Ninety per cent of symptoms affect the L5 or S1 roots. The symptoms in order of frequency are:

1. Those due to trauma or degenerative changes in the intervertebral discs or spinal joints producing pain and muscle spasm in the associated spinal dermatome (Figs. 12/7 and 12/8).
2. Those due to damage in muscles and ligaments produced by trauma, abnormal loading or bad posture. If close to the skin surface the signs may be localised but are usually similar to (1).
3. Those due to pressure of osteophytes or postero-lateral disc protrusion on the spinal nerves.
4. Those due to pressure of osteophytes or central disc protrusion on the cauda equina. The spinal cord terminates at the level of the second lumbar vertebra.

The use of the standard examination technique which is listed in Table 1, p. 240, will ensure that nothing is omitted.

SYMPTOMS (1) AND (2)
Changes which fall short of actual nerve compression cause local pain and produce an area of referred pain, often called lumbago, which is listed in Table 2. The pain is deep-seated and nagging, and may be associated with muscle spasm and reduced spinal motion.

SYMPTOMS (3)
Nerve compression produces similar or more severe pain but in

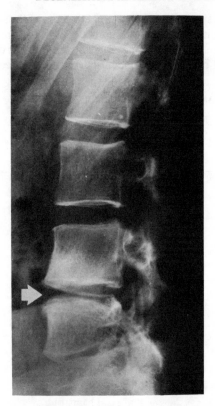

Fig. 12/7   A lateral radiograph of the lumbar spine showing degenerative changes with narrowing of the L4–5 disc, and loss of the lumbar curve due to protective muscle spasm

addition there are motor effects which are listed in Table 2 and altered, reduced or absent sensation in the areas shown in Figure 12/8. Plantar flexors and dorsiflexors are best tested with the foot on the ground with the patient standing or sitting respectively. There is muscle spasm, often with reduction in lumbar lordosis and mild lumbar scoliosis. It must be appreciated that there are individual variations in nerve distribution and the listed effects must be interpreted with caution.

Nerve compression is associated with nerve irritation detected by reduced straight leg raising with a positive Lasègue's sign or hip extension with the knee flexed (sciatic and femoral nerve stretch tests). Nerve compression symptoms in the distribution of the sciatic nerve, constitute sciatica, a term often abused by medical and lay people. The symptoms from a prolapsed disc are usually aggravated by straightening up from a stooping position far more than bending, lifting weights, coughing, sneezing and straining at defaecation. The pain is eased by rest, each patient having a preferred position.

TABLE 1   EXAMINATION OF THE BACK

Position	Musculo-skeletal system	Central nervous system	Referred pain
Standing	Inspection Range of back movement	Plantar flexor power	
Kneeling Sitting		Ankle reflex Dorsiflexor power	
Bending over table Sitting on table	Palpation	Knee reflex	
Lying supine	Range of hip movement	Straight leg raising	Abdominal examination
		Quadriceps and hamstring power Sensation on front of leg Plantar reflex	
Lying on left side		Right hip abductor power	
Lying on right side		Left hip abductor power	
Lying prone		Femoral stretch test Gluteus maximus tone Saddle anaesthesia	Rectal examination

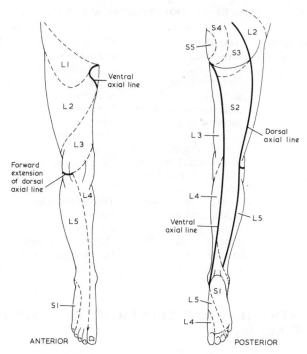

Fig. 12/8   The dermatomes of the lower limb

SYMPTOMS (4)

Cauda equina compression is a most serious condition. Involvement of all the nerves may occur with profound motor and sensory changes in the legs. Saddle anaesthesia and absence of buttock muscle tone are signs of S3–5 root damage. Further, involvement of the sacral nerves will produce additional motor and sensory changes but, more importantly, sphincter disturbances with retention of urine and faeces. Similar cauda equina symptoms may appear slowly with a spinal tumour or with spinal stenosis. In spinal stenosis, which is due to developmental or bony changes reducing the space available for the spinal cord, the compression symptoms may be exercise-related and may improve with rest, suggesting a vascular component to the symptoms which is not present.

Involvement of individual spinal joints, ligaments and muscles in inflammatory or traumatic processes will give rise to muscle spasm and pain in the distributions listed in Table 2.

TABLE 2   LUMBAR NERVE ROOT SYMPTOMS AND SIGNS

Spinal segment and root involved	Area of referred deep pain	Muscle weakness and wasting	Reduced or absent reflexes
L2	Upper buttock, groin	Hip flexors, adductors	
L3	Mid-buttock, anterior aspect of thigh	Hip flexors, adductors Quadriceps	Knee
L4	Lower buttock, round lateral aspect of thigh to anterior aspect of knee	Quadriceps Tibialis anterior	Knee
L5	Lower buttock, lateral aspect of thigh and calf	Tibialis posterior Peronei Toe extensors	Ankle
S1	Posterior aspect of thigh and calf	Calf and toe flexors Hamstrings, glutei	Ankle

INVESTIGATION AND TREATMENT OF LUMBAR SPINE LESIONS

The physiotherapist assesses the lumbar spine as described in Chapter 9. However, in the lumbar spine, psychological factors are probably more important as almost everyone has had backache at some time, and most people feel that backache is an inevitable result of the stresses of modern living. Backache is a major cause of loss of work but not all cases have significant pathological lesions in their spines. In other cases the backache may be related to an injury for which the patient is claiming compensation and in most cases this will complicate assessment. In many of these patients symptoms will not finally clear until adequate compensation has been received, usually three to four years later.

Investigations

Plain radiographs must be interpreted with caution as changes in the lumbar spine are very common with increasing age and bear little relation to symptoms. Oblique rather than lateral radiographs are required to demonstrate the apophyseal joints. A myelogram may be required to localise both root and cauda equina lesions (Figs. 12/9 and 12/10). Examination of the cerebrospinal fluid and other investiga-

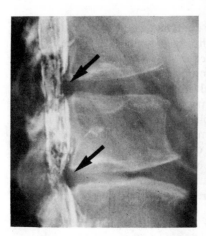 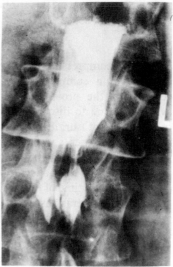

Fig. 12/9   A myelogram showing a disc protrusion at the level of L4–5 with a less marked protrusion at the L3–4 level

Fig. 12/10   A myelogram showing spinal stenosis with failure of the dye to extend below the middle of the fourth lumbar vertebra. The spinal stenosis is due to extensive degenerative changes which are clearly visible

tions are of little value except in excluding other conditions (Table 3). In some cases nerve conduction studies and electromyography may help to decide which nerves and muscles are involved.

Treatment

Most patients experience relief of a pain with clearing of the neurological symptoms and signs if a basic programme of treatment is followed.

DRUGS
The use of full dosage of a simple analgesic often supplemented by a muscle relaxant such as diazepam. Opiates may be required.

REST
Ideally the patient should have complete bed rest, with no pillows, on a firm mattress supported by boards for a period of up to three weeks. After an acute attack, patients should be encouraged to persist with such arrangements for sleeping each night; if necessary for ever. Most patients prefer a firm bed, once they have tried it.

In most patients it is unnecessary to proceed further, since symptoms will settle after a few days of this treatment.

SURGERY

Surgical decompression must be undertaken quickly in patients with cauda equina compression. This will require laminectomy and removal of the prolapsed material. In those with more chronic symptoms due to disc protrusion or osteophytes, unresponsive to other treatment, surgical removal of the compressing material may be required. In patients with very persistent symptoms, particularly if these are arising from the apophyseal joints, spinal fusion may be required. Some surgeons recommend spinal fusion as a primary procedure at the time of removal of the prolapsed material. However, these major operations must only be undertaken after careful assessment of the patient, as a disturbing number of patients continue to have symptoms despite apparently successful surgical treatment. (See Chapter 13.)

DIFFERENTIAL DIAGNOSIS OF BACKACHE

Although the conditions described above are the commonest causes of backache, the complaint is so frequently encountered in the general practitioner's surgery and in the orthopaedic clinic that other conditions must be remembered. It is easy for both patients and medical personnel to dismiss low backache as an inevitable consequence of the human race having adopted an upright posture. Table 3 lists some of the conditions which may cause low backache.

Vertebral fracture due to trauma, osteoporosis or neoplastic deposit is the only common cause of acute symptoms apart from acute disc protrusion and muscle or ligamentous tears. Further, there are age-related diseases in that osteochondritis (Scheuermann's disease) affects those under 15 years and neoplastic disease, osteoporosis and Paget's disease are uncommon in those under 50 years.

Assessment of low backache requires a full examination of the spine with the patient undressed, examination of the sacro-iliac and hip joints, measurement of leg length, a neurological examination and sufficient general examination to exclude the possibility of tumour (myeloma and secondary deposits from primary tumours in the lung, breast, kidney, prostate and thyroid glands are the commonest). Bowel and gynaecological diseases may cause backache and appropriate examination including rectal and vaginal examination will be required. The minimum radiographic requirements are an antero-posterior view of the lumbar spine and pelvis, a lateral view of the lumbar spine and a coned view of the lumbo-sacral junction. All patients over the age of 40 years should have a chest radiograph. The other relevant tests are shown in Table 3.

TABLE 3   COMMONER CAUSES OF LOW BACKACHE

Cause		Investigations	
		Radiological	Other
Congenital	Short leg		
	Sacralised L5	Diagnosis	
	Lumbarised S1	Diagnosis	
	Spondylolysis	Diagnosis	
	Spondylolisthesis	Diagnosis	
Traumatic	Prolapsed disc	Myelogram	
	Ligamentous tear		
	Fracture	Diagnosis	
Degenerative	Osteoarthrosis	Diagnosis	
	Hyperostosis	Diagnosis	
Inflammatory	Ankylosing spondylitis	Sacro-iliitis	ESR
	Reiter's disease	Sacro-iliitis	ESR
	Colitic arthritis	Sacro-iliitis	ESR
	Psoriatic arthritis	Sacro-iliitis	ESR
	Pyogenic osteomyelitis	Helpful	ESR, white cell count
	Tuberculosis	Helpful	ESR, white cell count
	Osteochondritis	Diagnosis	
Neoplastic	Secondary deposit	Helpful	Bone scan, alkaline phosphatase
	Myeloma	Helpful	ESR, bone marrow
	Spinal cord tumour	Myelogram	
	Primary bone tumour	Helpful	Bone scan, alkaline phosphatase
Metabolic	Osteoporosis	Changes	Calcium, phosphorus,
	Osteomalacia	Often diagnostic	Alkaline phosphatase
	Paget's disease	Diagnosis	Alkaline phosphatase
	Pyrophosphate arthritis	Diagnosis	
Postural	Pregnancy		
	Obesity		
	Occupational		
	Hip disease	Diagnosis	
	Scoliosis	Diagnosis	
Other	Gynaecological		
system	Renal	IVP	Local
disease	Rectal	Barium enema	examination

PHYSIOTHERAPY

Physical treatment for degenerative disease of the spine follows the principles laid down in Chapter 10, and should be preceded by an 'indications' examination and assessment by the physiotherapist as outlined in Chapter 9. It should be realised from the outset that treatment can only help alleviate symptoms, and will have little bearing on the disease-process and its ultimate prognosis.

CERVICAL SPINE

In acute exacerbation of disease affecting the cervical spine, rest may well be the initial treatment. The physiotherapist may supply a temporary collar (which is often made from Plastazote) for daytime wear to restrict movement, and a soft collar for support at night. The patient should be advised to avoid going into darkened rooms or out into the dark, and not to drive while wearing a collar. This is because the ability to judge distance is impaired due to loss of proprioceptive input from the cervical spine. The sleeping position should be discussed, and the number of pillows used adjusted as necessary. The patient can be shown how to make a 'butterfly pillow' by taking a soft, ordinary pillow and loosely tying the centre so that the two ends provide a support to prevent side flexion of the cervical region. The patient lies with his head and neck on the thin centre area with the two 'butterfly wings' supporting the neck. Postural advice for the head, neck and shoulders should also be given.

If pressure on a nerve root causes acute radicular pain in a patient with cervical spondylosis, relief of the pressure may be gained by the use of intermittent, sustained cervical traction. The patient is positioned so that the affected segment is in the mid-position of its range of flexion and extension, and traction is applied either manually or via a machine or pulley system. The pain should not be totally relieved as this often leads to an exacerbation when the traction is released. The pull may be maintained up to half an hour at a time and may be repeated more than once daily.

When the acute phase of pain has passed, passive mobilising techniques may relieve pain further and restore local movement. The patient should be given ergonomic advice (see p. 208), and have a home programme of gentle active movement and postural exercises to maintain a pain-free range of movement.

Heat in the form of hot packs, a hot water bottle or electrically heated pad, may help to relieve the pain of muscle spasm, as may massage to the neck and shoulder region.

Patients with more chronic pain of cervical origin may find relief from regional intermittent traction being used for its mobilising effect and relief of muscle spasm. Passive mobilising techniques which have a bilateral effect are very valuable, and more than one technique may be used in a treatment session. These may be followed by postural correction and active exercises to maintain the increase in range of movement. While these patients will seldom require the use of a collar, they will benefit from advice about sleeping positions and ergonomics.

THORACIC (DORSAL) SPINE

Degenerative changes in the thoracic spine are less common than in the more mobile cervical and lumbar regions. They are often the result of early disease, e.g. Scheuermann's disease in adolescence. If muscle spasm is prevalent some form of heat or massage may be used as a preliminary to mobilising exercises, and postural strengthening exercises. In many cases general passive mobilising may be valuable, but care must be taken.

Hydrotherapy provides an excellent medium to fulfill treatment aims. The heat promotes relaxation of muscle spasm, and the resistance, or assistance, of the water can be used for exercise as required. Swimming is excellent therapy, and the patient can be advised to continue it as an effective home activity.

LUMBAR SPINE

Lumbar spondylosis is a common condition which does not lead always to a disabling problem. It is a cause of low back pain in late middle-age and the elderly, and such patients may be helped by physiotherapy. Treatment will focus on relieving pain, which is usually of a chronic aching nature, and restoring functional movement. Heat and massage may be comforting but will not bring lasting relief. Passive mobilising techniques are valuable together with light, general back exercises. In men who are employed in heavy work, a corset may be supplied for working hours. Ergonomic advice and postural exercises should be given (see p. 208). Intermittent lumbar traction used as a mobilising technique can be valuable, as may hydrotherapy (as already mentioned). If a segmental level of instability due to a degenerate disc is shown to cause pain, the patient should have a course of stabilising exercises, particularly building up the abdominal muscles and re-educating postural control. All patients must be instructed in correct lifting and be given ergonomic advice.

Conservative management of prolapsed lumbar intervertebral disc

An acute disc prolapse must be accurately diagnosed, and most disc prolapses respond to conservative management. Surgery is restricted to those patients where there is evidence of severe nerve root, or cauda equina compression, or prolonged unremitting pain or disability which leads to complete inability to return to a working life.

Rest, either in bed or, if this is not possible, a plaster jacket, is required for three to four weeks. Simple analgesics may make the patient more comfortable while resting. Following this period, physiotherapy may be advised – this will always include advice on lifting.

Prolapse of a lumbar disc leads to referred pain down the leg due to nerve root compression. This nerve root pain may be worse distally and be shooting in nature. The treatment of choice to relieve such pain is intermittent lumbar traction, with the patient positioned accurately according to the segmental level. Great weight is not necessarily required and full relief of pain is *not* aimed for. Traction may be maintained for up to half an hour and may be repeated during the course of the day in severe cases, and should be carried out daily. It may take several days for prolonged pain relief to occur.

Such patients are not often left with marked loss of range of movement when pain is relieved, so mobilising exercises are rarely needed. Patients may need muscle strengthening exercises and re-education, particularly for the abdominal muscles. Postural control and correct lifting techniques should be taught as early as possible with regard to relief of pain. All patients should be given ergonomic advice. Swimming, preferably in a heated pool, is to be encouraged as an enjoyable activity to maintain spinal function.

BIBLIOGRAPHY

See pages 214 and 229.

Chapter 13

Surgery for Spinal Disorders – 1. Clinical

by J.P. O'BRIEN, MB, BS, PhD, FRCS(Ed), FACS

Spinal surgery is indicated in two definite categories:

Deformity including cord compression and congenital anomalies.

Pain.

The decision to intervene surgically is usually clear, in that the patient is severely disabled and unable to conduct his/her life normally. In both deformity and pain all the appropriate conservative measures will have been tried. The decision to operate is the final form of treatment. Seventy per cent of deformities and over 50 per cent of low back pain problems are idiopathic, that is, they have no known cause for the pain or deformity. The rationale of spinal surgery is to relieve the pain and correct the deformity. The surgeon faces two problems:

A. Making a decision about the precise pathological lesion which is producing the pain or deformity.

B. Deciding on the correct operative technique.

Two preliminary requirements are the formation of a multi-disciplinary team approach and the structuring of a comprehensive assessment of the patient.

THE MULTIDISCIPLINARY TEAM APPROACH

This is vital because most spinal problems are difficult to assess, needing clinical evaluation, physiotherapeutic assessment and various tests. They are also complicated in the adult by social, marital, employment and financial issues. It is often surprising how much greater the patient's real disabilities are when they have been carefully assessed by specialists in all the relevant fields, medical and paramedical. At Oswestry, meetings are attended by specialists from all appropriate disciplines to discuss the more difficult cases. Each specialist will have spoken to the patient and assessed him. By combining all this information a viable decision can be made. Team-work is essential if the total patient management is to be successful.

CAREFUL COMPREHENSIVE ASSESSMENT

For all forms of spinal disorders, detailed assessment involves:
1. A full clinical history, including a family history and completion of a Disability Index Chart (Fairbank et al, 1980).
2. A full physical examination with the patient standing in order that the physician can see if there is asymmetry; mobility is tested through a range of flexion, extension and rotation movements. The effect of movement on a deformity will be apparent and provide a clue to its flexibility. In cases of low back pain the anterior tenderness sign will confirm pathology in the lumbar spine (see p. 264).
3. Neurological examination: testing of reflexes, motor and sensory impairment.
4. Relevant tests may include, when appropriate, radiographs

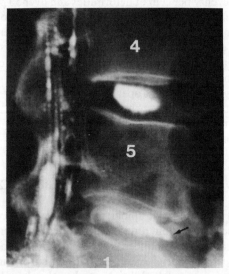

Fig. 13/1 Lateral radiograph showing discograms at lumbar 4–5 and lumbo-sacral levels. The upper disc is normal and the lower disc confirms disruption. The vertical streaking is the remnant of a previous radiculogram

(discograms (Fig. 13/1), facet arthrograms, radiculograms, tomograms, myelograms), respiratory function tests and gait analysis.

BACKGROUND INFORMATION

The motion segment

There are usually 23 motion segments containing discs in the spine (Fig. 13/2) making up a unique flexible multi-articulated structure protecting the spinal cord.

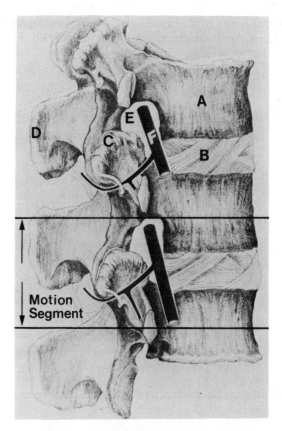

Fig. 13/2 Drawing to demonstrate the basic anatomy of the motion segment. A. Vertebral body; B. Intervertebral disc; C. Facet joint; D. Spinous process; E. Intervertebral foramen

Parts of the motion segment can be affected by a variety of pathological processes such as:

(a) Vertebral body, e.g. fracture
(b) Soft tissue, e.g. torn annulus fibrosus
(c) Nerve, e.g. compression.

In due course abnormalities in one segment, e.g. abnormal growth or loss of substance as in infection, will affect the adjacent segments. Locating the exact mechanisms of the motion segment that is at fault is crucial for diagnosis and treatment. Is the disc or the facet joint the primary problem or is it another entity?

Pain referral

The most confusing aspect of spinal disorders is the complex patterns of pain referral classically described by Kellgren (1939) (Fig. 13/3).

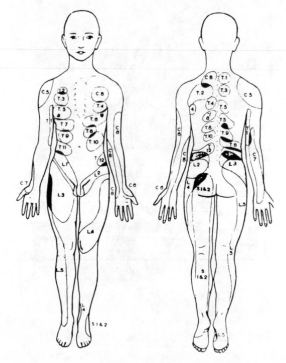

Fig. 13/3 Patterns of pain referral as demonstrated by Kellgren (1939). These patterns were produced by injection of minute quantities of saline into the interspinous ligaments at the various levels

1. Pain in the leg can be referred from any part of a motion segment in the lumbar spine and does not necessarily indicate nerve root compression.
2. Abdominal or chest pain may be referred from a source in the spine.
3. Real abdominal and cardiac lesions can have pain referral to the spine and this can be a cause of diagnostic confusion.
4. Groin pain is commonly referred from an involved lumbar motion segment and is often mistaken for uterine disease and results in a hysterectomy.
5. The outer half of the disc has a rich sensory nerve supply (Fig. 13/4) and tears of the annulus are common in domestic and

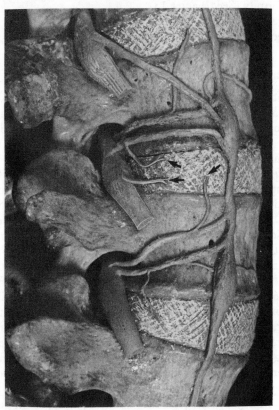

Fig. 13/4 Model to demonstrate the nerve supply of the disc. These small filaments can be seen with an operating microscope (Bogduk). They ultimately provide a rich sensory nerve supply to the outer half of the annulus fibrosus

industrial accidents. These will often produce leg pain but the radiculogram will be negative. This leads erroneously to surgical exploration in anticipation of finding a hidden disc lesion. This sequence of events is all too common and the increasing disability following a negative exploration makes a 'failed back surgery patient' one of the most afflicted sufferers in clinical medicine and they are too readily dismissed as psychosomatic cases.

TYPICAL AREAS FOR SPINAL SURGERY

(a) Trauma
(b) Deformity (See Chapter 15)
(c) Degeneration
(d) Infections and tumour (not discussed)

Trauma

The place of surgery in spinal injuries remains contentious.

In *spinal fractures*, gross instability will require stabilisation, the most popular method being double-Harrington rodding. It is vital that the spinal cord injured patient is handled in a special unit by a well-trained team of specialists.

Soft tissue injury is the most common cause of spinal pain. It is most disabling and difficult to diagnose because it is not apparent on a plain radiograph. A torn disc is unlikely to heal because of its poor blood supply, and continuing disability will necessitate fusion. The principle is that obliterating most of the movement within the motion segment will alleviate the pain.

The commonest site for disc injury is the lowest two motion segments, that is, lumbar 4–5 and the lumbo-sacral joints (Figs. 13/5 and 13/6). The thinnest part of the radius of the annulus fibrosus is posteriorly adjacent to the nerve root emerging from the intervertebral foramen. Continuing injury will tear more and more of the annular fibres; ultimately there will be a complete rent in the annulus allowing extruded nucleus pulposus to compress the nerve root thus producing the classical leg pain. This ruptured disc syndrome is confirmed by radiculography and will require posterior spinal surgery, ideally a 'fenestration' or interlaminar approach permitting access to the compressed inflamed nerve root and allowing the ruptured disc to be removed with care, thus decompressing the nerve root. This is the most common spinal operation but great care should be taken with the handling of the nerve roots because of the high risk

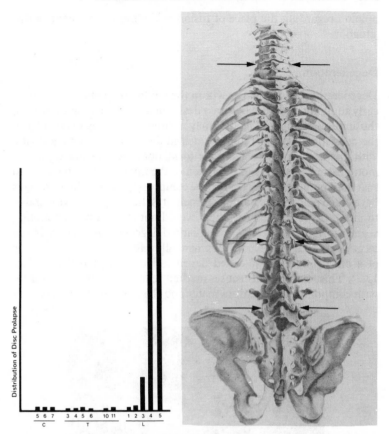

Fig. 13/5   Barograph to show the distribution of disc prolapse at the various motion segments in the spine. *Note* that the vast majority are confined to the lowest two segments

Fig. 13/6   Sketch of the axial skeleton to demonstrate the areas of the spine relatively susceptible to trauma (arrows). The rib cage provides basic stability to the thoracic spine

of nerve root scarring which appears to be associated with chronic intractable back and leg pain. Some patients seem more prone to the development of nerve root scarring than others.

In a ruptured disc, in biomechanical terms, there is instability of the motion segment and there are valid reasons why one should fuse this unstable segment. The incidence of chronic back pain several years after this operation is quite high but nonetheless there is divided opinion regarding the place of fusion of the motion segment in this situation.

Degeneration

Degenerative changes occur within the motion segment beginning in early adult life. The disc becomes desiccated and radial tears appear in the annulus fibrosus. The disc may narrow, producing overriding of the corresponding facet joints which in due course become arthritic with loss of cartilage, osteophyte formation, etc. Narrowing of the motion segment produces reduction of the intervertebral foramen so that the emerging nerve root may be compressed. When these changes have taken place in the motion segment it is therefore more vulnerable to minor degrees of injury which would not affect a normal motion segment. In the older age-group marked degenerative changes in the facet joints at the lumbar 4–5 segment allow forward shift of the body of 4 on 5 producing so-called degenerative spondylolisthesis (Fig. 13/7). This forward shift causes marked reduction of the spinal canal with compression of the dura mater and the nerve roots. It produces

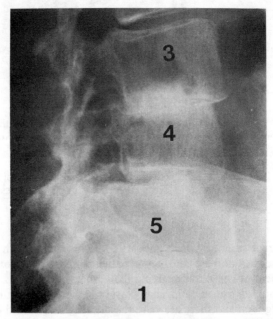

Fig. 13/7   Lateral radiograph to show degenerative spondylolisthesis at two levels in a 76-year-old female

an intractable back and leg pain which may require decompressive laminectomy to relieve the symptoms.

Another degenerative lesion which is being seen more commonly with an ageing population is associated with marked osteoarthritis of the facet joints producing large osteophytes which encroach on the space normally reserved for the spinal cord and nerve roots. In the cervical spine, osteophytes may encroach on the spinal canal and produce cord compression. In the lumbar spine these pathological changes produce 'spinal stenosis', which, if the symptoms of leg pain with walking become severe, will require decompressive laminectomy.

TABLE 1   SURGICAL PRINCIPLES

Cause	Principles of surgery
Compressed nerve root	Decompression (laminotomy)
Motion segment instability (trauma, disc degeneration, etc)	Stabilise the segment (fusion)
Deformity or displacement of the motion segment	Reduction of the deformity and stabilise (fuse)
Discogenic lesion	Remove the disc and stabilise the segment
Facet joint arthritis	Stabilise the segment to eliminate motion which causes the pain
Torn annulus fibrosus	Rest to encourage healing. If this fails, fusion required (segmental motion produces pain)
Spinal stenosis	Laminectomy
Infected vertebral body, e.g. TB spine	(a) Chemotherapy (b) Excision of the infected tissue (anterior approach); replace defect with bone graft
Tumour	Remove the tumour (perhaps two-staged procedure) stabilise with bone graft and metallic implants (irradiate if necessary)

THE PRINCIPLES OF SURGERY IN SPINAL DISORDERS

1. Surgery should only be embarked upon when conservative treatment has failed.

2. Surgery should only be undertaken after detailed preliminary investigations to define the precise pathological entity.
3. A brief summary of the surgical principles involved is shown in Table 1.

Case examples

1. A 76-year-old lady complained of severe pain in the back and both legs. Radiographs confirmed she had degenerative spondylolisthesis at lumbar 3–4 and lumbar 4–5 levels. Continuing pain made her virtually housebound. A decompressive laminectomy at both levels was performed, resulting in significant relief of back and leg pain (Fig. 13/7). It should be noted that this type of degenerative spondylolisthesis is most common at the lumbar 4–5, and two-level disease is quite unusual.

2. A 30-year-old female developed pain in her back and right thigh during pregnancy. Following delivery of her child, the pain continued and in fact became worse following a lifting injury several years later. There was clinical evidence of a lumbo-sacral joint lesion. Lateral radiograph demonstrated diminished height at the lumbo-sacral joint (Fig. 13/8).

It was confirmed by discography that the anatomical pain source originated in the lumbo-sacral disc. Because of continuing disablement and immobility an anterior lumbo-sacral fusion was done with removal of the disc and its replacement with bone graft from the left iliac crest. The patient's pain was relieved and she was able to carry out her normal household and social activities. A radiograph 12 months after surgery confirmed consolidation of the bone graft (Fig. 13/9).

RATIONALE OF STABILISATION

There are numerous techniques of fusion, for example, posterior facet joint fusion, fusion of the transverse processes, interbody fusion. What is surprising is that fusion in deformity and infection has a high success rate but in low back pain it remains a controversial issue. It is

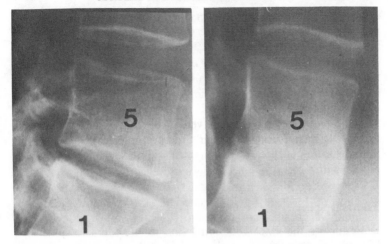

Fig. 13/8 Lateral radiograph of the lumbo-sacral joint which was identified as the level producing disabling back pain (see case report 2). *Note* the narrowing of the lumbo-sacral disc space

Fig. 13/9 Lateral radiograph demonstrating satisfactory healing of the bone graft following anterior lumbo-sacral fusion

not surprising that there are numerous techniques (over 20) for fusion in treatment of low back disorders.

The key factors are determining the exact pathological lesion and the precise motion segment which is causing the disability.

One of the greatest problems in clinical medicine is the failed back surgery patient. The commonest causes of failure are surgery at the wrong level and damage to nerve roots at the time of posterior exploration.

Cervical spine

The two commonest lesions requiring surgery in the cervical spine are: (1) disc disruption and (2) cervical spondylosis.

The point of practical significance is that cervical spinal lesions can produce pain radiating to the head, eye (visual disturbance), chest, shoulder, entire upper limb, fingers, thus being mistaken for migraine, coronary artery disease, frozen shoulder, etc.

The most common surgical procedures are:

Anterior cervical fusion: This involves disc excision and replacement with bone graft from the iliac crest. Postoperative immobilisation involves a soft collar until the bone grafts are healed clinically and radiologically

Less common is cervical spondylytic myelopathy (CSM) which produces local symptoms of pain as well as long tract signs (gait disturbance, etc) because of pressure by posterior osteophytes on the motor regions of the spinal cord.

The osteophytes may be removed at the time of anterior cervical fusion but many surgeons prefer to leave the osteophytes because immobilisation of them by fusion itself will cause the osteophytes to regress with time.

Thoracic spine

Deformity is the most common lesion in the thoracic spine (see Chapter 15). Pain from thoracic disc lesions does occur but it is quite infrequent and will often produce compression of the spinal cord. Accurate diagnosis is essential. Laminectomy for the treatment of the thoracic disc lesion has a very high incidence of paraplegia. The surgical treatment of a thoracic disc lesion is through an anterior approach, removal of the disc and stabilisation of the motion segment with a bone graft from the adjacent iliac crest.

REFERENCES

Fairbank, J.C.T., Couper, J., Davies, J.B. and O'Brien, J.P. (1980). The Oswestry low back pain disability questionnaire. *Physiotherapy*, **66**, 271–3.
Kellgren, J.H. (1939). On the distribution of pain arising from deep somatic structures with charts of segmental pain areas. *Clinical Science*, **4**, 35–46.

BIBLIOGRAPHY

Rothman, R.H. and Simeone, F.A. (1972). *The Spine*, 2nd edition, Vols 1 and 2. W.B. Saunders Co Ltd, Eastbourne.

Chapter 14

Surgery for Spinal Disorders – 2. Physiotherapy

by E. GOSS, MCSP

The types of patient found in an orthopaedic spinal disorders unit are varied. Many will have had previous surgery, for example a laminectomy, or perhaps a laminectomy followed by an exploration, and still be in their teens. Approximately two-thirds of patients will have low back pain and one-third some degree of spinal deformity.

The causes of back pain may be (1) congenital, e.g. hemivertebra producing a kyphotic deformity, or spina bifida producing a scoliosis deformity associated with low back pain; (2) acquired, e.g. infective tuberculosis or poliomyelitis producing both low back pain and deformity, or as a result of heavy work producing degenerative changes resulting in low back pain; and (3) due to trauma, e.g. fracture of the spine, or spondylolisthesis. The lumbar, thoracic and cervical spine may be affected individually or as a whole.

Physiotherapy aims to prevent postoperative complications and to help the patient regain independence and safe gross motor function, including transfers from bed to standing and to toilet, and gait training. Advice in back care and safe lifting is also important.

The philosophy underlying the physiotherapist's role is basically:
1. To reassure the patient.
2. To give the patient a general understanding of his back problem.
3. To give the patient confidence in himself and enable him to manage his back problem.
4. To give the patient and his family any advice which will enable them together to reduce the overall effect that the condition may have on lifestyle, including marriage, family and work.

McNab (1979) wrote '. . . Treat a patient – not a spine. Find out about the patient who has backache as well as finding out as much as you can about the back pain that the patient has.'

ASSESSMENT

A full assessment should always be carried out on every new patient, even though it may take up a lot of the physiotherapist's time. The past history, as accurate as possible, of the patient's back pain is very relevant. A thorough examination of posture, gait, pain patterns, disability, range of movement, neurology and muscle power should all be recorded. The height and weight are also important.

Pain patterns can either be recorded on a form (see Fig. 9/1, p. 192) or be photographed. Photography will also show the back contours, for example sway back or round shoulders, and will be useful for comparison – pre- and post-operation – of antero-posterior and lateral views. A scoliosis series – pictures to show the curve in all dimensions – will show the deformity and any pain.

If the photographic method of recording pain is to be used, the physiotherapist should start her palpation for pain and/or tenderness from the cervical spine and work distally. She should mark the pain patterns on the skin using mercurochrome for red and gentian violet for blue; bony, muscle trigger points or nerve pressure points are marked in red. The patient is then asked to indicate the pattern of referred pain which is marked in blue. The patient will usually outline the painful area quite accurately; if he cannot it may be easier to note where the finger passes over the skin and the patient asked to state if and when the sensation changes. Areas of sensitivity can then be marked as indicated above. This change in sensation will be a dermatome-type representation of the painful area referred from the 'red' tender spots already drawn. Figures 14/1 and 14/2 show pain patterns from cervical and lumbar lesions respectively.

Disability forms which are filled in by the patient can give good insight into his problems (Fairbank et al, 1980).

Range of movement is relevant depending on the painful episodes experienced by the patient. One method of measuring this is to palpate the posterior superior iliac spines, i.e. the dimples; mark this line, and extend it laterally to the left and right hip respectively. Place the tape measure with the 10cm mark on the line and your thumb on the 15cm mark; as the patient bends backwards the measurement will be between the 15 and 10cm mark. Side-flexion is measured in the same way using the lateral marks; the tape held on the right side as the patient bends towards the left, measures left side-flexion and is then repeated for the other side. This way of measuring is a modification of the Schober method (Schober, 1937).

Muscle power should be tested using the Medical Research Council

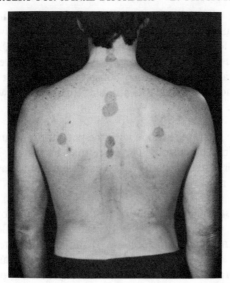

Fig. 14/1 Pain pattern from a cervical lesion

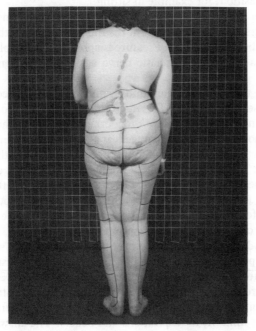

Fig. 14/2 Pain pattern from a lumbar lesion

(MRC) scale of grading muscle power (Oxford scale) to define associated limb weakness. If the patient has been bedbound or disabled for a long time disuse atrophy is quite common. A myometer reading of muscle groups is interesting to have but not essential.

Neurological examination may consist of testing reflexes, sensory changes, femoral and sciatic stretches, positive bowstring, and Babinski test.

Femoral nerve stretching is done with the patient prone and lifting the affected leg into extension. The knee may be flexed. If there is a positive femoral stretch pain will be experienced indicating femoral nerve irritation.

Sciatic nerve stretching is done in the supine position by lifting the affected leg with the knee fully extended into flexion, then dorsiflexing the ankle and forefoot. If the hip flexes to 90 degrees pain-free it is a negative straight leg raise. A crossed straight leg raise may also be present – when the unaffected leg is raised, pain is felt on the affected side of the back. If there is any doubt about the reaction of the patient to straight leg raising, testing should also be done in a different position, for example in sitting.

To test for a positive bowstring, the patient is in supine lying with the affected leg flexed to 90 degrees at the hip and the knee; the ankle is supported by the examiner. Pressure is applied to the popliteal fossa and pain is felt over the sciatic nerve again indicating nerve root irritation.

Anterior tenderness of the lumbar spine can be palpated and will indicate disc inflammation. This may be quite acute and produce back and leg pain. To test for anterior tenderness the patient should be in relaxed crook lying. Place the fingers at a perpendicular angle 2.5cm (1in) below the umbilicus and apply pressure gently to the lumbar spine. This will be approximately the lumbar 5 – sacral 1 area. Pain may be experienced slightly higher or to the left or right of the lumbar spine. If the patient is not relaxed, ask him to breathe out deeply. While performing this examination watch for a full bladder or tenderness due to abdominal symptoms or scars.

The social worker will interview the patient to prepare a social and, perhaps, a psychological report. The Minnesota Multiphasic Personality Inventory (MMPI) consists of hundreds of questions (399), some of which are repeated but asked in a different way, relating to the patient's home and upbringing, his relation to parents and friends, the way he sees himself, his aspirations and beliefs. The answers to the questions are tabulated on a special form and a graph drawn. The 10 sections assessed relate to hypochondriasis, depression, hysteria, psychopathic deviation, masculinity/femininity, paranoia, psychosthenia, schizophrenia, hypomania and social introversion. The social worker will report on the patient and advise as to the probable response to proposed surgery or further surgery and the general conditions relating to his/her back pain.

The ward nursing staff can provide valuable help in the assessment of the patient's disability. The following will be noted on the ward: walking time, sitting time, bed-rest positions, posture and pelvic tilt, exercise tolerance, pain tolerance and what tablets are needed during the day and at night, and the amount of sleep that the patient requires. A general opinion can be given as to the relationship between patient and staff, as well as patient to patient.

After the initial assessment of his pain and disability the patient may be put through a physiotherapy programme to see what improvement can be gained. Hydrotherapy is one of the easiest and most enjoyable forms of treatment; patients become more relaxed and confident, and exercise is easier due to the buoyancy, warmth and good feeling of the water.

Pre-operative physiotherapy

The aim of physiotherapy is to ensure that the patient is as fit as possible. This includes improving the chest expansion and vital capacity (which should be recorded in the notes), muscle power and general tone, circulation and endurance.

An explanation of the operation will be given by the doctor, and the physiotherapist will teach the necessary breathing and leg exercises to be done immediately postoperatively.

Following surgery, and once the patient is fully awake, chest expansion and foot and ankle movement are checked.

The postoperative management will differ according to the type of surgery.

GENERAL AIMS OF POSTOPERATIVE PHYSIOTHERAPY

The general aims of treatment are:
1. To keep the chest clear and expanding fully.
2. Maintenance of muscular power of the upper and lower limbs (but not pushing hip flexion if the patient has had a spinal fusion).
3. Relief of pressure.

4. Orientation, i.e. preparing for change of position from lying to sitting to standing by elevating the head end of the bed.

Preparation of the patient for getting out of bed includes strengthening exercises for the arms if crutches or sticks are to be required. A corset may be recommended and will be fitted by the physiotherapist who will ensure that the 'bones' are bent to the patient's lumbar spine. To put the corset on in bed the patient may bridge or roll.

There are two methods used for getting the patient out of bed:

1. The patient is turned into a prone position and gets out of bed feet first, with the hips supported on the bed. He keeps a straight back and comes upright using his hip and back extensor muscles with arm support. The bed height is important with this method.

2. The patient is turned on to the pain-free side; he slides his legs over the side of the bed and comes to sitting pushing up with both arms while the legs go down with gravity. The arms are then supporting the back in the sitting position. The patient moves forward, perching on the bed with his feet firmly on the floor. This method helps to overcome initial dizziness while the patient is still supported.

On the first time out of bed, re-education of balance with weight transference using arm support should be practised. If the patient is not dizzy a short walk helps regain confidence. The patient then progresses until he is independent with the help of one stick out of doors if necessary. Sutures are removed about 10–14 days post-surgery, when the patient is discharged either in a jacket, spica, corset or with no support. The orthotist may be asked to fit a corset or jacket to suit the particular patient's requirements.

Depending on the type of operation, the immobilisation period and the following mobilising will vary. The end goal is a return to work *and* relief of pain. Building-up of confidence and reassurance is essential to achieve independence for the patient.

Patients should be advised on activities of daily living by the occupational therapist and the physiotherapist. Each patient is given a progressive exercise programme which will include mostly isometric and relaxation exercises. A general advice form may be given. A follow-up appointment will be given to each patient at which time the spinal support, i.e. jacket or spica, may be removed and a mobilising programme started. Follow-up treatment will depend upon the surgeon's wishes.

SPECIFIC PHYSIOTHERAPY

One-level anterior spinal fusion

PRE-OPERATIVE

Before a spinal fusion the height, weight and vital capacity of the patient is recorded. He should be taught breathing exercises, general maintenance exercises for his arms, legs and trunk muscles and how to get out of bed following surgery (see p. 266).

POSTOPERATIVE

Day 1–3: Breathing exercises and general maintenance exercises. Do not flex the legs beyond 90 degrees.

Day 3–5: The patient is allowed up with an elasticated corset, plus walking aids, i.e. crutches or sticks, if necessary. This will be determined by muscle weakness of arms and legs, e.g. a patient with a leg affected by poliomyelitis may require a caliper on the affected leg and elbow crutches. (A good rule for the average patient without previous muscle weakness is to get up with two helpers supporting his arms on the first postoperative day, one helper and a stick the second day, then one stick and thus the patient is independent on the third.)

Day 5–10: Ambulation is gradually progressed with gait re-education, relaxation, posture correction and starting to use stairs.

Day 10–14: The sutures are removed and the patient is discharged in a support, either a jacket or a corset. The latter will be used if the back is stable and the patient has good muscle control, otherwise he may go home in a jacket or a spica made in whatever material is considered suitable.

The general aim is for the patient to be discharged without aids and be completely independent. He should be able to manage stairs, walk 100 yards and be able to sit comfortably for one hour. A stick may be given for use outdoors. If he goes home in a jacket it will be kept on for a minimum of three months and then changed to a corset. *Special* outpatient physiotherapy is *not* needed – only arm and leg strengthening exercises; *no* back exercises (other than isometric contractions). At the clinic follow-up, three months post-surgery, the patient will be advised to start swimming and do simple exercises depending on the consolidation of the fusion.

Two-level anterior spinal fusion

PRE-OPERATIVE

This will be the same as for the one-level fusion (see above).

POSTOPERATIVE

The patient is mobilised and allowed out of bed, wearing a corset, at approximately one week. The sutures are removed at 10–14 days; a plaster of Paris jacket is applied and worn for 3–6 months.

It should be noted that to immobilise the lumbo-sacral joint, the patient should be put into a single-hip spica. A jacket would be adequate for a lumbar 4–5 fusion, but a spica is required for a fusion at the level of lumbar 4 – sacral 1. If a spica is not advised for the latter (because the patient had abdominal distension or chest problems) then he would be discharged in an elasticated corset.

Posterior fusion with Harrington rods

PRE-OPERATIVE

This will be as previously described; in addition 'log rolling' is taught, as follows. The patient must *never* move the shoulders first and hips later thereby rotating the trunk. Head, shoulders, hips and legs flexed to a comfortable position, should turn all in one easy movement. The position of crook lying makes the movement easier. If log rolling is to be done with straight legs, then on rolling to the right the left ankle should be crossed over the right ankle to facilitate rolling without trunk rotation.

POSTOPERATIVE

General maintenance exercises are carried out in bed. If the back is stable, the patient may be (a) mobilised, when comfortable, in a corset or, (b) mobilised in a jacket after the sutures have been removed at 10–14 days. The jacket is worn for approximately six months.

If the patient is kept in bed for one to two weeks, it is useful to use a tilt table; this will help with circulation, chest expansion, head control and arm and leg movement using gravity. The patient may be transferred on to the tilt table either by lifting, via a sliding board, or by rolling from bed to tilt table.

Combined anterior and posterior spinal fusion with Harrington rods

POSTOPERATIVE

Week 1: The patient is nursed on a Stoke-Egerton turning-bed so that he log rolls only. Strong analgesics, e.g. papaveretum (Omnopon) or morphine, will be necessary for the first three days; they are given intramuscularly to facilitate movement and relaxation thereby reducing chest and urinary complications. The drugs will then be changed to mefenamic acid (Ponstan), or the same as he was taking pre-operatively, and gradually reduced. While the patient is being nursed in bed, urinals will be used for both men and women: bedpans are *never* used to prevent the back being strained; incontinence pads are used for bowel care.

Week 2: The patient can begin tilting and transfer into an ordinary hospital bed, such as the King's Fund type. He can be tilted for 10 minutes to start and progress to 30 minutes, which is the time needed for the patient to adjust to the vertical for the application of a plaster of Paris jacket.

Week 3: If the patient is stiff, or has had a long period of bed rest pre-operatively, hydrotherapy may be very beneficial. This would encourage free arm and leg movement and a more relaxed gait. Otherwise the patient tends to develop a stiff walk, which in turn leads to a stiff, painful thoracic and cervical spine with limitation of movement at the neck and the shoulders.

The patient is discharged in a single above-knee hip spica, plaster of Paris jacket or corset; if necessary, he will be supplied with aids through the occupational therapist. They may include dressing aids, e.g. a long shoehorn, aids for pulling up stockings or socks, or elasticated shoe laces; personal toilet aids such as a long back scrubber for reaching down to the feet; alterations in the house, e.g. grab rails in the toilet, raised toilet seats or the installation of showers. Provision of walking aids and wheelchairs may be arranged by different members of the team according to the procedure of the individual unit.

Anterior and posterior fusion two weeks apart

The immediate postoperative regime is as for the combined procedure (see above).

The patient remains on bed rest but carries out general maintenance therapy until a *week* after the second procedure. After that the tilt table is used; hydrotherapy may be advised especially as two operations may lead to a greater muscular weakness. A plaster of Paris support is applied prior to discharge and may be necessary for three to six months; if stable, a corset may be used.

With the above procedure the patient may become depressed due to the wait between operations; the stress and longer stay in hospital seems to slow down rehabilitation. The combined procedure appears to have quicker results in pain-free mobility when compared with the staged operations.

Laminectomy; discectomy

Once any infusion lines and drains have been removed the patient may be mobilised. A corset may be fitted if ordered by the surgeon. Strong isometric exercises and active back extension and abdominal exercises should be taught. Initially, sciatic stretch can be done in side lying and then in supine. The patient is discharged when the sutures have been removed and often continues as an outpatient.

If the laminectomy is done with Harrington rod fixation, i.e. for spinal stenosis, isometric exercises only are taught. The patient is then discharged in a jacket or corset.

If a nerve root decompression is done with a partial laminectomy, the patient is kept on bed rest for two weeks. He is then discharged either in a spica to rest the affected leg, or a spinal jacket or corset.

LIFTING AND BENDING

Correct lifting should be taught to all back patients during their time in hospital before and after surgery. Prior to surgery, patients will have managed at home perhaps making beds while kneeling or ironing for short periods seated. They will already have adapted to their activities of daily living. They would tend to leave lifting to other people in the household or move objects one by one instead. Low cupboards and high shelves have probably been avoided as much as possible.

After admission patients find they have a locker in which to put their possessions. Usually the largest space for clothes is at the bottom, so they must bend to get at slippers for everyday use. Correct lifting is taught by putting the strongest leg behind the other leg and bending the knees as if genuflecting. The back remains straight. The knee of the back leg then rests on the floor so that the position is stable. The patient is then safe to use his arms.

When lifting an object off the ground, the weight should be clasped tight to the chest. The stronger back leg then pushes up while the front leg controls the movement, the back remaining straight. If the legs are together, then bending down and rising is unstable and the patient is likely to wobble. If the object being lifted is an awkward shape or heavy, it should be lifted in stages. First from the floor to a table or chair placed directly in front of the object, and then carried away. Do not turn or twist while lifting.

Therefore, to bend the knees and keep the back straight is the ideal way to lift, but not all people have strong quadriceps or pain-free knees. In some cases, it may be easier to bend forwards from the hips on the stronger leg and counterbalance with the other leg extended. This is the way a patient in a single-hip spica would have to bend. If the arms are free they can be used for support.

When lifting light objects such as clothing, it is much easier to use a 'helping-hand' aid with perhaps just a slight bend of the knees. Most of these aids have a magnet on them so are useful for moving things like pins and other objects out of the way.

COMPLICATIONS FOLLOWING SPINAL SURGERY

Complications that may follow surgery include deep vein thrombosis, pulmonary embolus, paralytic ileus (this is most likely to occur immediately postoperatively when an abdominal approach has been used), associated stiffness of the thoracic spine, neck and shoulders, wound infection, neuralgia and graft site pain. If a plaster of Paris support is worn then particular care must be taken of the skin.

FITTING CORSETS, PLASTER JACKETS AND HIP SPICAS

Corsets

Corsets are used for supporting the abdominal and back muscles in patients with low back pain, e.g. the overweight patient with poor abdominal musculature; a patient who has been recumbent and is to be mobilised; or a person whose work demands lifting and where the extra support of a corset would be beneficial. They may also provide the support needed following some spinal surgery (Fig. 14/3).

Corsets can be obtained 'ready-made' either by hip or waist measurement. They vary in type of material, depth, amount of support, e.g. bones or metal struts, and types of fastening. A corset which is mostly made of elasticated fabric can be pulled tight and thus give a very firm support. Some suppliers make male and female corsets which vary in hip measurement and so give a better fit. If the patient is not suitable for a ready-made corset, he will require one made to measure. This may be for coccygeal pain when the corset needs extending to the gluteal fold; or after thoracic surgery when the corset should be extended to the shoulders with shoulder straps.

The measurements required to make a corset are: waist; hips at the widest region; xiphisternal notch to groin anteriorly; and the lower border of the scapula to mid-buttock posteriorly with arms by the

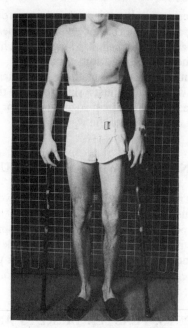

Fig. 14/3   A well-fitting corset

side. The metal struts used in the corset should be exactly moulded to the contours of the patient and inserted. After a spinal fusion the back contour will very likely alter and should be checked if the corset was fitted prior to surgery. After spinal surgery, especially with posterior instrumentation, the lumbar curve flattens and so lengthens the spine; there is a similar effect on the thoracic curve. Some corsets have pads inserted for extra lumbar support and warmth.

Applying a spinal jacket (plaster of Paris or other material)

Jackets may be applied for patients with low back pain and/or following surgery. For a patient with stability of the spine postoperatively, the jacket can be applied with the patient standing; if necessary traction may be given by application of a head-halter apparatus. This ensures a comfortable jacket with good correction.

If the spine is unstable in standing or following Harrington rod instrumentation for scoliosis, the patient must have a jacket applied before weight-bearing. It is then applied with the patient supported, in lying, on a special frame such as the Abbot frame.

A three-point pressure for a plaster of Paris or other material jacket, is required: anteriorly at the sternum or below the nipple curve; at the symphysis pubis; and posteriorly in the lumbar area. The plaster should be trimmed so that there is no pressure while sitting, arm movement is full and the patient independent for toilet purposes. Skin care is very important; cream and powders soften the skin and should not be used, instead surgical spirit or soap and water should be used to clean and toughen the skin.

CARE OF THE PLASTER

Depending on the material used, the plaster may be waterproof or not. Plaster of Paris is still the most useful because it conforms to the body shape, but it is not waterproof. Elasticated plaster of Paris (Orthoflex) used with Soroc is very durable and gives a good tight fit. Hexalite, Baycast and Scotch cast are other materials used; they are not so easy to mould or apply, but they are waterproof.

Other orthoses may be used and/or adapted for the following conditions:

The Boston brace is made of polythene for patients with scoliosis or low back pain. It is more convenient as the brace may be removed for toilet purposes and is made to measure from a plaster of Paris cast (Fig. 14/4).

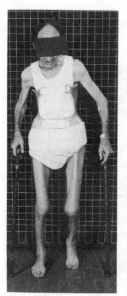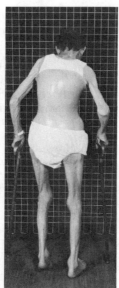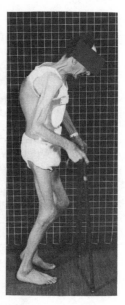

Fig. 14/4 An adapted Boston brace: anterior, posterior and lateral views

The Jewitt brace is made of metal alloy and leather and is used for thoracic support perhaps following surgery to stabilise the thoracic spine after removal of an hemivertebra.

The Milwaukee brace is also made of metal alloy and leather and is used to support scoliosis patients with a curve suitable for splinting (see Fig. 15/12, p. 286).

Braces may be specially lined with sheepskin as an extra safeguard if the skin is sensitive as with a spina bifida patient who has undergone posterior spinal surgery.

REFERENCES

Fairbank, J.C.T., Couper, J., Davies, J.B. and O'Brien, J.P. (1980). The Oswestry low back pain disability questionnaire. *Physiotherapy*, **66**, 271–3.
MacNab, I. (1979) *Backache*. Williams and Wilkins Co, Baltimore.
Schober, P. (1937). Lendenwirbelsäule und Kreuzschemeren. (The lumbar vertebral column and backache.) *Müenchener Medizinische Wochenschrift*, **84**, 336.

BIBLIOGRAPHY

Cailliet, R. (1981). *Low Back Pain Syndrome*, 3rd edition. F.A. Davis Co, Philadelphia.
Keim, H.A. and Kirkaly-Willis, W.H. (1980). *Clinical Symposia*, **32**, 6.
MacNab, I. (1979). *Backache*. Williams and Wilkins Co, Baltimore.
Maurice-Williams, R.S. (1981). *Spinal Degenerative Disease*. John Wright and Sons Limited, Bristol.
Moll, J. and Wright, V. (1980). *Measurement of Spine Movement*. In *The Lumbar Spine and Back Pain*, 2nd edition (Jayson, M.(ed)). Pitman Books Ltd, London.
White, A.A. and Panjabi, M.M. (1978). *Clinical Biomechanics of the Spine*. J.B. Lippincott Co, Philadelphia.

Chapter 15

Spinal Deformities

by J.P. O'BRIEN, MB, BS, PhD, FRCS(Ed), FACS
and V. DRAYCOTT, MCSP, ONC

SCOLIOSIS

Scoliosis comes from the Greek meaning 'a curvature of the spine'. It is now used specifically for lateral spinal curvatures in excess of 10 degrees. The pathological description is clear: scoliosis is seen as deformed vertebrae when the vertebral body shifts towards the convexity of the curve and the spinous processes deviate to the concave side (Fig. 15/1). If the deformity involves the thoracic spine, the result is a diminution in the entire volume of the thoracic cage leading ultimately to respiratory impairment. The spinal deformity will be reflected in distortion of the spinal canal itself which may be responsible for spinal cord compression, particularly in congenital curvatures.

Scoliotic deformities are classified according to their magnitude, direction, location and aetiology. Ninety per cent of scoliosis is so-called 'idiopathic'; treatment thus remains empirical and speculative. There are, however, two general points: (1) Usually the younger the patient at the onset of the curvature, the worse the prognosis for the deformity; and (2) Curves which are rapidly deteriorating and/or are painful usually need surgical treatment.

SCHOOL SCREENING

Prevention is better than cure and the recently popular school-screening programmes, which were initiated in North America more than 20 years ago, usually involve the survey of normal schoolchildren between the ages of 10–14 years. This is the most vulnerable age period for scoliosis precipitated by the growth spurt.

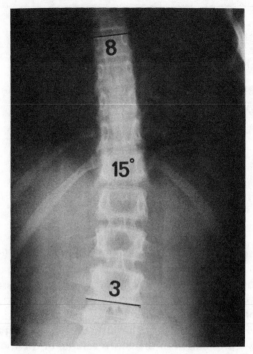

Fig. 15/1   Radiograph demonstrating typical slight idiopathic scoliosis

The first school-screening programme in the United Kingdom was initiated in Oswestry in 1976 and the overall results compared exactly with those in North America. Normal schoolchildren between the ages of 10–14 are submitted to the forward-bending test (Fig. 15/2). A positive incidence of approximately 3 per cent is observed. The school-screening programme is carried out in schools by the visiting community nurses or physical education teachers, who are trained to assess asymmetry of the spine and trunk with the child bending forward.

Those with a so-called positive 'forward-bending test' are asked to attend the appropriate spinal clinic at the hospital for further examination and possible radiograph of the spine. This school-screening programme is carried out annually and children are followed up until the end of the growth spurt. School screening has been largely responsible for the earlier detection of adolescent idiopathic scoliosis leading to a large number of children being treated by brace therapy and fewer requiring spinal surgery.

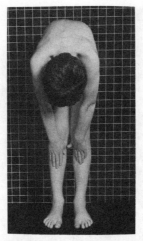

Fig. 15/2 The forward-bending test. This picture shows a 'positive' result. *Note* the asymmetry across the shoulders, and the uneven rib hump

Team-work

Often an appointment to attend a spinal clinic is a traumatic event in a family and considerate management of the family and child by all members of the assessment team can affect the whole co-operative framework vital to successful treatment. Most families are uninformed about scoliosis and need reassurance, education and full explanation of all the steps in the initial conservative treatment. Many spinal centres have tried to overcome the parents' doubts and difficulties by the provision of a brochure which provides simple explanations and helps to reassure parents and child.

THE CURVE IN SCOLIOSIS

Types

There are three main types of scoliotic curve which account for most cases of scoliosis:

    idiopathic
    paralytic
    congenital.

However, there are numerous lesser known causes of scoliosis, the most common of which is neurofibromatosis and others, for example, such as metabolic bone disease, osteogenesis imperfecta, etc.

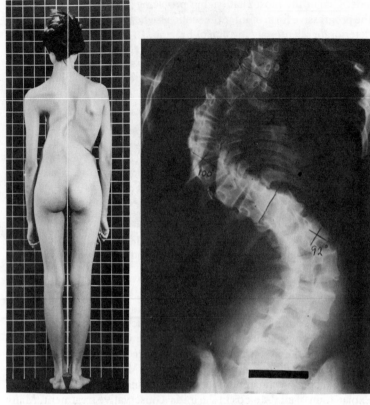

Fig. 15/3 Patient with idiopathic scoliosis

Fig. 15/4 Radiograph demonstrating an idiopathic double scoliosis

Idiopathic scoliosis (Figs. 15/3, 15/4)

This is the largest group of scoliosis and, as the name implies, there is no obvious reason for the appearance of the curvature. The sub-groups of idiopathic scoliosis are classified according to the age of onset of the curvature:

INFANTILE (ONSET BETWEEN BIRTH AND 3 YEARS)
This is common in the UK but rare in North America. In 85 per cent of these infants there is spontaneous resolution of the curve without treatment. The majority are male and the curve is convex to the left

side. One of the most challenging problems in scoliosis treatment is the progressive form of infantile scoliosis where the curve continues to deteriorate relentlessly in spite of bracing. In many of these patients, early surgery is required to prevent inevitable deterioration.

JUVENILE (AGE OF ONSET BETWEEN 3 AND 10 YEARS)

As a group they have a poor prognosis because they have had a longer period of growth and development in which to deform and deteriorate (spinal deformity tends to deteriorate maximally during the growth spurt).

The management of these patients, if the curvature is advanced enough, will usually be bracing in the hope of delaying fusion should it be required. Fusion of the spine at an early age does eliminate growth over the fused segments and will result in a shortened stature at maturity; nonetheless, it is sometimes essential to proceed with fusion to prevent severe deformity.

There is currently an encouraging surgical development in the form of subcutaneous rodding of these immature curves *without* simultaneous fusion. This requires occasional lengthening of the rods so that the spine is kept straight and vertebral growth is allowed to continue with the child held in a well-fitting brace. Although it has only been in practice for several years, the results are promising for such a difficult problem.

ADOLESCENT (AGE OF ONSET 10 TO 20 YEARS)

With increased effective school-screening programmes there is earlier detection of scoliosis in this age-group resulting in a larger number of them being treated by bracing and fewer requiring surgery.

ADULT (AGE OF ONSET OVER 20 YEARS)

Scoliosis may occur as a result of disc degeneration in the older age-group. Mild scoliosis, if already present, is said to deteriorate at the rate of about 1 degree per year. An acute deterioration (6–7 degrees in a year) is occasionally seen associated with pregnancy.

Adult patients often have several other problems not seen in the younger age-groups. Severe pain in lumbar scoliosis may be the reason for which the patient seeks medical attention. Scoliosis in the adult is associated with an increased incidence of respiratory impairment and a higher rate of complications if surgery is required.

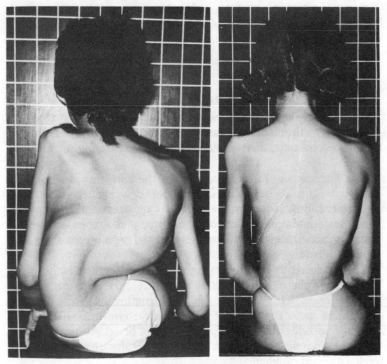

Fig. 15/5 (*Left*)   Pre-operative picture of a girl with paralytic scoliosis. *Note* the severity of the curve and the high degree of pelvic obliquity

Fig. 15/6 (*Right*)   Postoperative picture of a girl with paralytic scoliosis. This dramatic correction was achieved by combined posterior and anterior surgery with instrumentation and fusion

Paralytic scoliosis (Figs. 15/5, 15/6)

The three commonest causes of paralytic scoliosis are:
    poliomyelitis
    cerebral palsy
    spina bifida.

Post-poliomyelitis scoliosis. The vaccines of Salk and Sabin have dramatically reduced this disease, although it is still very common in many parts of the Third World. Twenty-five per cent of children affected with paralytic poliomyelitis will develop scoliosis, which is a serious problem as it is inevitably progressive (muscle imbalance) and it has the associated problems of pelvic obliquity, limb paralysis, severe deformity and respiratory impairment.

Cerebral palsy has a commonly associated scoliosis due to the muscle imbalance, and surgery should be considered if it will improve the child's level of function.

Spina bifida scoliosis is common. The curvature is complicated by the associated anaesthetic skin below the neurological deficit and in some cases with a paralytic bowel and bladder.

Congenital scoliosis (Fig. 15/7)

Most congenital curvatures are apparent and visible at birth. Some milder congenital anomalies, however, may not appear until much later, usually at the time of the adolescent growth spurt. There is a high incidence of associated genito-urinary abnormality and lesions

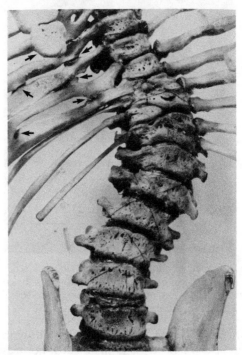

Fig. 15/7 Specimen showing congenital scoliosis. *Note* the multiple anomalies of spine and ribs (arrows)

within the spinal canal such as fibrous bands, diastematomyelia, etc. The use of a brace in these curves is ineffective and if progression of the curve has been demonstrated surgery will be required.

The curve

1. The extent of the curve is recorded in degrees and measured by the Cobb method (Fig. 15/8). It is commonly regarded as significant if it measures over 10 degrees and most surgeons nowadays regard all curves measuring over 60 degrees as an absolute indication for surgery. Complications with respiratory impairment are usually apparent with thoracic curves over 60 degrees.

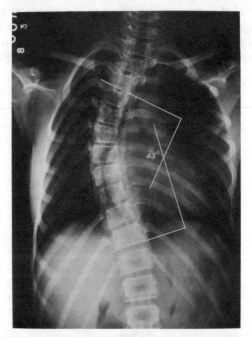

Fig. 15/8 Cobb method of measuring the angle of scoliosis. The end vertebrae of the curve are the last ones tilting towards the concavity of the curve. The angle is measured at the intersection of two straight lines drawn across the end vertebrae

2. Curvature can be convex to the left or right side or in the case of a double curve it will be left- and right-sided. For reasons not fully apparent 90 per cent of adolescent curves are convex to the right side and are most commonly seen in females.

3. Scoliotic curves are named from the apex of the curvature namely:
   Cervical scoliosis apex between C1 and C6
   Cervico-thoracic scoliosis, apex at the cervico-thoracic junction
   Thoracic scoliosis, apex between thoracic 2 and thoracic 11 levels
   Thoraco-lumbar scoliosis, apex at the thoraco-lumbar junction
   Lumbar scoliosis, apex between lumbar 2 and lumbar 4 levels
   Lumbo-sacral scoliosis, apex at the lumbo-sacral joint.
A curve may thus be described as 'idiopathic, right-sided thoraco-lumbar scoliosis measuring 60 degrees'.

CURVE PROGRESSION AND THE ILIAC APOPHYSIS
Scoliosis deteriorates most rapidly during the period of spinal growth. The cessation of spinal growth coincides with completion of growth in the iliac apophysis (Fig. 15/9). It usually takes about one year between the time the iliac apophysis appears at the front of the iliac crest on the radiograph until the time it completes its growth in the posterior part of the iliac crest. This is known as *Risser's sign* and the various stages of appearance of the apophysis are known as Risser 1, 2, 3, etc, indicating the stage of spinal immaturity. Risser '5' indicates complete fusion of the iliac apophysis and this coincides with the completion of spinal growth which usually indicates the end of significant rapid deterioration in the deformity.

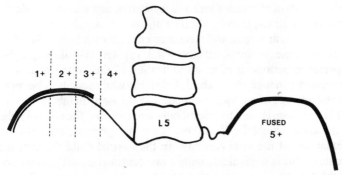

Fig. 15/9   Risser method of assessing maturity of the spine

CLINICAL MANAGEMENT – CONSERVATIVE

The assessment of the patient with scoliosis will include a detailed case history with physical examination, appropriate radiological examination of the spine and myelography when indicated (all cases with congenital scoliosis).

Observation

If the curve is mild (say less than 20 degrees) then a half-yearly clinical appointment for radiographs and clinical photographs will be adequate in the first instance.

Brace management

Brace management will be decided when the curve is of the appropriate aetiology and not severe enough to warrant surgery. Bracing may in some cases be used to hold the child's spine until he is at a more suitable age for surgery. When the curve is not suitable for bracing or when the brace is not tolerated by the patient, or, occasionally, when he refuses to wear the brace, then surgical correction and fusion will be required.

PHYSIOTHERAPY

Assessment

This consists of charting a series of measurements which include vital capacity, chest expansion, exercise tolerance, weight, total height, sitting height, arm span and measurement of the rib hump. When the thoracic spine is involved the vital capacity is of the utmost importance because it gives an indication of the impairment of the respiratory function of the child. Often the vital capacity is below the normal average of an equivalent child of the same height.

The *arm span* is used to give an indication of what the normal height of the child would be if scoliosis were not present, thus allowing comparison of the vital capacity. In the normal child the arm span measurement is equivalent, within one centimetre, to the total body height, thus the discrepancy between those measurements will give an indication of the approximate height lost in the curve.

The *rib hump* is measured by means of a gauge in a thoracic curve or, conversely, the depth of the valley in a low thoracic or lumbar curve (Fig. 15/10). The measurement is taken by placing the gauge over the child's back in a forward bending position and also in prone lying. The outline of the contour produced is then traced on to graph paper as a record (Fig. 15/11). It is interesting to note that the degree of truncal asymmetry is not specifically related to the lateral curvature of the

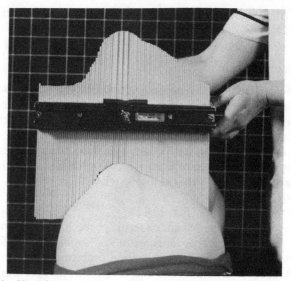

Fig. 15/10   Use of gauge in the measurement of rib hump. The illustration shows the measurement of the 'valley' in the lumbar region (ribs not involved in the curve)

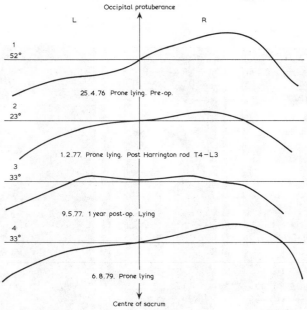

Fig. 15/11   Graphs showing the measurement in a right thoracic 5–12 scoliosis of the rib hump over three years

spine. All of these measurements are repeated at regular intervals and any marked change should be reported to the surgeon.

Treatment by bracing

The choice of treatment is dependent upon various factors such as the age, degree of curvature and the general condition of the child. Conservative treatment is usually instituted if the lateral curvature is less than 40 degrees, or in particularly young children in whom spinal fusion is to be deferred until a later age. This takes the form of the wearing of a Milwaukee or Boston brace depending upon the site of the curve, combined with specific exercises.

THE MILWAUKEE BRACE (Fig. 15/12)

Milwaukee brace care demands a team approach where the orthotist, physiotherapist, orthopaedic surgeon and social worker all see the patient to help solve social and medical problems as they arise. It is important to stress to the child and the parents that the wearing of a Milwaukee brace will not 'cure' the scoliosis but, combined with an active exercise programme, it will prevent, in most cases, deterioration of the curve.

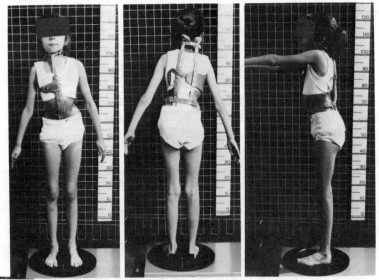

Fig. 15/12   The Milwaukee brace: anterior, posterior and lateral views

A negative cast is taken by the orthotist of the child's pelvis, together with appropriate measurement of the upright bars, occipital and throat pads. Once the brace is completed the child is fitted with it and appropriate exercises taught. The exercises are aimed at reducing the lumbar lordosis, so often seen in scoliosis, strengthening the abdominal muscles and increasing the vital capacity. These are printed as a hand-out and given to the child and the parents. A typical set of exercises used would be as follows:

MILWAUKEE BRACE EXERCISES

All exercises are to be done 10 times.

Exercises should be held for a count of five seconds.

Exercises should be done on a firm surface (floor) and done slowly.

1. Pelvic tilt, back lying with knees flexed.
   (a) Keep the shoulders flat on the floor and breathe regularly.
   (b) Tighten the buttocks.
   (c) Force the small of the back into the floor by tightening and pushing the abdominal muscles backwards (roll the points of the pelvis up towards your face).
   (d) Hold for five seconds, then relax.
2. Pelvic tilt, back lying with knees straight.
3. Sit-ups with pelvic tilt (out of brace).
   (a) With knees bent, feet on floor, tilt the pelvis and hold the tilt.
   (b) With elbows straight, or arms folded across chest, roll up and touch forehead to knees.
   (c) Unroll slowly down again.
   (d) Release the tilt and relax.
   Initially the feet may be stabilised.
   Progress to a partial sit-up without feet being held.
4. Modified bicycle exercises.
   (a) Tilt the pelvis and hold.
   (b) Do not raise the legs up over hips, but do bicycle movement with legs.
5. Pelvic tilt in the standing position.
   (a) Pinch a 10 pence piece between your buttocks. This will put you in a good pelvic tilt.
   (b) Now try to walk without letting the coin drop.
   (c) Keep shoulders back, head erect.
   Make this a good posture habit. Do several times.
6. Deep breathing exercises in back lying position (out of brace).
   (a) Divide the chest into three parts, upper, middle and lower.
   (b) Breathe in deeply, then breathe out completely in each part.

7. Back extension – lying on stomach (out of brace).

   (a) Place pillow under waist to prevent 'hollow' back.

   (b) Arms are down at sides, palms down.

   (c) With knees held down, tilt the pelvis and hold for the rest of the exercise.

   (d) Pinch shoulder blades together (keep palms down). Raise arms, shoulders and head about 4 inches (head in straight line – nose pointing to the floor – chin tucked in).

8. Push-ups with pelvic tilt.

9. Hip-flexor stretch (out of brace).

   (a) Lying on your back on firm surface – bed or table.

   (b) Hang one leg over edge – to the side.

   (c) Hug opposite leg to your chest. Pull with both arms to keep knee to chest.

10. Hamstring stretch.

   (a) Lie on your back on the floor with one leg through a doorway.

   (b) Opposite leg should be up on door jamb (to point of tightness).

   (c) With knee straight, push the 'up' leg down against the door jamb as hard as you can – as though you could move the whole wall. Hold for five seconds.

   (d) Relax leg, slide further forward through doorway, lifting the 'up' leg higher without bending the knee. This stretches the muscles behind thigh and knee.

11. Derotation: this should be performed many times throughout the day.

   (a) Gently hold front brace upright, elbows up at shoulder level and pointing forward.

   (b) Tilt pelvis and hold throughout exercise.

   (c) Inhale deeply, expanding backward against the posterior uprights with chest wall. 'Arch like a cat.' (The thoracic pad will press against the rib hump and help to derotate the spine. Also the thoracic valley should fill out.)

12. Active correction of the major curve – again performed many times during the day.

   (a) Standing, hands on hips, tilt the pelvis.

   (b) Shift away from the pad and hold for five seconds. (Avoid hollow-back, twisting your body or pulling shoulders forward.)

   (c) Use a full-length mirror to practise shifting and walking in a corrected position.

In some hospitals, the child is often admitted for a period of five days in order to attain perfect fitting of the brace and ensure proficiency in doing the exercises. The brace should be worn for 23 hours a day, being removed only for bathing. All normal physical activities are encouraged and, where possible, should be increased. Obviously body-contact sports should be avoided for the opponents' benefit! Every effort should be made by the members of the team to make the patient feel completely normal in the brace; fashionable clothing combined with the services of a proficient orthotist ensures that the brace is virtually unnoticeable. The patient should be seen at regular intervals when the brace is checked and re-adjusted as necessary. Radiographs are repeated at six-month intervals in and out of the brace in an erect position. Once skeletal maturity is almost complete, the patient is weaned gradually from the brace over a 12-month period. Eventually the brace is worn at night only, until the spine is absolutely mature and further curve progression arrested.

CLINICAL MANAGEMENT – SURGERY

Surgical procedures for scoliosis

INDICATIONS FOR SURGERY
    Cord compression
    Progression of the curve
    Pain
    Respiratory impairment
    Cosmetic

(a) *Cord compression* associated with spinal curvature is most commonly seen in kyphotic deformities (these will be discussed later). A compressed cord may be seen in severe congenital deformities. The cord must be surgically decompressed if lower limb function is to be preserved and this will sometimes require staged surgical procedures. Decompressing the cord is the first stage, followed several weeks later by correction of the deformity and fusion of the spine.

(b) *Progression of the curve* is most commonly seen in the adolescent growth spurt, and as a result of disc degeneration in the older patient. The curve will become biomechanically unstable and progression will continue.

(c) *Pain* is commonly seen in scoliosis, most frequently in the adult lumbar curve. It is essential in the investigation of these patients that the anatomical source of pain be identified before attempts at correcting the deformity are undertaken.

(d) *Respiratory impairment* is most common with thoracic scoliosis and paralytic deformities. Surgical correction and fusion of the spine in these patients is often done, not so much to improve the lung function as to prevent its further deterioration.

(e) There is invariably a *cosmetic* factor in all cases of scoliosis. The thoracic scoliosis with severe rotation and, therefore, a marked rib hump is the most deforming. Double curves and lumbar scoliosis are the least disfiguring.

THE USE OF PRELIMINARY TRACTION

There are two forms of spine traction: skeletal and non-skeletal, depending on whether pins are used in the skull and lower limbs or pelvis to achieve strong traction. It is important to remember that traction not only stretches and corrects the deformed spine but it also stretches the spinal cord and therefore when traction is used it must be monitored with regular neurological assessment.

The various forms of *spinal skeletal traction* include halo-femoral traction, halo-pelvic traction (Fig. 15/13), halo wheelchair traction; the latter because it is well tolerated by the patient is becoming increasingly popular. The non-skeletal traction system most common is that developed by Dr Yves Cotrel (see p. 296).

With halo-femoral traction, it is essential that the lower limb joints be put through a full range of joint motion each day, especially the hip joints, in order to prevent avascular necrosis. Strong forces being applied to the hip joints distract the joint, probably interfering with its blood supply and over a period of several weeks this is likely to produce avascular changes in the femoral head with resulting hip stiffness and significant disability.

Pre-operative skeletal traction should only be used when indicated because of the risks involved. In lesser degrees of deformity there is little to be gained with preliminary traction. A typical example of a case which would benefit with preliminary traction would be a paralytic scoliosis measuring 100 degrees associated with pelvic obliquity.

Methods of surgical fusion of the spine include:

POSTERIOR FUSION ONLY (Without correction) (Fig. 15/14)

This may be considered when correction of the curve is regarded as possibly dangerous, for example, some mild curves with diastematomyelia (a bony spur within the spinal canal). Most surgeons would prefer to fuse the spine and to use internal fixation, for example, a Harrington rod without gaining correction, but with the use of the rod as an internal splint to encourage healing of the bone grafts.

Fusion without internal fixation may be considered in the young

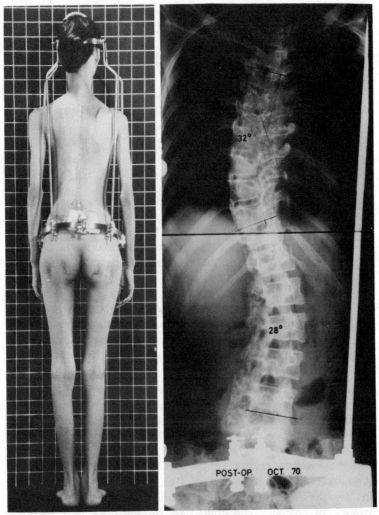

Fig. 15/13 (*Left*)   Patient in corrective halo-pelvic traction: nowadays only used for severe fixed spinal curves

Fig. 15/14 (*Right*)   Radiograph showing posterior fusion in the same patient, a 14-year-old female *cf* Figs. 15/3, 15/4

child under 7 or 8 years where the implants themselves are too large for the soft neural arches. In these cases, the surgeon may consider fusing the spine and then obtaining correction one to two weeks after surgery by a plaster technique using the traction table.

POSTERIOR INSTRUMENTATION AND FUSION OF THE SPINE

This is the most commonly accepted form of treatment for idiopathic scoliosis and the implant most commonly preferred is that designed by Harrington.

The principles of posterior fusion are as follows:

(a) A subperiosteal dissection to expose the entire length of the deformed spine.

(b) Insertion of hooks one or two levels above and below the spinal deformity.

(c) Removal of autogenous bone graft from the posterior aspect of one iliac crest.

(d) Removal of the facet joints over the length of the spine to be fused and the addition of the supplementary bone graft.

(e) The addition of the Harrington rod using safe, corrective forces.

(f) The function of the spinal cord can be checked by the so-called 'wake-up' test or by the increasingly popular spinal cord monitoring equipment.

(g) Application of a plaster of Paris jacket (using a traction table) until the spinal fusion is confirmed to be solid both by clinical and radiographic means. This usually means six to nine months in a plaster jacket, changing the jacket at about three months.

Other forms of posterior instrumentation have been designed, including a turnbuckle system which pre-dated Harrington's instrumentation, and was designed by the late Mr Frank Allan of Oswestry.

LUQUE INSTRUMENTATION

A new method gaining popularity is the Luque instrumentation which involves the use of two malleable rods and multiple wires affixing each lamina to the rods. The multi-level fixation does away with the necessity for postoperative plaster of Paris immobilisation; this has a very real benefit in patients with respiratory insufficiency such as those with muscular dystrophy.

COMBINED ANTERIOR AND POSTERIOR FUSION

For the more complex cases, such as paralytic scoliosis with pelvic obliquity, a combined anterior and posterior instrumentation is used; and sometimes if the curvature is severe preliminary halo-femoral traction may be used. The anterior correction and fusion is done, employing the screw and cable technique of Dwyer (Fig. 15/16) and this is supplemented two weeks later by an extensive posterior fusion with a Harrington rod. The Dwyer operation involves the radical removal of the intervertebral discs and this mobilises the curve significantly so that greater correction of the deformity is obtainable than by a posterior instrumentation alone. The combined Dwyer and Harrington rod technique is particularly successful when pelvic obliquity is associated with the deformity and this is commonly seen in paralytic scoliosis (Figs. 15/15, 15/16).

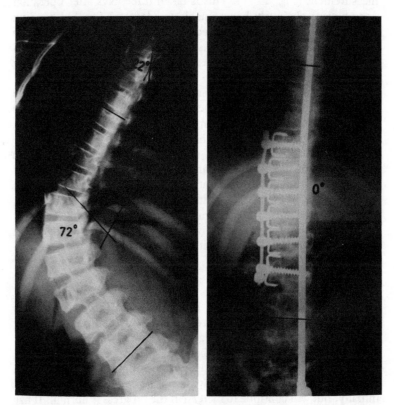

Fig. 15/15 (*Left*)   Radiograph showing pre-operative paralytic scoliosis in a 12-year-old male

Fig. 15/16 (*Right*)   Radiograph of same patient as 15/15 showing correction of the paralytic scoliosis by combined anterior and posterior instrumentation and fusion using a Harrington rod and the Dwyer screw and cable instrumentation

PHYSIOTHERAPY

In children where the prognosis of the curve is poor, surgical intervention is necessary (see p. 289).

PRE-OPERATIVE CARE

Pre-operatively the routine assessment, as described earlier, should be repeated and recorded. It is in the surgical cases that the measurement of the rib hump in prone lying is most relevant as a comparative measurement (Fig. 15/11). This is taken three days after operation – the patient obviously being unable to adopt the forward-bending position. Pre-operative localised breathing exercises should be taught, and in the more severe cases the patient should be introduced to, and taught how to use, the intermittent positive pressure breathing (IPPB) apparatus.

A full neurological assessment should be made prior to the operation in order to have a baseline postoperatively. Cord damage may occur during the operation, most certainly as a result of ischaemia from excessive stretching on the vessels during distraction. The patient should be taught foot and ankle movements and static contractions of the quadriceps and gluteal muscles as these should gently be encouraged postoperatively. Team-work is vital in such cases as the onset of any change in neurology may be insidious and it may well be the nurse who is bathing the child or making the bed who becomes aware of the change. Any such change should be reported at once, no matter how insignificant it may seem.

POSTOPERATIVE CARE

Postoperatively any respiratory problems which may arise in the simple posterior fusion cases are largely due to respiration being inhibited by pain. Sufficient analgesics combined with frequent visits from the physiotherapist to encourage deep breathing, is usually sufficient to prevent any postoperative complications. The vital capacity should be recorded daily; it will be considerably decreased initially, but will continue to increase if the progress is normal. It has been found, however, that it is often 18 months postoperatively before the pre-operative vital capacity is regained.

In cases where an anterior approach has been made through a thoracotomy incision, the patient will return from the surgery with a chest drain inserted, and will require more intensive chest physiotherapy including vibrations, and assisted coughing. Great care should be taken, however, not to be too vigorous in treatment because of the fusion.

The patient is nursed in bed, being log-rolled (see p. 268) by the nursing staff. Respiratory care and gentle lower limb activities are continued during this time. The rib-hump measurement is also taken, in prone lying, on approximately the third day postoperatively, and is seen to have decreased dramatically in most cases (Fig. 15/11). This measurement, together with the others mentioned, is repeated at regular intervals throughout the patient's growing life. However, in some of the patients, despite maintaining correction of the lateral curve, the rib hump seems to re-appear, and in some cases, become greater than originally. The cause of this is as yet unknown.

The patient becomes ambulant once the plaster of Paris jacket is dry. He is taught to get out of bed by rolling into the prone position and 'coming up' backwards, thus using the back extensor muscles as added splintage and support. To get back into bed, he should approach the bed forwards and go down on to it in a prone position. Initially, while in hospital, the nursing staff should be aware of this method, and be taught how to supervise the patient getting in and out of bed, at meal times and visits to the bathroom, etc. Once the patient is completely independent he may be discharged and it is at this time that he must be told to go home, return to school, where appropriate, and to lead a perfectly normal life. Body-contact sports, horse riding, etc, are obviously not suitable at this stage. As these patients are often adolescent it is important to reassure them about their appearance in the plaster of Paris jacket and advise and encourage them accordingly. The jacket is worn for a minimum of six months when a radiograph is taken to determine whether the fusion is solid. If this is so, the plaster jacket may be removed and normal life resumed.

The treatment described relates to the most common form of scoliosis, i.e. adolescent idiopathic scoliosis. Until recently the myopathic neuromuscular type of scoliosis, because of its severity, has rarely been treated. However, it is now possible to treat some of these patients by means of the Luque instrumentation (p. 292). The problems are varied, ranging from gross respiratory insufficiency pre-operatively, to alteration of posture and sitting balance in a wheelchair postoperatively. It has been found by experience that it is vital to have close co-operation with the local wheelchair suppliers and technicians, as alterations to arm heights, back and head rests, and even controls in motorised chairs, are necessary immediately postoperatively. As a result of the technique it is possible to sit the patient out of bed on the first day postoperatively to avoid prolonged bed rest; *but* there is a dramatic change in the trunk height and general posture. It may be necessary to use a soft cervical collar for the first few days as head control is often impaired due to the change in position. Once the patient has adapted to his new position, and in no way must he have been deprived of any previous function such as self-feeding, it has been found to have improved the respiratory function as well as his general outlook on life.

COTREL TRACTION
This is an autodynamic, self-elongation traction. It consists of a head halter, with a pelvic portion and foot pieces attached to the head halter via an overhead frame.

The patient is attached to the apparatus in a position of back lying with the knees flexed (crook back lying). As he extends the knees so traction is exerted upon the spine (remember the foot pieces have been attached overhead to the head halter).

Ideally, the patient spends most of the day on traction, but where this is used at home he should use it for at least two hours a day. It should be used at least 15 minutes in each hour. At night the head halter should be attached to about 5kg (10–11lb) of traction over the head of the bed; the head of the bed being elevated and the patient's body-weight providing the counter-traction.

KYPHOSIS

A kyphosis is less common than scoliosis but in some types it is more dangerous because it is very likely to progress, and in some instances to compress, the spinal cord with resulting paraplegia.

The general shape of a kyphosis may be:
1. A gradual round back deformity as with ankylosing spondylitis, or
2. Acute or hunchback deformity as with tuberculosis of the spine (Figs. 15/17, 15/18).

A simple classification of kyphosis is as follows:

GRADUAL CURVATURE

Adolescent deformities

These include adolescent kyphosis which is the result of wedging of the vertebral bodies during the phase of growth and is usually confined to the thoracic spine. Another type which is fairly common is

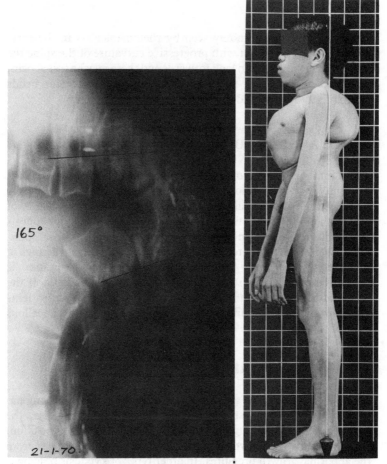

165°

21-1-70

Fig. 15/17   Lateral radiograph of a 15-year-old male with severe tuberculous kyphosis. *Note* vertebral body destruction and cord compression at the apex of the deformity

Fig. 15/18   Photograph of the patient whose radiograph is shown in 15/17

Scheuermann's disease which is most commonly seen in the thoracic spine and is obvious in the adolescent with a round back deformity which on the radiograph demonstrates abnormal changes in the vertebral growth plate.

Ankylosing spondylitis

This syndrome is commonly seen by rheumatologists in the early phases of the disease but with progressive curvature of the spine the patient loses the ability to look forwards and there may be spinal pain, progressive height loss and loss of balance as the patient bends progressively further and further forward.

ACUTE ANGULATION

The commonest causes of acute angulation of the spine (hunchback deformity) are tuberculosis of the spine and congenital kyphosis. Actually any pathological process causing destruction or absence of part or all of the vertebral bodies will produce a kyphosis (a kyphosis by definition is shortening of the anterior column of the spine – vertebral bodies and intervertebral discs). Finally there is a range of syndromes which may produce kyphosis; the most common is probably senile osteoporosis where there is gradual collapse of the vertebral bodies with an increasing curvature, and in these patients there may be quite significant pain from collapse of the cancellous bone of the bodies.

THE SURGICAL TREATMENT OF KYPHOSIS

This will vary primarily with the cause of the deformity. Bracing has been shown to be most effective in Scheuermann's disease, the appropriate brace holding the thoracic spine in an extended position, thus unloading the growth plates and allowing them to recover from the abnormal growth pressures. In other types of kyphosis bracing is not effective.

SPINAL CORD COMPRESSION

A progressive kyphosis is particularly likely to compress the spinal cord (Fig. 15/17). For this reason, if surgery is contemplated, myelography is essential in planning the operation.

In the whole field of kyphotic deformity it is the congenital and tuberculous lesions which are most likely to lead to severe problems because of spinal cord involvement. The principles of treatment of these acutely angled kyphotic deformities are:

(a) Detailed preliminary investigation including respiratory function tests and myelography.

(b) Spinal cord decompression through an anterior surgical approach when compression has been indicated with preliminary investigations.

(c) Correction of the deformity if this is safe and feasible. This may mean gradual, controlled traction over several weeks using some system already referred to under the section on scoliosis.

(d) Final stabilisation of the spine using bone grafts in order to preserve the correction of the kyphosis obtained with traction.

These deformities are most commonly seen in the thoracic spine where there will be inevitable impairment of respiratory function and where the spinal cord is most vulnerable. This group therefore presents one of the biggest problems in spinal deformity.

PHYSIOTHERAPY

Kyphosis may be described as an exaggeration of the normal thoracic curve, and may be postural or structural in nature.

Postural kyphosis is a general involvement of the thoracic spine and is most often due to habitual bad position. This condition is most commonly seen at the period of rapid growth into adolescence; predisposing causes include defective sight or hearing, bad seating or lighting in schools which impose the poor posture upon the patient. The adolescent girl may suddenly become very conscious of breast development and so try to hide this by developing a 'round' back. The treatment involves correcting the underlying causes by communicating with the school and checking the sitting position of the child, altering it where necessary, and combining it with a course of intensive physiotherapy.

The aims of physiotherapy should include muscle strengthening exercises for both the abdominal muscles and the back extensors. Mirror work should be encouraged so that the patient is made aware of his poor posture. It is often found that the hamstring muscles are tight, associated with an increased lumbar lordosis, and these should be stretched where possible. In many cases it is possible to get the co-operation of the school and the exercises may be included in the general programme of physical education.

In more severe cases it may be necessary to prescribe a Milwaukee brace for the patient, adapting it by applying posterior pads on the posterior upright bars as opposed to the lateral pads as used in cases of scoliosis. Should a Milwaukee brace be necessary the appropriate exercises are taught and performed in the brace (see p. 287).

Structural kyphosis may be due to tuberculosis of the spine, congenital wedging of the vertebrae, and epiphyseal changes in the vertebral body growth plate (Scheuermann's disease). The latter condition is most common in adolescence and is localised to the lower thoracic region. The patient is most often a boy of 13 to 16 years, tall and thin, complaining of backache. Radiographs will show the growth plate abnormality, and treatment will be bracing with a Milwaukee brace. The initial assessment should include measurement of height, weight and respiratory function – the latter is important as some boys develop tight pectoral muscles. An additional measurement could be a spondylograph (see p. 356). All measurements should be repeated at regular intervals. It is hoped that the well-fitting brace will help to protect the spine from pressure stresses until the epiphyseal plates are fully developed and, combined with an exercise programme, enable posture to be improved.

Postoperative physiotherapy

In the case of congenital wedge vertebrae surgery is indicated. Because the procedure involves a thoracotomy, physiotherapy will be directed towards preventing respiratory complications developing. In addition, if the patient has halo-femoral traction in situ, twice-daily movements of the lower limbs and neck should be carried out. At all times a careful watch must be kept for any neurological changes. The second stage, to fuse the spine in a corrected position, will require the same physiotherapy as previously described on page 267.

SPONDYLOLISTHESIS

An unusual deformity in adolescents is spondylolisthesis or dislocation of the lumbo-sacral joint. All degrees of forward shift of the body of lumbar 5 on the first sacral body may occur, but spondylolisthesis refers mainly to severe slips, usually due to congenital maldevelopment of the neural arch of lumbar 5. The end result is a grotesque posture, kyphosis at the lumbo-sacral joint and significant anterior trunk shift. There are often serious neurological problems because of the compression of the nerve roots at the lumbo-sacral level. Some of these problems may have minimal deformity and little pain; others are severely disabled with pain and severe deformity. The surgical treatment generally recommended for severe spondylolisthesis of lumbar 5 in the adolescent is fusion in situ, in other words,

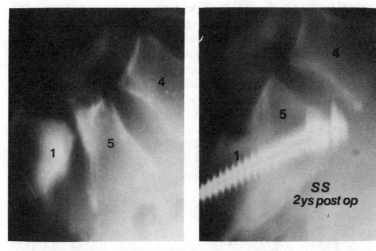

Fig. 15/19 (*Left*)   Pre-operative lateral radiograph showing severe
spondylolisthesis (Grade 4) in a 12-year-old male

Fig. 15/20 (*Right*)   Postoperative lateral radiograph showing reduction and
fusion of the spondylolisthesis to maintain the correction

accepting the deformity and obtaining stability through arthrodesis.
Recent efforts in Oswestry have been aimed at safe correction of the
deformity, reduction of the dislocation and fusion of the lumbo-sacral
joint. This new surgical technique includes the following stages:

1. Laminectomy of lumbar 5 with simultaneous lateral fusion of
   lumbar 5 to the sacrum (McPhee and O'Brien, 1979).
2. A period of skull-femoral traction lasting 10 to 14 days with regular
   detailed neurological observation because of the possible risk of
   injury to the lumbo-sacral nerve roots.
3. When reduction has been achieved, removal of the lumbo-sacral
   disc through an anterior approach and its replacement with bone
   graft from the iliac crest (Figs. 15/19 and 15/20). The available
   evidence suggests that the spine then grows straight.

Clinical features may be minimal with the patient complaining of only
slight low back pain; on examination it is often possible to palpate the
'step' due to the forward displacement. Surgical measures are
commonly advised. In severe cases this takes the form of fusion after
some degree of reduction of the slip has been obtained. It is in these
cases that physiotherapy is important.

   Skull-femoral traction is applied after the initial laminectomy, and
the reduction is achieved by hyperextension combined with a

longitudinal pull (Fig. 15/21). The degree of elevation of the trunk platform is determined by radiographs. Regular neurological observations are necessary, watching for any symptoms produced by stretching of the femoral nerve or cauda equina lesions. Gravitational oedema can be a problem, and support stockings should be worn as well as intensive ankle and knee movements being encouraged. The traction is removed twice daily for vigorous exercises to be given to the lower limbs – hip flexion beyond 60 degrees must be avoided.

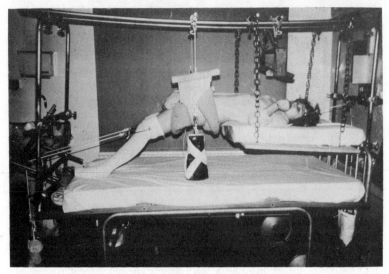

Fig. 15/21 Traction used to reduce a spondylolisthesis prior to spinal fusion

Isometric contractions of the glutei and active extension of the knees should be encouraged. Neck movements should be given. Once sufficient reduction has been achieved an anterior spinal fusion is performed. Postoperatively the patient is log rolled (see p. 268) for about 10 days, after which a plaster of Paris jacket is applied and the patient mobilised. The jacket is worn for a minimum of six months or until the radiograph shows fusion of the bone graft.

BIBLIOGRAPHY

Benson, D.R., DeWald, R.L. and Schultz, A.B. (1977). Harrington rod distraction instrumentation. Its effect on vertebral rotation and thoracic compensation. *Clinical Orthopaedics and Related Research*, **125**, 40.

Blount, W.P. (1973). *The Milwaukee Brace*. Williams and Wilkins Co, Baltimore.

Hancox, V. (1981). Cotrel traction for patients with scoliosis. *Physiotherapy*, **67**, 3, 71–2.

James, J.I.P. (1976). *Scoliosis*, 2nd edition. Churchill Livingstone, Edinburgh.

Lindh, M. and Bjure, J. (1975). Lung volumes in scoliosis before and after correction by the Harrington instrumentation method. *Acta Orthopedica Scandinavica*, **46**, 934–48.

Manning, C.W. (1974). Scoliosis. *Physiotherapy*, **60**, 1, 9–13.

McPhee, I.B. and O'Brien, J.P. (1979). Reduction of severe spondylolisthesis. A preliminary report. *Spine*, **4**, 4, 430–4.

Moe, J.H. (1972). Methods of correction and surgical techniques in scoliosis. *Orthopedic Clinics of North America*, **3**, 1.

Moe, J.H., Winter, R.B., Bradford, D.S. and Lonstein, J.E. (1978). *Scoliosis and Other Spinal Deformities*. W.B. Saunders Co Ltd, Eastbourne.

Newman, P.H. (1974). Spondylolisthesis. *Physiotherapy*, **60**, 1, 14–16.

Nordwall, A. and Willner, S. (1975). A study of skeletal age and height in girls with idiopathic scoliosis. *Clinical Orthopaedics and Related Research*, **110**, 6–10.

Robin, G.C. (1973). *Scoliosis*. Academic Press, London.

Zorab, P.A. (1969). *Scoliosis*. William Heinemann Medical Books Limited, London. (Out of print, obtainable in medical libraries.)

Chapter 16

Rheumatoid Arthritis and Juvenile Chronic Arthritis

by D.J. WARD, MB, FRCP
and M.E. TIDSWELL, BA, MCSP, ONC, DipTP

Several classifications of rheumatological disorders have been attempted but none is entirely satisfactory. There are over 180 synovial joints in the body and almost as many diseases can affect them. For the purpose of this section it is proposed in the following four chapters to discuss those conditions which are most commonly encountered by the physiotherapist.

RHEUMATOID ARTHRITIS

This is a common disease affecting approximately 1.5 million people in the United Kingdom. It occurs worldwide but is more common in some countries than others. Descriptions of the disease only started to appear towards the end of the 18th century; although several studies suggest that isolated cases were described previously, there is a lack of definite evidence and it remains likely that rheumatoid arthritis is a disease of relatively recent times.

The diagnosis is based mainly on clinical grounds and may be difficult to make in the early stages. Although helpful the rheumatoid factor test is not specific. The American Rheumatism Association drew up a list of criteria for the diagnosis of rheumatoid arthritis and although helpful, problems do arise especially with early cases and those classed as 'possible' or 'probable'. Patients in the latter classes progress to more typical rheumatoid arthritis, to normal health or into a different disease altogether.

AMERICAN RHEUMATISM ASSOCIATION CRITERIA FOR THE DIAGNOSIS OF
RHEUMATOID ARTHRITIS
  1. Morning stiffness.

2. Pain on motion or tenderness in at least one joint.
3. Swelling of one joint due either to soft tissue or effusion or both.
4. Swelling of at least one other joint with an interval free of symptoms no longer than three months.
5. Symmetrical joint swelling (same joint).
6. Subcutaneous nodules.
7. Typical radiographic changes which must include demineralisation in periarticular bone as an index of inflammation.
8. Positive test for rheumatoid factor in serum.
9. Synovial fluid showing poor mucin clot formation when added to dilute acetic acid.
10. Histopathology of synovium consistent with rheumatoid arthritis.
11. Characteristic histopathology of rheumatoid nodules.

Symptoms or signs must be present for at least six weeks to satisfy criteria 1 to 5. Rheumatoid arthritis may be classed as 'classical' (seven criteria required), 'definite' (five criteria) or 'probable' (three criteria). The requirements for a diagnosis of 'possible' rheumatoid arthritis are any two of the following present for at least three weeks: morning stiffness, history of joint pain or swelling, subcutaneous nodules, elevated ESR or C-reactive protein.

It is necessary to set these criteria against a list of exclusions such as:
Diffuse connective tissue disease, e.g. systemic lupus erythematosus (SLE), systemic sclerosis, dermatomyositis, polyarteritis nodosa, mixed connective tissue disease
Gout and crystal arthropathies
Infectious arthritis
Spondyloarthropathies
Osteoarthritis
Sarcoidosis, and many other less common arthropathies.

It must be remembered that the disease has such a varied presentation and course that many have questioned the possibility of several different disease entities. It may well be that there are several different initiating factors and/or different ways in which the disease expresses itself, this being determined by the individual patient's genetically controlled immune response.

Aetiology and pathogenesis

The cause of rheumatoid arthritis is still unknown. Much is known about the immunological and inflammatory changes but the initiating factor has not been isolated. It is thought that an antigen(s), possibly microbial, enters the body and leads to the formation of antibodies. Immune complexes are formed (antigen plus antibody) and these lead to the development of inflammation in the synovium. At its junction with cartilage and bone, the synovium organises into an invasive front (pannus) with liberation of enzymes capable of eroding cartilage and bone. The normal mechanisms which inhibit inflammation and degradative enzymes are overwhelmed in a narrow zone just in front of the advancing pannus.

Other changes occur – the proteoglycan content of cartilage diminishes making it more susceptible to pressure and, in adjacent bone, osteoclasts are activated leading to demineralisation and increased susceptibility to degradative enzymes.

We have already said that rheumatoid arthritis is common and it follows that the initiating agent(s) must also be common, so why should some not get the disease? There is an increased incidence of it in first degree relatives but not in spouses, suggesting the importance of a genetically determined host response, i.e. disease susceptibility. There are still many questions to be answered, e.g.:

1. What is the nature of the initiating agent?
2. Is there more than one such agent and would this explain the diverse nature of rheumatoid arthritis?
3. Why is the arthritis so persistent? Does the initiating agent, or parts of it, remain in tissues relatively protected from the body's immune response? (e.g. cartilage). Is it in continuous supply? (e.g. from the gut). Is it not dealt with in the same way as most antigens, either because of a failure of the immune system or because the body's own protein is being altered by the disease process and is no longer being dealt with as self-protein? (i.e. it becomes antigenic).
4. Do genetic markers (e.g. HLA-DRw4 in RA) reflect an individual's susceptibility to disease and the manner in which it will be expressed? Again a possible explanation for the different clinical patterns of disease.

Many other possibilities have been considered but discarded. Endocrine imbalance, metabolic disease, environmental factors and many others have not satisfactorily explained the disease. Although not causative it is generally agreed that stress (emotional or physical) can influence the disease adversely.

Pathology

Normal synovium consists of thin areolar connective tissue with an often incomplete surface of synovial cells. In the early phase of inflammation venules and capillary loops dilate and leucocytes pass into tissue spaces and eventually into the synovial fluid. Chronic inflammatory cells (plasma cells and lymphocytes) pass into the synovial tissue later. The synovial membrane becomes oedematous, vascular and cellular. The vascular changes include focal areas of necrosis; the lining synovial cells multiply and become several layers thick. Thus there develops the thickened synovial membrane of rheumatoid arthritis. The chronic inflammatory cells are thought to have a role in continuing the immunological → inflammatory chain and, indeed, rheumatoid factor can be isolated from them.

At this stage, no harm has befallen the cartilage or bone but eventually a process of erosion (Fig. 16/1) and degradation will supervene: thus we have an initial reversible phase which can go on to cause irreversible damage. Sometimes the disease itself does not seem to be sufficiently aggressive and will halt before this critical phase. If not, there will be progression to varying degrees of joint destruction with loss of cartilage and bone leading to deformity, subluxation, secondary degenerative change and the possibility of fibrous ankylosis.

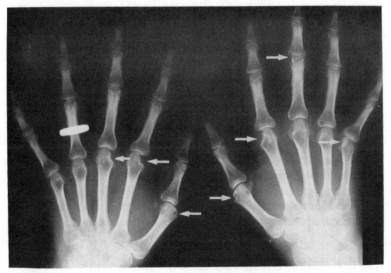

Fig. 16/1   Radiograph showing early erosive changes in the hands

Tendon sheaths behave in the same fashion as synovium and proliferative granulation tissue here (Fig. 16/2) may cause tendon rupture or attenuation.

Vasculitis is commonly found in rheumatoid arthritis and indeed may be responsible for many of the changes seen. It is responsible for

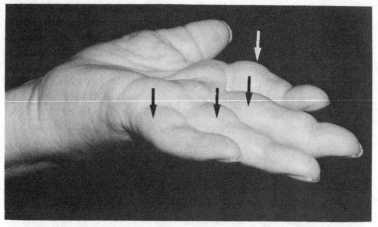

Fig. 16/2   Flexor tendon sheath distension due to rheumatoid arthritis

peripheral neuropathy, various skin and visceral lesions, and may also be an early feature of rheumatoid nodule formation. Essentially there is inflammatory occlusion of small blood vessels and there is evidence that soluble immune complexes may be involved in the process.

Subcutaneous nodule formation is seen in about 23 per cent of patients. The nodules are commonly found along the extensor aspect of the forearm; other sites may be noted – usually over areas subjected to pressure and overlying a bony prominence. Similar nodules can occur in viscera, e.g. lung. Histologically there is an acellular necrotic centre surrounded by radially palisading histiocytes and around these lies fibrous connective tissue. Both nodule formation and vasculitis are related to the finding of rheumatoid factor in the blood and usually a worse prognosis (see Fig. 16/5).

The capsule of the joint and peri-articular tissues are often stretched. Muscle wasting and osteoporosis are common findings.

Clinical features

The onset of the disease is most commonly between the ages of 35 and 55 though it can occur at almost any age. Women are affected more than men in a ratio of 3:1. The actual onset is most often subacute or chronic, but may be acute or episodic. Occasionally patients present with prodroma such as malaise, carpal tunnel syndrome, weight loss, etc.

Theoretically any synovial joint may be affected but for unknown reasons not all are in any one patient. Wrists, hands, metatarso-phalangeal joints and knees are involved early. The spine (except for the neck), sacro-iliac joints and distal interphalangeal joints are clinically spared. An important feature is the symmetry of the disease (e.g. involvement of both hands). Morning stiffness of several hours' duration is a common early symptom. Rheumatoid arthritis is a generalised and systemic disease usually with anaemia, frequently muscle wasting, osteoporosis and sometimes with extra-articular features. There may be weight loss. Pain, stiffness and limited function are the main complaints. Peripheral joints become swollen due to a combination of synovial hyperplasia (synovitis) and excess fluid in the synovial cavity (effusion). They demonstrate increased heat and on examination are often tender with restricted movement. Eventually, if there is progressive erosion of cartilage and bone combined with weakened ligaments, tendons and muscles, deformities occur and secondary osteoarthritis may develop. Fibrous ankylosis is sometimes seen.

INDIVIDUAL JOINTS

Cervical spine: Involvement often leads to subluxation in an antero-posterior plane. This is more common at the atlanto-axial level but more dangerous at the sub-axial level (usually not below C4 on C5) (Fig. 16/3). Lateral radiographs of the neck include flexion and extension views to demonstrate such lesions. Less commonly, upward subluxation may occur with danger to the medulla.

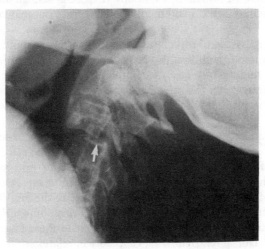

Fig. 16/3 Radiograph showing sub-axial subluxation in rheumatoid arthritis

As a result of neck involvement there may be root symptoms and signs, pain in the neck with radiation to the occiput, upper motor neurone lesions with varying degrees of para- or tetraplegia and vascular symptoms due to kinking of the vertebral arteries (visual upset, transient hemiparesis, vertigo, etc). The patient may be in danger from intubation during anaesthesia, from sudden braking during car journeys and from over-zealous physiotherapy. A collar usually helps root symptoms but occasionally fusion may be necessary if there is evidence of progressive upper motor neurone signs.

Temperomandibular joints: Apart from pain, limitation of movement may lead to difficulty in eating. Disease at this site can result in diagnostic difficulty. Pain arising from the neck, ear, temporal artery, sinuses and teeth may cause confusion.

Cricoarytenoid joint: This joint is not commonly involved but when it is, hoarseness of voice results and there is always the danger of developing stridor. Rarely tracheostomy may be required indicating how important it is to be aware of the possibility of this joint being affected.

Shoulder and shoulder-girdle: Several joints may be affected (sterno-clavicular, acromioclavicular, etc) but the most obvious one is the glenohumeral. In addition there is often disease of the rotator cuff. Basic activities such as dressing, feeding, attending to personal hygiene may be impaired, especially if there is also elbow involvement. Swelling is not a commonly noted feature but may occur.

Elbow: Apart from difficulties resulting from inability to flex, rotational movements are also impaired. Lack of full extension is a common finding but rarely of importance except when carrying shopping bags, etc. Occasionally there may be direct entrapment of the ulnar nerve in its groove.

Wrists: Pain here will impair the function of the whole hand. As with the hand it is common for the dominant side to be affected most. Dorsal subluxation of the distal end of the ulna not only makes rotational movements painful (for instance turning taps, door knobs, or the like) but also puts the extensor tendons to the fourth and fifth and sometimes the third fingers in danger (Fig. 16/4). Rupture of these tendons will result in inability to extend these fingers except passively. Dorsal tenosynovitis, especially in relation to the extensor retinaculum, may also lead to attenuation and rupture. Carpal tunnel

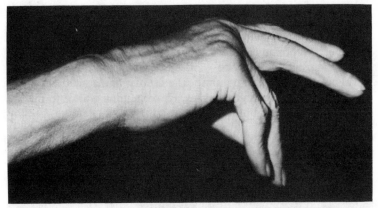

Fig. 16/4 Ruptured extensor tendons to the fourth and fifth fingers related to the subluxed lower end of ulna

syndrome is common. Eventually there is a tendency to palmar subluxation often with ulnar deviation.

Hands: Metacarpophalangeal and proximal interphalangeal joint involvement is frequent and an early feature. Palmar subluxation and ulnar deviation are common late features at metacarpophalangeal level (Fig. 16/5). The ulnar deviated hand may be aesthetically displeasing but can remain a good unit functionally. Attempts to prevent or correct ulnar deviation meet with little success.

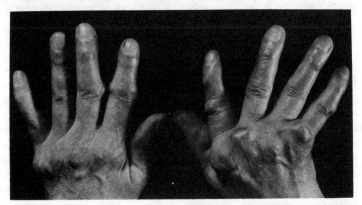

Fig. 16/5 Rheumatoid arthritis of the hands showing (a) ulnar deviation at the metacarpophalangeal level of the right hand; (b) soft tissue swelling of the metacarpophalangeal joints; (c) nodule formation; (d) vascular lesions of the nail beds

Various deformities may occur at proximal interphalangeal joint level, e.g. swan neck and button-hole (Fig. 16/6). At first swan neck deformity (flexion deformity at metacarpophalangeal level, hyper-extension at proximal interphalangeal level and flexion at distal interphalangeal level) may be overcome, but when fixed, power grip is lost. Flexor tendon sheaths may be the site of granulation tissue in the hands and weakness of grip ensues. Flexor tendon nodule formation may lead to triggering of the fingers.

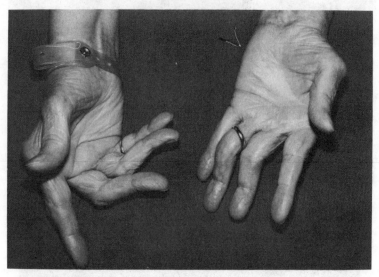

Fig. 16/6 Rheumatoid arthritis of the hands showing: *right hand*, button-hole deformities (Boutonnière's) and *left hand*, swan neck deformities

Hips: Hip involvement occurs in approximately 40 per cent of patients but is not usually an early feature. Difficulty with transfers, walking, climbing stairs, etc, may be encountered; sexual problems could be important. Pain from the hip is often referred to the knee. Sometimes trochanteric bursitis adds to the pain pattern. Radiologically the typical deformity is that of protrusio acetabuli, the eroded head of femur pushing its way centrally into the acetabulum and indeed sometimes through it. (*cf* The upward subluxation typical of osteoarthritis.)

Knees: The early occurrence of synovial swelling and effusion make the knee joint especially suitable for synovectomy, either chemical or surgical. The presence of effusion alone may not signify the development of severe destructive change, but continuing synovial hyperplasia in addition usually leads to deformity, instability and secondary degenerative change. The deformity is usually flexion and valgus. Rarely varus deformity (the hallmark of osteoarthritis of knee) may occur on one side and valgus on the other giving rise to a 'wind-swept' deformity (Fig. 16/7).

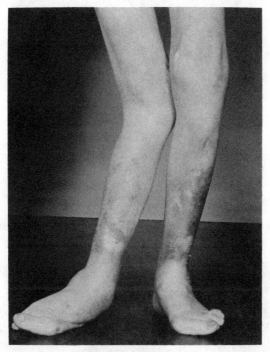

Fig. 16/7 Rheumatoid arthritis of the knees showing the wind-swept deformity. Skin changes on the shins are due to long-term corticosteroid therapy

It is important to look for the presence of popliteal (Baker's) cysts, which may be small or large (Figs. 16/8, 16/9). They result in a tight feeling behind the knee when walking or climbing stairs and are of particular importance if they rupture. Sudden calf pain with oedema of the leg and a positive Homan's sign exactly mimic the findings in deep vein thrombosis, and many patients are still treated inappropriately with admission to hospital and anticoagulants. Arthrography should demonstrate a ruptured cyst but this author would always combine it with venography since a ruptured cyst may occur with, or lead to, deep vein thrombosis.

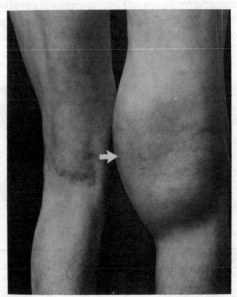

Fig. 16/8   Rheumatoid arthritis affecting the knee showing a Baker's cyst

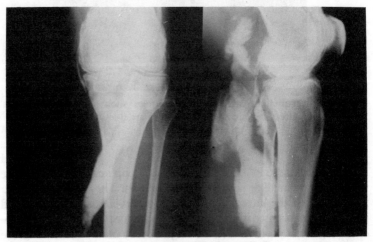

Fig. 16/9   Arthrogram of the left knee joint showing a ruptured Baker's cyst (AP and lateral views)

Hind feet: Ankle joints are usually spared but more distal joints are not. Pain on walking, especially over uneven ground is a common complaint. The usual deformity to develop is that of the valgus foot and this becomes more likely if there is attenuation or rupture of the posterior tibial or long plantar flexor tendons just posterior to the medial malleolus. The presence of a valgus deformity of the knee and foot each increases the potential worsening of such deformity at the other site and emphasises the need to take all the limb into consideration when contemplating treatment at any one joint.

Metatarsophalangeal joints: Disease here may be present without symptoms in the early stages and it may be important to have radiographs even though there are no complaints. Frequently, however, the patient has pain and complains of a sensation of walking on pebbles. Subluxation commonly occurs, resulting in an increase in the depth of the forefoot such that ordinary shoes either will not fit or result in pressure lesions both dorsally and under the heads of the metatarsals. The forefoot is often increased in lateral width as well, hallux valgus deformity being common.

EXTRA-ARTICULAR FEATURES
Apart from weakness, general malaise and weight loss, the following deserve consideration:

Nodule formation: (see p. 308)

Vasculitis: Necrotic nail-fold lesions (see Fig. 16/5) are not necessarily as bad a prognostic sign as the nodular necrotic lesions in the hands and vasculitic lesions elsewhere. Other manifestations of vasculitis are peripheral neuropathy (usually sensory, symmetrical and in the feet), purpura, leg ulcers, ischaemic or even gangrenous digits and indeed almost any organ may be affected although, surprisingly, the kidneys escape. Obviously infarction of the gut is a surgical emergency but occurs very rarely and in practice one is most often faced with either a neuropathy and/or the skin changes obvious to the eye as mentioned above. It is important for the physiotherapist to be aware of the hazards of heat treatment in the presence of neuropathy and she may find the management of leg ulcers one of the most difficult and unrewarding tasks in rheumatology.

The presence of both vasculitis and nodules may influence the decision with regard to drug treatment in particular the second-line or disease-modifying drugs (p. 325).

Ocular: There are a number of changes that occur in the eyes. The most common complaint is that of dryness or grittiness and this is part of the sicca component of Sjögren's syndrome. Less commonly there may be a dry mouth in addition. More severe problems present themselves with severe inflammatory disease such as scleritis. The side-effects of drugs may be manifest in the eyes, for example the cataracts associated with long-term corticosteroid therapy, the retinal changes with antimalarial drugs and the corneal deposits of gold.

Central nervous system: It is perhaps useful to summarise the neurological problems which may occur. Nerve root, upper motor neurone, and transient cerebral and cerebellar lesions may occur with neck disease. Carpal tunnel syndrome is common. Direct nerve involvement at elbow and knee is less common. Mononeuritis multiplex or peripheral neuropathy are seen with vasculitis.

Pulmonary: Pleural effusion is by no means uncommon and the fluid has features similar to joint fluid. The presence of pulmonary nodules may lead to problems of differential diagnosis (e.g. from multiple secondary deposits or from carcinoma if a solitary nodule). Fibrosing alveolitis and interstitial fibrosis (usually of mid- and lower zones) sometimes occur, and may give rise to dyspnoea. In addition, such changes may present a problem with regard to general anaesthesia.

Cardiac: Pericarditis is common but does not give rise to problems in most cases. Occasionally pericardial effusion may give rise to tamponade and require urgent aspiration. Constrictive pericarditis is rare, but a surgical emergency. Granuloma may form and interfere with the conducting system of the heart or lead to incompetence of the aortic valve. Such changes are uncommon.

Alimentary: The most frequent problems arise with drug therapy. Most drugs are capable of causing indigestion, but in addition the non-steroidal anti-inflammatory drugs are prone to cause blood loss, either occult or as manifest by haematemesis and melaena. An iron-deficiency anaemia added to the anaemia of the disease itself is a very common finding.

Renal: There seems to be an increased incidence of urinary tract infection, especially in females. Added to this, there is the possibility of analgesic nephropathy, leading to renal impairment after many years of analgesic consumption, and amyloidosis leading to nephrotic syndrome.

Haematological: Rheumatoid arthritis is often accompanied by a normo- or hypochromic, normocytic anaemia. Usually the level of haemoglobin does not fall below 10.0g/100ml unless there is an added iron-deficiency anaemia (with a microcytic picture) most often related to peptic ulceration and/or drug therapy. Macrocytic anaemias occasionally occur. The platelet count (normal 200–400×10⁹/litre) is sometimes elevated in relation to disease activity and may be depressed as a side-effect of certain drugs such as gold and penicillamine. The ESR and acute phase reactants are elevated. The white cell count is rarely elevated except in the presence of infection or associated with corticosteroid therapy.

Muscle: Muscle wasting is common especially in the vicinity of inflamed joints or as a result of nerve involvement (e.g. carpal tunnel). Corticosteroid therapy enhances muscle wasting. In a very few cases, actual inflammation of muscle (myositis) may occur.

Bone: Peri-articular osteoporosis is common in relation to inflamed joints. Apart from this, there is an overall loss of bone density. Additionally, osteoporosis is a common long-term side-effect of corticosteroid therapy (Fig. 16/10). This aspect is obviously impor-

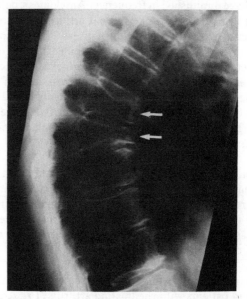

Fig. 16/10 Radiograph showing vertebral collapse due to osteoporosis following corticosteroid therapy for rheumatoid arthritis

tant in relation to joint replacement (poor 'bone stock') and physiotherapy. The wedging of plasters in the correction of flexion deformities may, for example, lead to micro-fractures.

Depression: There is true depression associated with rheumatoid arthritis in some cases, but more common is the depression associated with the frustration created by inability to perform normal daily tasks and the worry about what will happen in the future.

Oedema: Many patients with rheumatoid arthritis have oedema. This is usually due to factors including anaemia, decreased use of pump muscles due to immobility, the presence of a low serum albumin, sometimes associated with amyloidosis, and intercurrent cardiovascular disease.

COMPLICATIONS
Amyloidosis describes the cheese-like material deposited in tissues (especially of the reticulo-endothelial system in liver, spleen and kidneys) as a result of long-term infection or inflammation. At one time it was more commonly associated with chronic tuberculosis and osteomyelitis but with the introduction of suitable antibiotics these conditions have diminished in frequency. Amyloidosis occurs in up to 10 per cent of patients with rheumatoid arthritis and possibly even more frequently with longer duration of disease. It does not present as a clinical problem in anything like this number but will occasionally be a problem most commonly presenting as nephrotic syndrome (heavy proteinuria, low serum albumin and gross oedema). Diagnosis can be made in 75 per cent of cases by rectal biopsy, and in a higher percentage by renal biopsy though the latter is a more dangerous procedure. There is no specific treatment although chlorambucil has been used in children.

Sepsis: Septic arthritis must always be considered when there is an exacerbation of symptoms in any joint and especially with regard to total joint replacements. Sometimes the findings are minimal but often there is pyrexia, a drop in blood pressure and a leucocytosis. Joint aspiration and blood cultures should always be undertaken under such circumstances.

Intercurrent infections are said to be a reason for diminished life expectancy in patients with rheumatoid arthritis. *Pressure lesions* and *traumatic leg ulcers* are frequently encountered in patients who are very immobile.

Iatrogenic disease is one of the commonest 'complications' to occur. By this is meant the occurrence of disease induced by treatment. Obviously drugs must be held responsible for much of this but physical and surgical measures also play their part.

Laboratory investigations

Unfortunately there is no specific test for rheumatoid arthritis. The *rheumatoid factor test* is helpful but not diagnostic. It may be carried out as the SCAT (Sheep Cell Agglutination Test) or a variety of latex tests (less specific). The SCAT is positive in 70 per cent of those patients who have definite or classical rheumatoid arthritis and usually signifies a poorer prognosis if positive in the early stages of the disease. Vasculitis and nodule formation are often associated with a positive test.

Anaemia is common. Levels of *haemoglobin* down to 10.0g/100ml are not unusual. If iron deficiency is superadded (due to drugs, peptic ulcer, etc) the level may fall much lower.

The *ESR* is elevated. In some laboratories other acute phase reactants may be studied, e.g. plasma viscosity, C-reactive protein. Regrettably such tests do not always parallel the disease activity in its broadest sense. *Serum albumin* is often lowered (with or without the presence of amyloidosis) and *globulins* (especially gamma globulins) elevated. Immune complexes formed of gamma globulins may be demonstrated but the measurement of such complexes is extraordinarily difficult. The *white cell count* is usually normal unless the patient is receiving corticosteroids or there is infection present. The *platelet count* may be elevated in association with active disease. *Liver function tests* may be abnormal and in some patients the alkaline phosphatase reflects disease activity.

Joint fluid is usually much less viscous than in osteoarthritis. The SCAT may be positive and there is often a high protein concentration. The white cell count is elevated and may even reach levels up to 10×10^9/litre. Around this level, however, the possibility of infection arises and whenever a joint is aspirated fluid must always be sent for culture. This is the only way in which infection, as we know it, can be identified.

Radiology

Before cartilage and bone destruction has occurred, there is soft tissue swelling, (due to synovitis and/or effusion) and peri-articular osteoporosis. Later there is narrowing of joint space, due to cartilage loss, erosion of bone, cyst formation, deformity and sometimes secondary degenerative changes.

What is the value of radiology? It may assist in the diagnosis. It gives a factual record of disease progression. It may help in determining whether or not synovectomy is feasible or whether joint replacement is indicated and if so in what form. It is essential to assess the state of the cervical spine and also in the case of surgery, cardiovascular and respiratory status. Specialised techniques include arthrography, myelography (for neck lesions), arteriography and radio-isotope studies. CAT scanning should prove of great value in studying neck and other lesions.

Course and prognosis

It is common practice to think of rheumatoid arthritis as a severe, crippling disease, and indeed this is the picture seen all too frequently in hospital. However, the prognosis in over 50 per cent of patients is really very good.

Course: Episodic → Remaining a mild disease

                    → Insidious progressive disease

        Partial or complete remissions

        Progressive disease → Rapid

                    → Intermediate

                    → Slow

It would appear that in some patients synovitis occurs but does not necessarily progress to cartilage and bone destruction. In others, such destruction may occur with no, or minimal, clinical synovitis. Yet again, in some, destructive change may be a feature in the early phase of the disease only, whereas in others it progresses relentlessly over many years. The concept of variability is important. The disease varies from patient to patient and even in the same patient at different times. Any assessment of prognosis and plan of management must take this into account. How aggressive is the disease? At what stage is it aggressive? For how long is it aggressive? Yet another variable is the responsiveness of patients to disease-modifying drugs – some are, some are not. As can be seen, it is extremely difficult to give a prognosis in each individual case and extremely important for regular assessment in any programme of management. A better understanding of the many variables should result in a more accurate prognosis being possible and a more logical and appropriate plan of management being made.

Some pointers to prognosis do exist. Patients with an acute onset fare better than those starting insidiously, and males, especially young ones, better than females. The presence of the rheumatoid factor in the serum early in the course of the disease, nodules, vasculitis, ocular involvement, and Felty's syndrome usually indicate a poor outlook. As our knowledge of tissue typing increases, our ability to pick out those with a good or bad prognosis and those who will respond to drugs could improve. Generally life expectancy is less than normal due to intercurrent infection, amyloidosis, renal disease, etc.

SOME POINTS TO REMEMBER
1. Diagnosis is based mainly on clinical grounds and may be difficult to make in early stages.
2. There are different types of onset.
3. The clinical picture varies from patient to patient and from time to time in the same patient.
4. Not all patients develop severe deforming disease and the prognosis is good in over 50 per cent of patients.
5. Patients rarely develop evidence of disease in every synovial joint – some joints are more commonly affected than others.
6. Systemic and extra-articular features may be prominent.
7. There may be associated features as in Sjögrens syndrome (dry eyes and sometimes dry mouth) and Felty's syndrome (spleno-megaly, leucopenia and leg ulcers).

Management

Any plan of management must be tailored for the individual and be based on a total knowledge of the disease, its variability, the total environment of the patient and regular assessment. We have already discussed the disease and its many variables in terms of manifestations and course. What about the patient? Where is his house/bungalow/flat and what are the physical limitations imposed by it both inside and out? Is the spouse alive, well, interested in helping, already permanently intent on caring in every respect or, if no spouse, where, if any, are the relatives? Are neighbours helpful, where are shops etc? How much can the patient do for himself? How much does the patient want to do? It is always emphasised that a patient who has taken years to sink into a state of dependency is not going to mobilise and achieve independence in a few weeks. How much improvement is possible anyway? How much can be prevented? Is hospital admission required? What help might be available from social and community services and from local councils? What is the situation with regard to employment?

Fortunately most patients do not require such in-depth study but many do. In such cases a one-off assessment is not sufficient. The disease changes, other diseases may be superadded and the environment and/or the patient's ability to cope with it may also change. Regular assessment is the ideal basis upon which to form any co-ordinated programme of management and this is why a team approach is essential. We are concerned with the relief of symptoms, the halting or slowing down of the disease, the prevention or correction of deformity, an attempt to enable the patient to cope with his/her environment and, if not, then to make changes in that environment such that independence is maintained. It remains an unfortunate fact that many patients are referred late rather than early in the course of the disease.

PROGRAMME
1. Regular assessment
2. Education of patient
3. Physical measures:
   physiotherapy
   occupational therapy
   nursing
   community services
   DRO
   local council
   provision of aids, appliances, splints, orthoses, surgical shoes, etc
4. Drug therapy
5. Surgery

REGULAR ASSESSMENTS
As outlined above and often made by an occupational therapist.

EDUCATION OF PATIENT
He needs someone to spend time explaining the nature of the disease. What is it and what can be done for it? What can the patient do to help? How much time should be spent at rest and what activity or exercises should be undertaken? When and for how long should splints be worn? Will the disease affect offspring? These and many other questions require answers and we are often guilty of not giving our patients enough time. We can also help by dispelling the fears and anxieties often present in the minds of patients and their relatives.

PHYSICAL MEASURES
Knowing what the patient cannot do is a good starting point. If a patient is unable to negotiate a step to the toilet, the physiotherapy

should be aimed at training him to do so. If this were to prove impossible, then the step should be removed or ramped. The first objective is to make the patient able to cope with the environment. If not possible, then the environment should be modified. Similarly a first objective may be to teach a patient to comb his hair with an ordinary comb. If this is not possible only then should a long-handled comb be tried. Aids and appliances must be appropriate, and outside hospital their use must be ensured. As this is a changing situation, speedy provision of aids is essential; the gap between hospital and home must be avoided. If a suitable milieu is provided in hospital this should, as closely as possible, be copied in the patient's home environment when he returns there. Splints and surgical shoes are of obvious importance; of equal importance is that they fit and are used properly.

The community services including general practitioners, health authorities, social services, local authorities, voluntary organisations, works' doctors and employers may all be involved. A patient is not just treated in hospital. He has to be prepared for an existence outside hospital and to achieve this the hospital and community services must be co-ordinated.

Of course there are other objectives apart from teaching or enabling a patient to cope. Relief of pain, correction or prevention of deformity, the improvement of muscle power, the use of orthoses and so forth all need to be considered.

Drug therapy

At one end of the clinical spectrum, patients with mild disease may require no more than occasional analgesia. At the other end, in the case of progressive disease, more potent drugs may be used in an attempt to halt or slow down the aggressive nature of the disease.

In using drugs, the following points should be taken into consideration:
1. The objective to be attained.
2. The regime should be as safe as possible, i.e. the use of the least toxic drug and in the smallest dose necessary to achieve the objective.
3. Anti-rheumatic drugs cause more iatrogenic disease than any other group of drugs.
4. The more potent drugs (e.g. gold, penicillamine) are often the most potentially toxic and their use must be constantly monitored.

It is common practice to divide drugs into categories but the headings for these categories vary considerably.

GROUP A (ANALGESIC DRUGS TAKEN ON AN 'ON DEMAND' BASIS)
These include paracetamol, low dose salicylate, codeine, dihydrocodeine, dextropropoxyphene, diflunisal and occasionally pentazo-
cine (Fortral) and buprenorphine (Temgesic).

GROUP B (NON-STEROIDAL ANTI-INFLAMMATORY DRUGS TABLE 1)
Many of these act only to give pain relief. In animals, however, and
sometimes in man, they do exert an anti-inflammatory effect and some
are even claimed to modify the course of the disease though such
claims must be treated with caution. This type of drug is taken
regularly and should be administered for a two- to three-week period
before being changed on the basis of lack of effect. It may then be
replaced by another one for a further two- to three-week period. The
search is for a member of this group which will help the patient
symptomatically without causing upset. Unfortunately there is no
way of knowing which patient will respond well to which drug and
which patients will experience unwanted side-effects. It is 'trial and
error', though some are more likely to give rise to adverse effects than
others.

As a rule only one of this group should be used at a time. Some of
these drugs are long acting and if taken at night may give relief from
early morning stiffness. Indomethacin is a good example of this and a
long-acting form taken at night can be used in conjunction with a
different drug taken during the day.

As well as giving relief these drugs also possess unwanted adverse
effects for some patients. The most common side-effect is on the
gastro-intestinal tract and indigestion is a common complaint. They
may also be responsible for slow blood loss due to superficial gastric
erosion giving rise to anaemia and may lead to massive haemorrhage.
Their use is contra-indicated in patients with peptic ulcer. One of the
most difficult situations arises when a patient has either perforated a
peptic ulcer or bled from it. Drugs are stopped and the patient may be
left with little or nothing to relieve his pain.

Other side-effects may occur and tend to vary from one drug to
another. Although perhaps infrequent, there is a possibility of renal
damage with long-term use (analgesic nephropathy).

The patient should continue with these drugs only if he is convinced
that his symptoms of pain and stiffness are improved. It may be
necessary to withdraw the drug and note any worsening of symptoms.
The patient sometimes does this himself when he forgets to renew a
prescription. If he experiences more pain and stiffness under these
circumstances then it is worthwhile continuing the drug.

TABLE 1 NON-STEROIDAL ANTI-INFLAMMATORY DRUGS

Approved name	Proprietary name
azapropazone	Rheumox
benorylate	Benoral
choline magnesium trisalicylate	Trilisate
diclofenac	Voltarol
fenbufen	Lederfen
fenoprofen	Fenopron
flurbiprofen	Froben
ibuprofen	Brufen
indomethacin	Indocid
ketoprofen	Alrheumat; Orudis
naproxen	Naprosyn; Synflex
phenylbutazone	Butazolidin
piroxicam	Feldene
sulindac	Clinoril
tiaprofenic acid	Surgam
tolmetin	Tolectin

GROUP C (DISEASE-MODIFYING DRUGS)
Many different headings have been used for this group which show delayed onset of clinical effect, usually two months or longer, and potentially have greater toxicity. Monitoring is mandatory.

Main drugs antimalarials – chloroquine (Avloclor)
                            – hydroxychloroquine (Plaquenil)
              gold (Myocrisin)
              D-penicillamine
Others   cytotoxic drugs – azathioprine (Imuran)
                                        cyclophosphamide
                                        chlorambucil
              levamisole
              dapsone
              sulphasalazine (Salazopyrin)
              phosphonates (?)

These drugs should be used when the disease is early, aggressive and progressive.

Antimalarials: Chloroquine phosphate (Avloclor) 250mg; hydroxy-chloroquine sulphate (Plaquenil) 200mg. Either of these compounds may be used, chloroquine being given once a day and hydroxychloro-quine twice or three times a day. Any benefit is not usually seen for at least two months and treatment is usually continued for nine months. (This could be prolonged if an alternate-day regime is established.) If effective, a total of three courses may be given with a three-month interval between each course.

The main danger is that of retinal damage which may be irreversible and lead to blindness. It is because of this that regular ophthalmo-logical supervision is advisable, especially after the first course. Skin eruptions may occur and occasionally indigestion, especially with chloroquine.

Gold: This is given as sodium aurothiomalate (Myocrisin) intramus-cularly. Following a test dose of 5mg, 50mg is given weekly. Usually 400mg is required before any effect is seen. If after 600mg no benefit has been observed, it should be discontinued. Otherwise it may be given to a total of 1 gram and thereafter continued with a maintenance dose of 50mg every month. This regime is somewhat arbitrary and modifications may be made in individual cases.

The most common side-effects are: a rash usually preceded by itching, renal damage and bone marrow depression. While on weekly injections, the urine must be tested each week for protein, and blood tests to include white cell count and platelets at fortnightly intervals. Thrombocytopenia (low platelet count) is the commonest blood abnormality to occur. Any trend towards this, the presence of proteinuria or the occurrence of a rash are all indications for stopping gold therapy. Other side-effects can occur but are less common.

D-penicillamine: This is administered orally starting with a low dose, usually 125mg daily. At intervals of several weeks the dose may be increased by increments of 125mg to 500mg or sometimes 750mg daily. With such a regime it can take many months for any beneficial effect to occur. Strict monitoring is again essential and is similar to that used for gold. Apart from renal and haematological effects, rashes are common both early and late in the course of treatment and gastro-intestinal symptoms are frequent especially loss of taste and nausea.

Other drugs in this group are used less often. All must be monitored.

GROUP D (CORTICOSTEROIDS)

These may be given orally, by parenteral injection or by intra-articular injection. There is no doubt that cortisone, in whatever form, does improve symptoms dramatically in most patients. Unfortunately there are side-effects after long-term use. There is no evidence that the ultimate outcome of the disease is influenced by corticosteroids although for a time the quality of life is vastly improved. As a rule the development of side-effects is related to the amount of cortisone given and it is important, therefore, to give the smallest dose possible to achieve a clinical response. By mouth, the drug of choice is prednisolone. Every attempt should be made to keep the dose at 5mg or less per day except for a temporary increase during an exacerbation.

Corticosteroids may be considered in those patients who have not responded to other drug regimes and whose quality of life is very poor. They may also be considered for socio-economic reasons and in the elderly. Other possible indications include severe systemic disease, scleritis, Felty's syndrome and the more dangerous forms of vasculitis. Very rarely should steroids be used in the young. Every attempt should be made to withdraw the drug if it seems appropriate.

Short term there is little to choose between a course of prednisolone by mouth or ACTH (or Depo-Synacthen) by injection. This probably applies to long-term therapy as well except for a slight difference in the incidence of various side-effects.

There are different ways in which corticosteroids may be used. It is helpful to exhibit prednisolone or ACTH for a two- or three-month period when a long-acting drug (Group C) is introduced, to cover the period taken for the latter to be effective. Similarly a short course can be useful during an exacerbation of disease and dangers should be few.

Pulse therapy using 1 gram of methylprednisolone via an intravenous infusion on each of three successive days has been claimed to induce remission but further trials are required.

Although the side-effects of corticosteroids are legion, those most frequently encountered in rheumatology are: thin skin, usually associated with thin bones, easy bruising and laceration, 'mooning', weight gain, fluid retention, sepsis, and gastro-intestinal lesions. The danger of suprarenal insufficiency during stress or infection is ever present.

Because there are different drugs with different actions we need to ask when do we use which? Early in the course of the disease, one of the non-steroidal anti-inflammatory drugs should be used in conjunction, if necessary, with a simple analgesic taken on demand. If other than indomethacin (Indocid) is used the latter may be added at night time in long-acting form (Retard) by mouth or as a suppository. Assessment of the effect of this regime should be made after two weeks and if not successful or if causing side-effects, a different non-steroidal anti-inflammatory drug should be used; it may be necessary to make several changes before finding a drug which is helpful and not causing adverse effects.

If the disease is aggressive and progressive, then it will be necessary to consider the use of one of the slow-acting drugs of Group C. These drugs should be introduced early in treatment and, if possible, before significant damage to cartilage and bone has occurred. They are of little value in patients who have severe deforming arthritis of many years' duration. If a slow-acting drug is introduced it is sometimes helpful to use a short course of corticosteroid (say for two months) to cover the period taken for the drug to work. Intra-articular steroids may also be given during this period.

Should the disease still progress and quality of life be severely impaired, then longer-term corticosteroid therapy may have to be considered.

GROUP E (INTRA-ARTICULAR THERAPY)

The use of intra-articular steroids has been the source of much debate. Overall there is little evidence to support the concept that they are dangerous. Obviously, repeated frequent use is to be avoided partly because some of it will be absorbed into the circulation and act like systemic steroid, partly because it is an invasive technique (though with care, infection is highly unlikely), and partly because one should be thinking of an alternative more definitive form of treatment. Various preparations are available. Indications include:

1. Treatment of an acute exacerbation in a joint.
2. As an adjunct to physiotherapy, either in serial splinting or when the maximum improvement obtained by the physiotherapist still leaves a joint with an unacceptable painful limitation of movement.

Tendon sheaths and soft tissues may also benefit from local steroid injections. As a rule the effect of intra-articular corticosteroids is short-lived, and various other substances have been used in an attempt to ablate synovial granulation tissue (chemical synovectomy). These alternatives are only likely to be effective in the relatively early stage of the disease before cartilage and bone destruction have occurred. Radioactive materials are most often used in this country (e.g. radioactive yttrium for knees, radioactive erbium for smaller joints). They should be avoided in the young. Other substances have been tried and of these osmic acid has proved useful for knee synovitis.

Finally let me reiterate that each patient must be considered as an individual. What is the current situation? What is likely to happen? How can help be given? – and in what way? What does the patient want? What about relatives? – what do they want to give and how able are they to give it? And so we go on to think about the patient as a whole: the total environment must be considered every time we think anything about a patient. What guidance? What drugs and when? What surgery and when? What physiotherapy and when? There is a right time for each aspect of management. There is no uniform approach that applies to every patient. Think! *You* must know what each patient needs – always based on a knowledge of the disease and this concept of total environment. All round assessment is essential, otherwise you will find yourself in a wilderness, not knowing which way to go.

PHYSIOTHERAPY

As there is no cure for rheumatoid arthritis, successful management of the disease is assessed by the quality of life achieved by the patient throughout the period of disease activity and the degree of function retained as the disease process comes to an end. A well-adjusted, independent patient will have been assessed, advised, counselled and treated by different professional groups during the course of the disease. Professional responsibility for physical rehabilitation falls to physiotherapists and they are closely concerned with patients at all stages of the disease. A disadvantage of this long contact is that some patients may use the physiotherapist's professional expertise as a mental and physical prop and not gain maximal therapeutic value from physiotherapy.

Figure 16/11A shows the fulminating course of the disease with periods of exacerbation and remission, and these will produce progressive deterioration of the musculo-skeletal system with consequent reduction in the patient's physical capacity. Physical treatment which is continued irrespective of disease activity, becomes associated with this progressive deterioration by the patient who may even blame treatment for the exacerbation which, predictably, will occur. Figure 16/11B indicates the patient's varying function in line

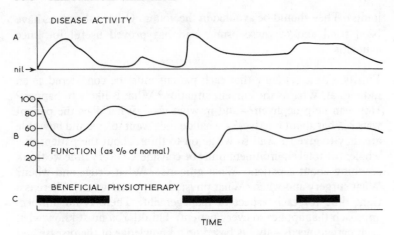

Fig. 16/11 Schematic representation of the fulminating course of rheumatoid arthritis

with the established disease pattern, showing sharp falls in the level of physical performance at onset and during the early part of acute phases. Functional levels will improve as the joint activity reduces, rising to a peak some time after the termination of the exacerbation; each successive peak is lower than the previous one. This peak of functional independence is maintained for some time, and then the slow decline in performance preceding the next sharp fall is recognised.

Physiotherapy will be of most benefit during acute phases, and should be continued until no further improvement in function is observed. It should then be withdrawn (Fig. 16/11C) and the patient expected to be self-reliant until the next acute phase, or the slow performance slip, produces specific problems which can be aided by a course of treatment. Using this approach, the patient will associate physiotherapy with relief of distressful symptoms and improvement in function. Therapist and patient will find courses of treatment rewarding and the patient's attitude will be more positive, knowing help can be obtained should the need arise.

Although joint pathology follows a predetermined course, no two patients will be affected in quite the same way. The mode of onset, joints affected, pattern of the disease and the patient's response will all influence the ultimate prognosis and contribute to the unique nature of every patient. As no two patients are identical, schemes of treatment will also require individual tailoring to the needs of the patient as determined by assessment. Because the disease fluctuates frequently causing patients' needs to change rapidly, treatment programmes must be flexible.

Before an appropriate treatment programme can be devised, adequate assessment is essential: this will provide information on the patient's physical and functional levels of performance at the time of examination. Problems are identified and, if they will respond to physical treatment, goals are set, treatment planned and implemented. Pre-treatment assessment provides a baseline for evaluation of the effectiveness of physiotherapy and frequent reassessment to monitor progress is required. Changes can be introduced to the programme when necessary.

Before considering specific areas of assessment, it is appropriate to identify the four places where patients will meet physiotherapists.

IN-PATIENT ADMISSION

Inflamed joints must be rested and this is best achieved by admission, when possible, to a specialised unit where patients are not subjected to the turmoil of a busy general medical ward. More often than not the acute rheumatoid arthritic patient *will* be admitted to a general medical ward. Hospital admission removes the patient from the social and economic pressures of home and ensures that there will be adequate rest. With rest he will improve and this will encourage him to co-operate with treatment. Initially patients are often depressed and being with others with similar problems can be helpful. As the active phase of the disease subsides, activity can be introduced under controlled conditions, monitored carefully and its effects evaluated.

Subsequent admissions will be for specific acute phases when a period of rest, reassurance and reassessment is considered necessary. On all occasions the physiotherapist's role is one of assessment, treatment and advice for the patient in all aspects of his physical and functional activity. A complete physical assessment should be made on each admission so that a picture may be built up of the patient and be available for comparison. Several sessions may be required for the initial assessment, and only on completion can treatment objectives be decided and then implemented. A full assessment should also be made prior to discharge, and any changes noted.

OUTPATIENT ATTENDANCES

Patients may be referred to the physiotherapy department for the management of particular problems or for tailing-off treatment after a period in hospital. Again accurate assessment is necessary before and during treatment, and prior to discharge.

OUTPATIENT CLINIC ATTENDANCE

Assessment of a steadily deteriorating joint, or a check on a particular aspect of the patient's capability may be undertaken.

DOMICILIARY VISITS

To obtain a complete picture it helps if patients can be seen in their homes and, if possible, at work so that advice may be given for a continued independent life.

ASSESSMENT

Charts may be used to record the assessment findings; they have the advantage of saving time and avoiding duplication of examination. Because the patient's condition can change from day to day and, indeed, during the day, it is necessary to indicate (1) the time at which the patient was assessed; (2) whether any new drug regime has been introduced; or (3) whether exercise has influenced the measurements.

A summary of the physiotherapy assessment findings should be placed in the patient's notes for reference by other members of the therapeutic team. This summary could include posture, gait, degree of independence in the activities of daily living, any associated problems, and an outline of the treatment given.

Pain

Standard methods of testing are used to measure factors such as joint movement, muscle strength or respiratory function but pain is more difficult to quantify. Self-assessment by the patient is a valuable indicator to gauge the effect of the pain on the patient's performance. The pain felt is localised on a body image chart (an example is shown on p. 192) and quantified by the patient at each site identified. Pain is graded at the sites identified between the extremes of 'no pain' and 'extreme pain' using some form of scale.

Following the patient's subjective assessment the physiotherapist can gain objective information by determining if there is pain on pressure at rest, on passive or an active movement. If pain occurs during movement, is it constant at all points of the range? If it varies, how does it vary? Is it a factor causing limitation of movement and what will produce relief?

Swelling

Although comparisons should be made between both sides of the body
(unless the disease is only unilaterally active) this does not provide a
baseline. Not only should circumferential measurements of joints be
taken, but an attempt should be made by palpation to determine the
source of the swelling. Excess synovial fluid is soft to the touch and
compressible; thickened synovium presents with a firm, though
soggy, feel; and calcification produces hard nodules or ridges. Where
joints are not easily measured, such as the tarsus and carpus, volume
displacement measurements can be taken (Fig. 16/12). In both the
direct and indirect methods the limb to be measured is immersed into
the container to a predetermined level.

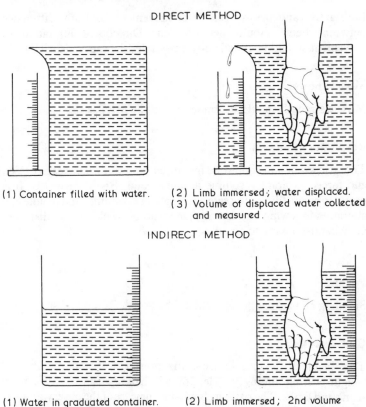

DIRECT METHOD

(1) Container filled with water.

(2) Limb immersed; water displaced.
(3) Volume of displaced water collected
    and measured.

INDIRECT METHOD

(1) Water in graduated container.
    1st reading taken.

(2) Limb immersed; 2nd volume
    reading taken. 2nd—1st gives
    volume of immersed limb.

Fig. 16/12   Volume displacement measurements of joints

Skin condition

The general texture and condition of the skin is observed: any skin lesions, subcutaneous nodules or alterations in the texture of the nails and hair are noted. Local erythema over affected joints with an associated rise in temperature may be evident.

Deformity

When recording deformity it is important to note whether it is fixed or correctable by passive means.

Joint range

Both active and passive ranges of movement (and any difference between them) should be recorded. Directional limitation of movement should be noted and, if possible, the cause identified.

Muscle power

Muscle strength should be graded using the MRC scale.

Respiratory function

Thoracic excursion should be measured, and the vital capacity (VC) and forced expiratory volume in one second (FEV_1) recorded. It is useful to assess the resting rate and depth of breathing, and to note any alteration following a set activity, for example walking a set distance, or rising from lying to standing.

Posture

Standing and sitting posture should be noted.

Gait analysis

This includes the use of aids; the presence of abnormalities of weight-bearing, timing, step length, width of base; and posture of the trunk and limbs. The patient should be unaware of the observations so that a natural gait is recorded; the Benesh notation (McGuinness-Scott, 1982), clinical photographs or video recording are suitable methods for this purpose.

Activities of daily living

A considerable amount of information will have been collected by this stage of the assessment which will be meaningless, unless it is related to the ability of the patient to cope with the activities connected with daily living. This part of the assessment should be done in co-operation with the occupational therapist and should include observation of the following: transfer from bed to chair and vice versa, from chair to standing and return to sitting, the ability to manage slopes, stairs and uneven ground, washing, getting in and out of the bath, managing the toilet, etc.

Hand function

A separate assessment of this is essential. As well as including the daily activities already mentioned, the physiotherapist should note how able the patient is to support weight through the upper limb. This is important for it will influence the choice of walking aids.

TREATMENT

Successful management of the rheumatological patient depends on meticulous assessment. For each patient the diversity of symptoms and their effect on his quality of life, personality and ability to co-operate must be taken into account when planning treatment. The *principles* of treatment for the affected joints remain constant: it is the *techniques* which may require adaptation to be effective in different areas.

Principles

1. Relief of pain.
2. Prevention of deformity.
3. Correction of deformity.
4. Maintenance and restoration of joint range.
5. Maintenance and improvement of muscle tone.
6. Maintenance of optimum function.

PAIN

Pain and arthritis are inextricably linked. A cycle of activity which develops between arthritis, depression and pain must be broken before the patient's condition will improve. An arthritic pathology induces depression which, in turn, produces pain, or augments what is already present. Depression lowers the pain threshold, so pain is magnified and conventional analgesics become less effective. Not surprisingly this disease has been described as 'the long pain'. There is a positive side to pain, namely to provide a natural protection against harmful overuse of affected joints.

Control of pain by physiotherapy is directed primarily at reducing protective muscle spasm.

1. Applications of heat that have been found to be clinically effective are infra red irradiation, hot packs (wet or dry) and paraffin wax. Short wave diathermy (SWD), by increasing the intrascapular engorgement, will increase pain if inflammation is present, and therefore is less effective.

2. Cooling the area using ice-towelling techniques or ice-cube massage over the affected joints will relieve pain, provided the cooling is sufficiently prolonged to reduce the conduction velocities of nerves supplying the muscles in protective spasm.

3. Interferential current may be used as a treatment of affected joints. A strong analgesic effect will be gained by using a 100Hz current, but 90–100Hz is more beneficial as accommodation of the nerves is reduced. Membrane permeability is increased with improved absorption, healing and blood supply to the part by using a frequency of 50–100Hz.

   Care must be taken when treating acutely inflamed joints as excessive movement may cause damage once the protective pain and muscle guarding are eliminated.

4. Acutely affected joints which are more painful on movement will respond favourably to isometric contractions around the joint(s).

PREVENTION OF DEFORMITY

In the early stages pain, swelling and protective muscle spasm encourage the patient to assume postures that will anticipate deformity. Later there is adaptive alteration of the fibre length of peri-articular structures, and inequality of muscle power contributing to deformity and, subsequently, alterations in bone shape. Constant monitoring of the disease activity with specific attention to joints affected is required. To prevent deformity occurring, postural awareness, exercise, and passive stretching of structures or splintage may be employed.

Postural awareness not only involves the recognition of a faulty *general* posture with its tendency to tolerate progressive flexion due to weakness of anti-gravity muscles, but also specific *local* postural abnormalities of affected joints. Correct posture in bed, in a chair and in standing and walking should be taught and the patient instructed to spend some time each day in lying, either supine or prone.

General exercise on land or in water will improve the strength of anti-gravity muscles and should be encouraged. The muscle groups which are particularly at risk are the back extensors, glutei and quadriceps. Specific exercises to prevent an imbalance of muscle power developing around affected joints will help retain normal alignments.

Passive stretching of tight structures must be specifically directed towards stretching the structure at risk, e.g. the flexor aspect of the joint capsule. Accurate anatomical knowledge is essential in order to apply the stretch longitudinally to the structure.

Splintage is valuable, particularly when joints are acutely affected. Resting splints will reduce the protective muscle guarding which encourages deformity. They should be worn at night and for predetermined periods during the day. Made usually of plaster of Paris (POP), they should be well-fitting, padded over bony points to avoid pressure and be easy to apply. The following points should be remembered:

Hands: The wrist should be held in a neutral position or in a few degrees of extension; the metacarpophalangeal joints should be just off full flexion; any ulnar drift (deviation) should be corrected; the interphalangeal joints in about 5 degrees of flexion. The thumb should be slightly abducted from the palm and in opposition. It should be able to support the tips of the fingers.

Knees: The knee should be splinted allowing about 5 degrees of flexion. A back-slab is applied which extends from just distal to the ischial tuberosity to just proximal to the heel.

Ankle and foot: The splint should extend from the level of the neck of the fibula to the tips of the toes. It should hold the ankle at 90 degrees (plantigrade) and control any valgus or varus deviation.

CORRECTION OF DEFORMITY

Before embarking on a regime to correct a deformity, the physiotherapist needs to be reasonably certain that function will be improved. Following correction, either by conservative or surgical methods, the muscles involved in holding the corrected position will need to be strengthened so that the deformity does not recur.

Joints which are held in a deformed position develop convex aspects where soft tissues are lengthened, and concave aspects where soft tissues are shortened (Fig. 16/13). Methods of correction include:

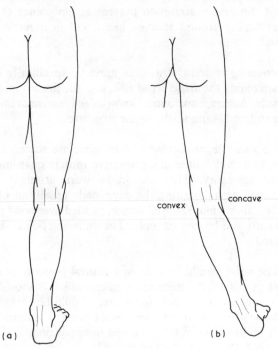

convex   concave

(a)   (b)

Fig. 16/13 Posterior view of leg: (a) normal alignment; (b) valgus deformity of knee (genu valgum)

Serial plasters (POP): A POP cast is applied, well padded, over the deformed joint. After 2–3 days it is split on the concave side and separated as far as possible using the uncut POP on the convex side as a hinge. Wedges are inserted to maintain the achieved position and the whole part secured by a POP bandage. The procedure can usually be repeated once before the entire plaster has to be replaced (Fig. 16/14a, b, c, d).

Serial splinting: A resting splint is made for the joint. It is removed for specific exercise to the lengthened muscles enabling them to improve

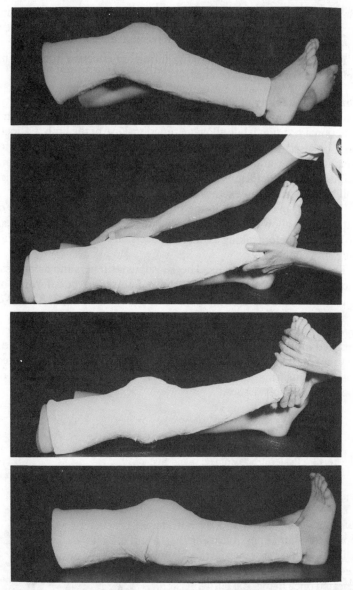

Fig. 16/14 (a) Patient with a knee flexion deformity in a plaster of Paris cylinder; (b) the splint around the knee leaving a hinge anteriorly – correction has been effected, posterior aspects of the plaster separated; (c) correction maintained, awaiting a plaster bandage completion to hold the cylinder in a new position; (d) the completed cylinder with correction of the deformity

the joint position and maintain control of the newly achieved position. As definite improvement is gained it will be necessary to make a new splint.

Both serial plasters and serial splinting are effective in correcting deformities of the wrist or knee.

Orthoses: Instability of a joint leads to loss of function and deformity. To overcome this an orthosis may be prescribed to hold the joint in a functional position while allowing functional use of the limb. Calipers may be used to control an unstable knee, correcting the line of weight-bearing and controlling any tendency to flexion, rotation, valgus or varus deformity. The incorporation of a hinge at the knee will allow flexion and extension.

The wrist may be held in the functional position of 10 degrees of extension to allow the patient to evaluate for himself the effects of an arthrodesis, before taking a conscious decision to accept surgery (Fig. 16/15).

The incorporation of flanged heels, valgus stiffeners and metatarsal pads, etc into shoes can help to stabilise joints, correct deformity or re-align weight-bearing through the leg (see Chapters 1, 2, 3 and 4).

Dynamic splints: These are particularly useful following hand surgery. Resisted muscle work is possible with associated joint movement. At rest the splint holds the affected joints in a corrected or over-corrected position, ensuring that deformities do not progress because of shortening of soft tissues.

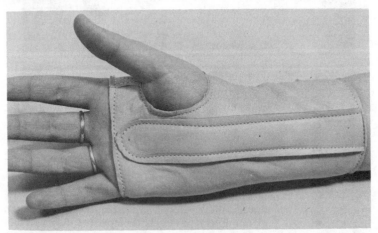

Fig. 16/15 A functional wrist support. Made in soft leather with a removable metal strut anteriorly which can be adjusted to give greater or less support

MAINTENANCE OF JOINT RANGE

During normal daily activities few, if any, joints are put through a full range of movements. This does not cause problems in the normal joint but in one with inflammatory disease progressive loss of range will occur. It is essential therefore to put all joints through a full range of movement each day; as passive movements will increase protective muscle spasm, active-assisted movements should be given.

Restoration of lost range: In joints where there is a significant limitation of movement, treatment objectives will be directed towards restoring the range to normal. It is necessary to identify the factor(s) producing restriction and to encourage active movement into the previously lost range. Where the tissue shortening is severe, serial plaster or skin traction may be used to provide a prolonged stretch (see p. 112). Less severe shortening may respond to passive stretching, e.g. hip flexion caused by a tight ilio-inguinal ligament may be alleviated by a period of prone lying each day.

Protective muscle spasm will be reduced by active exercise. Proprioceptive neuromuscular facilitation (PNF) techniques of slow reversals, hold-relax, contract-relax, and repeated contractions may be found of value. Hydrotherapy will be beneficial providing warmth which will aid relaxation, and the supportive effect of buoyancy which will reduce the pain and muscle spasm induced by exercises involving weight-bearing of affected joints. Protective muscle spasm around unstable joints attempts to stabilise them, but in so doing will restrict movement; providing appropriate splintage will release muscles to perform movement. Any range of movement regained must be under the voluntary control of the patient as an unstable joint will be more detrimental to the patient's function than one with a limited range of movement.

MAINTENANCE AND IMPROVEMENT OF MUSCLE POWER

A feature of rheumatoid arthritis is weakness of muscle associated with wasting. To overcome this the patient will need to carry out regular exercise and, as with all treatment regimes, the exercises need to be tailored to the individual. Guidelines can be indicated for their application.

1. Exercise should be within the patient's tolerance and should not cause an increase in pain. If there is residual pain after exercise, associated with an increase in joint symptomology, the amount should be reduced at the next treatment until the optimum requirement is found.

2. Progression of exercise will tend to be slow but should be noticeable (to the patient). Resisted exercise will be most effective in improving the strength of muscle, and PNF techniques are useful.
3. When joints are acutely inflamed, rhythmic stabilisations can be used to exercise the muscles with minimal joint movement. As the inflammation subsides slow reversals, hold-relax and repeated contractions may be used to improve muscle power.
4. Postural mechanisms will need to be re-educated; trunk muscles strengthened by mat work; resisted walking used to strengthen lower limb musculature.

Pool therapy allows graded exercise by using the buoyant effect of the water to assist, and then resist, muscle contraction. It is a form of recreational exercise which can be continued by patients who have access to a warm pool. Bad Ragaz pool exercises are most effective. The rheumatoid patient will require a water temperature of about 36°C (96.8°F), and should not be immersed for more than 20 minutes. Although this type of treatment is enjoyable, it is also tiring and patients must have an adequate rest afterwards.

The use of cooling paraffin wax to provide an increasing resistance for the intrinsic muscles of the hand may be helpful.

The use of dead weight or mechanical resistances offered by springs or pulley circuits is not to be recommended for these patients. Vulnerable joints can be traumatised by such techniques because the resistance is not automatically adjusted to the patient's performance. Exercise sessions should be brief and the patient allowed to rest afterwards. Several short sessions in a day are more beneficial than one long session. Patients should be given a scheme of exercises for home use; they should be taught carefully and frequent checks made to ensure that performance levels remain acceptable.

MAINTENANCE OF OPTIMUM FUNCTION
The whole management of rheumatoid arthritis centres around the maintenance of the patient's independence, as well as providing the best quality of life within the restrictions imposed by the disease. When performance is deteriorating intervention can enable particular lost skills to be regained and independence prolonged. In some instances alternative ways to independence may be achieved by skilful physiotherapy or by the provision of aids by the occupational therapist.

Independence does depend largely on keeping mobility; gait disturbances which occur early in the disease will inhibit the patient's activities and have a marked effect on his overall performance.

Walking aids may be required in conjunction with other forms of treatment to preserve the actual ability to walk. The use of conventional aids such as sticks, elbow crutches and walking frames is dependent on the patient being able to tolerate weight-bearing through the upper limb joints. As these joints seldom escape involvement the selection of an appropriate aid can present problems. If there is inability to support weight through the dorsiflexed hand then sticks, elbow crutches and pulpit walking frames are inappropriate. Patients with limited wrist extension tend to support their weight on the first metacarpophalangeal joint, or in the web between the thumb and index finger; this strains the joints of the thumb and the aid is less effective. Forearm support (gutter) crutches, which allow the weight to be supported by the ulnar border of the forearm, should be used. The overall height and position of the forearm support and hand grips can be adjusted to suit the patient. Straps with Velcro fastenings keep the forearm in position and enable the crutch to be lifted without the use of the hands. Patients who have active disease in the elbow and shoulder joints will be unable to use this type of crutch, but poor *hand* function is not a contra-indication.

Although some weight relief can be gained unilaterally by using a single crutch on the contralateral side, far more benefit is gained by using two. To provide greater support and more stability, a gutter Rollator may be used – that is a frame with small wheels at the front, into which gutter supports are set.

JUVENILE ARTHRITIS

Up to the age of 16 there are several types of arthritis affecting children.
1. Rheumatoid arthritis starting in the young. This is typical of the adult form, but usually worse. Most commonly it affects girls, often between the ages of 8 and 16. It has a bad prognosis.
2. Arthritis associated with psoriasis, inflammatory bowel disease (ulcerative colitis or Crohn's), infection (Yersinia, rubella, etc) or even Reiter's. *Remember*, arthritis may occur before psoriasis and colitis make their appearance.
3. Ankylosing spondylitis. This usually occurs in boys, especially between the ages of 12 and 16. Peripheral arthritis is more often seen in the young. Later, the typical changes of ankylosing spondylitis become more obvious.
4. Diffuse connective tissue diseases. These include systemic lupus

erythematosus (SLE), dermatomyositis, systemic sclerosis and polyarteritis nodosa. Joint symptoms may occur and be prominent early in the course of the disease.

5. Infection. This group includes tuberculosis, and other chronic infections. Even the common virus infections seen in children may be associated with arthralgia and arthritis.

After excluding the above conditions and others not mentioned, we are left with a group of children who have arthritis but are not classified.

In 1897 George Frederick Still described some features pertaining to these children; this was called Still's disease. Understanding of this condition has led to a better definition of juvenile chronic polyarthritis. This is dependent on the type of onset of the disease, i.e. (1) systemic; (2) polyarticular; or (3) oligo-articular.

The systemic features are those described by Still. Malaise, weight loss, fever (typically rising in the evening and normal in the morning), rash (usually erythematous, salmon pink, evanescent and often associated with a rise in temperature or induced by external heat such as bathing), lymphadenopathy, splenomegaly, pericarditis; – in fact, a child looking and being very ill with a multitude of systemic features. All too often this child, with only minimal joint problems, is investigated in great depth before the correct diagnosis is considered. Approximately half of such children will develop a chronic arthritis.

Those with polyarticular onset often continue to have active joint disease until their late teens. Physiotherapy has an important part in the preservation of the integrity of joints until the active phase of the disease has passed.

Children with few joints involved often have a good prognosis with one exception – they are more likely to have iridocyclitis, an inflammatory disease of the eye which can lead to blindness. This is especially likely to be present if there is a positive anti-nuclear antibody (ANA) test. All children with juvenile chronic poly- (or oligo-) arthritis should have ophthalmological checks – eye disease is seldom recognised by either the child or the parent until it is advanced.

The management of these children is specialised. Drug treatment resembles that for adult rheumatoid arthritis but corticosteroids should not be used unless the ocular state demands it. Chlorambucil has been shown to help those children who develop amyloidosis.

Children with severe arthritis and eye involvement are especially prone to depression if, in addition to their existent problems, they are faced with dwarfism associated with (a) their arthritis and (b) corticosteroid therapy. Treatment, even more than with adult rheumatoid arthritis, requires total understanding, and parents, child, doctors, physiotherapists, occupational therapists, teachers, careers advisors should all be involved.

PHYSIOTHERAPY

Long-term management of children is complex involving co-ordination of activity between hospital, home and school to ensure that the child receives maximum benefit from therapeutic procedures with the least disruption of family life and education.

Physical procedures vary little from those used in the treatment of adults and the key to success is the rapport built up between the patient, parents and therapist. Parents need to understand the implications of the diagnosis and co-operate fully with the therapist to ensure that the affected child grows and develops physically, mentally and socially within acceptable norms.

Assessment

Details of assessment are as previously discussed (p. 332) and here some of the predicted findings are indicated. Distribution of joint involvement differs between children and adults, with children commonly displaying symptoms in knees and hips, as well as wrists, ankles, hands and neck. The child will respond to pain by becoming withdrawn, adopting antalgic postures and restricting movement in parts that are painful. Contractures, producing deformity, will develop if inflamed joints are held immobile (Fig. 16/16). Lack of movement reduces the stimulus to growth of the skeleton, leading to retardation.

Treatment

Parents have to be educated to co-operate fully with the different professional groups involved in the treatment of the child. Careful positioning to avoid contracture and deformity developing may be augmented by resting splints during the active stages of the disease. Contractures that have developed may be reduced by serial plasters, and a programme of activity to exercise muscles and joints in full range, or within the pain tolerance is necessary to maintain muscle tone and mobility. Muscle groups on which to concentrate are the extensors of the spine, hips and knees which, if combined with exercises to shoulder retractors, will avoid flexed postures and poor

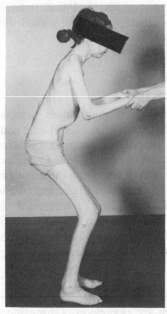

Fig. 16/16 Severe deformities and muscle wasting in juvenile chronic polyarthritis

gait patterns developing. Water is a useful medium and children respond well to pool treatments, gaining relief from pain and protective muscle spasm by immersion in the warm water. Buoyancy provides assistance or resistance to movement and weight-bearing activities such as walking are able to be re-learnt. Once any initial fear of the medium has been overcome, children gain confidence and enjoyment from exercises in the pool and will work well as individuals or in groups.

Gait analysis and correction, if required, are essential with particular emphasis laid on gaining heel strike and normal heel-toe sequence during stance phase (see Chapter 2). Any tendency to limping, walking on flexed knees or other gait abnormality should be eradicated and posture corrected.

Where resting splints are used, joints should be placed in functional positions; function may be improved by a light, working splint to provide stability of one or more affected joint to enable easier performance of daily activities. An example of this is a wrist support which will make writing easier.

Monitoring the child's progress should be continued until the disease has run its course. This could be many years ahead. In successful management, treatment becomes incorporated with family routines, and it is hoped that the child emerges in adulthood with the capability of leading a near normal life.

REFERENCE

McGuinness-Scott, J. (1982). *Benesh Movement Notation*. Chartered Society of Physiotherapy, London.

BIBLIOGRAPHY

See page 409.

Chapter 17

The Spondyloarthropathies

by D.J. WARD, MB, FRCP
and M.E. TIDSWELL, BA, MCSP, ONC, DipTP

In this group are included:
    Ankylosing spondylitis
    Arthritis associated with psoriasis
    Reiter's syndrome and reactive arthritis (Salmonella, Yersinia)
    Arthritis associated with inflammatory bowel disease (ulcerative
        colitis and regional ileitis)
    Behcet's syndrome   ⎫ Not described
    Whipple's disease   ⎭

Involvement of the spine and sacro-iliac joints to a greater or lesser degree is the common factor. When this occurs, there is a high incidence of HLA B27 positivity on tissue typing. Peripheral arthritis varies and is usually most obvious in psoriatic arthritis. Clinical overlap sometimes occurs among members of this group (e.g. between psoriatic arthritis and Reiter's syndrome, and between ankylosing spondylitis and the arthritis associated with inflammatory bowel disease). Ocular inflammation is common to a number of these entities, as is evidence of bowel disease. Features of one disease may be seen in other members of the group, and this concept of overlap is an important one.

ANKYLOSING SPONDYLITIS

Typically this occurs in young men, usually starting in the third decade of life. It is an inflammatory condition affecting the spine, sacro-iliac joints and sometimes, especially in the younger patient, peripheral joints. There is a strong association with the histocompatibility antigen HLA B27. Peripheral joint involvement has been said to occur in up to 60 per cent of patients. The large joints (shoulders and hips) are the most commonly affected, but in the young patient (say between 12 and 20) a more florid peripheral picture may characterise the presentation with the axial features only becoming predominant at a later stage. In the older male, however, there may be no evidence of arthritis apart from the back. In a small number of cases, peripheral arthritis may become apparent after many years of spinal involvement (in some cases this is due to rheumatoid arthritis occurring in addition to the spondylitis, i.e. there are two diseases present, but it is believed that there may be a form of ankylosing spondylitis associated with the late onset of peripheral arthropathy as part of the disease).

Aetiology

There is a genetic predisposition for the disease as demonstrated by the finding of HLA B27 antigen in over 90 per cent of patients. However, some 7 per cent of the normal population are also B27-positive indicating that there must be an environmental factor to trigger the disease in susceptible individuals. In this respect there has been some evidence to suggest abnormalities in the intestinal bacterial flora of patients suffering from ankylosing spondylitis and this could be the source of an initiating factor.

Some 50 per cent of offspring will also carry the HLA B27 antigen but only one in five will develop the disease.

Pathology

There is involvement of synovium, articular capsule and ligaments where attached to bone. Peripheral joint changes are similar to those seen in rheumatoid arthritis, i.e. a non-specific synovitis, but there may be subtle differences such that joint destruction and erosion are not so severe in ankylosing spondylitis.

Inflammation at the site of attachment of ligaments to bone is known as *enthesopathy* and is characteristic of ankylosing spondylitis. It occurs especially in the spine and around the pelvis resulting in tufting of bone often along the iliac crests and from the femoral tuberosities as well as the spine.

As a result of the inflammatory change in the spine, reactive bone formation occurs and bridging takes place between the vertebral bodies, usually from the edge of one body to that of the next along the outer layers of the disc; this is known as marginal syndesmophyte formation. Less commonly the syndesmophytes grow beyond the opposite vertebral rim to lie alongside the vertebral body (non-marginal syndesmophytes). Anterior and posterior longitudinal spinal ligaments are also involved, the end result being spinal fusion (bamboo-spine) (Fig. 17/1). Any number, or all, of the vertebrae may be involved except perhaps for the atlanto-axial junction where subluxation may occur (Fig. 17/2). A common early site for syndesmophyte formation is around the dorso-lumbar region.

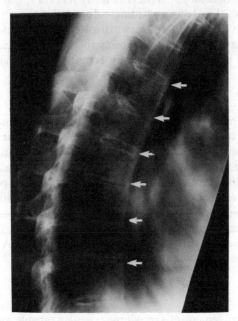

Fig. 17/1 Radiograph showing bony fusion in ankylosing spondylitis

Changes in the sacro-iliac joints eventually lead to fusion. Other changes may be found in the symphysis pubis (erosion) and the manubrio-sternal joint. Ankylosis of costovertebral joints results in a grossly diminished respiratory excursion.

With the exception of atlanto-axial subluxation, neurological sequelae are rare until late in the disease. After years of ankylosis, however, stress fractures may occur, usually starting in the posterior arch and sometimes passing through the disc space. If severe and acute, pain and neurological abnormalities may be obvious at the beginning, but often it is a slow process, the small fracture in the posterior arch developing into a pseudarthrosis. Such an event should be suspected in a patient with long-standing ankylosis if there is a recurrence of pain after years of asymptomatic disease. Isotope scanning and tomography should identify the lesion.

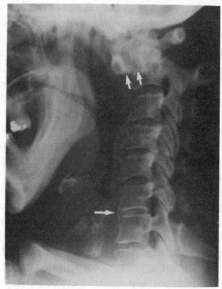

Fig. 17/2 Radiograph showing atlanto-axial subluxation in ankylosing spondylitis. *Note* anterior calcification

It has been said that the disease is much more common in men than in women (surveys varying from 9:1 to 4:1) but of late it has been suggested that it is much under-diagnosed in women. Despite the latter claim, in clinical practice there is still a marked male preponderance. Perhaps in women it is a milder disease and takes longer to develop. Whereas rheumatoid arthritis may be a relatively recent disease, ankylosing spondylitis has existed for thousands of years.

Signs and symptoms

The onset of ankylosing spondylitis is often insidious. Low back pain is the dominant symptom and is associated with stiffness. Occasionally pain occurs first in other parts of the back, or the patient may present with sciatic-type pain. In the young, peripheral joints may be the first affected. Not infrequently, the patient seeks medical advice at a stage when extensive back involvement has already occurred, often with postural deformity. Pain at sites of tendon insertion may be a problem (e.g. the heel and pelvic girdle). Less commonly, iritis may be the presenting feature. The back symptoms are made worse by resting and improved by mild exercise. Morning stiffness is common.

Loss of the normal lumbar lordosis is one of the first signs although there may be spinal stiffness due to muscle spasm. Eventually bony ankylosis leads to a fixed back all too often with a dorsal kyphos. The head appears to be pushed forwards; there is rounding of the shoulders; diminished distance between the lower costal cage and iliac crests antero-laterally; and a need to stand with hips and knees flexed in order to see forwards (see Fig. 17/4). Early, it will be noticed that the skin does not stretch over the lumbar interspinal spaces when the patient bends forwards. Movement can be gauged by placing one's fingers on the spinous processes of successive vertebrae and noting how much separation occurs when the patient tries to flex. Lateral flexion should also be checked since this is impaired in ankylosing spondylitis but not in the case of prolapsed discs. Various methods of measuring limitation have been used. Finger-tip to floor distance and occiput to wall distance are no longer thought to be of much value. The Schober indices of forward and lateral flexion may be helpful (see p. 262). Chest expansion is usually measured and found to be diminished. In an attempt to compensate, there is increased diaphragmatic movement and a ratio between chest expansion and diaphragmatic movement may be of more value than the former alone. Spondylograms are still requested (see p. 356).

Pain is often elicited when pressure is applied to bony points around the pelvis and sometimes with pressure on the manubrio-sternal angle. Stressing the sacro-iliac joints can also result in pain during the early stages of the disease in the presence of sacro-iliitis.

Course

The disease may abort at any stage. Dorso-lumbar and sacro-iliac involvement is more common than total spinal fusion.

Back pain is the most obvious symptom. This may continue for many years but it is not uncommon for the symptoms to settle and remain in abeyance for 10 years or more. There may then be a return of pain and it is then that the possibility of fracture and pseudarthrosis must be considered.

The eventual posture will depend upon the degree of spinal fusion and the success or otherwise of physiotherapy and postural exercises.

Complications

There are a number of complications, the most common being iritis. Inflammatory eye disease occurs in 20 per cent of patients and may even be the presenting feature of the disease. Urgent treatment with topical corticosteroids is required.

Neurological involvement occurs either as a result of atlanto-axial subluxation or fractures as previously described.

Cardiovascular problems occur infrequently (e.g. aortic incompetence).

Impaired respiratory excursion is counter-balanced by increased diaphragmatic movement such that lung function may be almost normal. Occasionally apical fibrosis occurs but does not cause much of a problem.

As with rheumatoid arthritis, amyloidosis causing renal failure may be a long-term result.

Investigations

Haematological abnormalities are mostly non-specific and of little help. The ESR may be raised, and similarly changes in plasma viscosity and C-reactive protein occur. Tissue typing is not routinely carried out. It must be stressed that a positive result for HLA B27 is *not* diagnostic; however, occasionally where a diagnosis is proving difficult a negative result would make one look very carefully for an alternative explanation for symptoms.

Radiological changes occur in the sacro-iliac joints (erosions and sclerosis), but these can be difficult to interpret in the young patient during the early stage of the disease. The lumbar vertebrae become 'squared' losing their anterior concavity as seen on a lateral view. Syndesmophyte formation is often first seen at the dorso-lumbar junction but may eventually involve most of the spine. Calcification of the anterior and posterior ligaments and fusion of the posterior facet joints are also demonstrable in well-established cases. Tufting of bone is common along the iliac crests, inferior pubic rami and around the femoral tuberosities.

Isotope scanning using technetium may be helpful in determining the site and degree of inflammation and may also be of value in detecting pseudarthroses.

Treatment

Not all patients require much in the way of analgesic therapy but none the less most seek pain relief at some stage. Simple analgesics or non-steroidal anti-inflammatory drugs are commonly prescribed. It is usually stated that these should be sufficient but there are a few patients whose pain is unrelieved by such drugs. In the past, radiotherapy was used in such cases but it is now recognised that blood dyscrasias can result from such treatment. Very occasionally radiotherapy may be considered for the treatment of a *localised* area when pain is *very* severe. Again, the use of corticosteroids is not favoured although a short, reducing course is unlikely to be harmful and may tide a patient over an acute exacerbation.

The disease-modifying drugs (gold, penicillamine, etc) have not proved helpful in ankylosing spondylitis.

Physiotherapy is aimed at maintaining back posture. Apart from this, it is characteristic of the disease that patients find their symptoms improve with exercise. Regular exercise programmes throughout the day are essential but can only be carried out within the limits of pain. Hydrotherapy is excellent and the patient should be encouraged to go swimming regularly providing he does so only in warm water. Beds should be firm and only one pillow used.

Patients must be assessed frequently. Deterioration in measurements may indicate the need for hospital admission, a short course of steroids, reappraisal of exercise programmes, etc. The possibility of hip disease causing further problems with posture must always be borne in mind. Flexion deformities of hips are common.

In the acute stage, rest may be essential. Relief of pain has to be achieved, after which a programme of exercises instituted to maintain posture and mobility and prevent deformity occurring. At the same time attention must be paid to conditions both at home and at work. Encouragement is required at all times and many are helped by joining a society composed of patients with ankylosing spondylitis. An explanation of the disease, the management and the prognosis will do much to allay fears and increase the prospect of total co-operation by the patient.

Occasionally surgery may have to be considered. In the case of severe hip disease, total joint replacement will relieve pain and make the quality of life better. With a fixed kyphotic back, however, the patient will still walk and stand with hips and knees flexed and, unfortunately, the hip flexion may become fixed due to the tendency to form new bone around the prosthesis. Spinal osteotomy has been carried out in some cases but there is the danger of causing neurological damage. Fusion of a pseudarthrosis may also be considered, and atlanto-axial dislocation may call for fusion. In the latter two cases splintage may be all that is required and these are the only occasions when immobilisation may be considered.

The patient with a sedentary job has more chance (and quite a good one at that) of staying at work until retirement than a patient doing manual work. The DRO may be able to help. Attention to posture at work is of the utmost importance, and prolonged sitting should be avoided.

PHYSIOTHERAPY

Assessment of the patient with ankylosing spondylitis is essential before an appropriate programme for the management of the disabilities resulting from the disease can be drawn up. Movement in affected joints must be retained and the patient needs to be taught the importance of exercise for them. He must be totally committed to a daily exercise programme for the duration of the disease and beyond in order to minimise the effect of the disabilities caused by the progressive spinal ankylosis and associated loss of thoracic mobility. Most frequently the patient will be treated as an outpatient. He will require periods of admission during acute phases or when surgical intervention to reduce the effect of disability is advocated, for example the insertion of prosthetic replacements for peripheral joints.

Assessment

As the spinal joints are principally affected the assessment will concentrate on this area taking into account the patient's general posture, spinal position, spinal mobility, thoracic mobility and respiratory function. It will also be necessary to identify any involvement of peripheral joints and to assess function.

GENERAL POSTURE

To assess posture adequately the patient should be observed in standing and sitting. As spinal mobility decreases and the lumbar curve is lost the thoracic curve gradually becomes exaggerated. Hips and knees may be flexed to maintain an acceptable distribution of body-weight. Loss of the cervical curve causes the patient to hyperextend the atlanto-occipital joint and protrusion of the jaw is apparent. Observation from different positions will enable any deviation from the normal to be noted.

SPINAL POSTURE

The most significant deviations from a normal spinal posture result from the loss of the secondary spinal curves with the elimination of first the lumbar and, later, the cervical lordosis. The thoracic curves are exaggerated and the patient's spine becomes progressively rounded. As lateral deviations are comparatively rare, the most

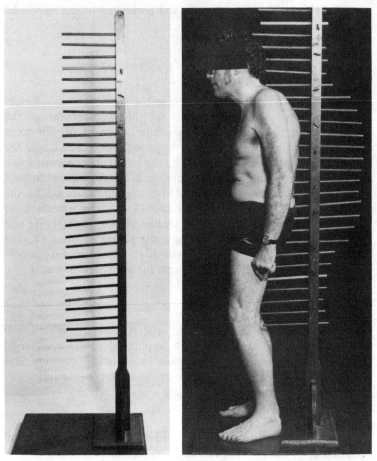

Fig. 17/3(*Left*) Spondylometer

Fig. 17/4 (*Right*) Patient with ankylosing spondylitis being measured with a spondylometer. *Note* the typical posture

appropriate method of recording spinal posture is the spondylograph. *Method*: The patient stands on the base of the spondylometer (Fig. 17/3), close to the upright in the most erect posture he can assume, heels should touch the base of the upright (Fig. 17/4). Rods spaced at 5cm (2in) intervals on the upright are adjusted to make light skin contact over the vertebral spines and locked in position. Measurements of the patient's overall height, level of the vertex, seventh

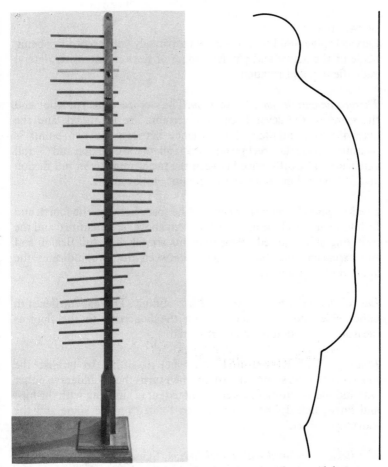

Fig. 17/5 (*Left*)   Outline of the patient's posture on the spondylometer

Fig. 17/6 (*Right*)   Spondylograph trace of patient shown in 17/4

cervical vertebra, posterior superior iliac spines and the head of the fibula are taken. The distance of protrusion of the rods from the upright is measured and these readings are transferred to graph paper thus plotting the anteroposterior curves of the patient's spine (Figs. 17/5, 17/6). Spondylographs should be plotted annually and they provide a record of progress of the disease. Serial clinical photographs may be used to augment the spondylographs if facilities are available.

SPINAL MOBILITY

Cervical spine mobility is measured separately with recordings being made of the active and passive ranges of flexion, extension, lateral (side) flexion and rotation.

Thoraco-lumbar flexion and extension: The sacrococcygeal junction and the spine of the seventh cervical vertebra are identified, and the overlying skin marked. The distance between the two points is measured in (1) the erect position, (2) full forward flexion and (3) full extension. The difference between the measurements in full flexion and full extension indicates the amount of movement.

Lumbar spine flexion and extension: The space between the fourth and fifth lumbar vertebrae and a point 10cm above, are identified and the overlying skin marked. Measurements are taken in full flexion and full extension and the difference between the two indicates the amount of movement.

Lateral flexion: This is measured in standing. The patient flexes to either side and the distance from the fingertips to the floor is measured. Rotation must be prevented.

Rotation: This is measured either (1) in sitting to localise the movement to the spine; the patient then turns the shoulders to either side and the amount of movement noted; or (2) in lying with the hips and knees flexed; the pelvis is then rotated on the spine and the movement noted.

Hip flexion combined with spinal flexion: Standing erect, the patient then flexes forward allowing his hands to reach straight downwards. The distance between the fingertips and the floor is measured. This movement has a functional purpose for the patient, e.g. sitting on a chair, going up and down steps, and being able to reach his feet to put on shoes and socks.

Assessment of peripheral joint mobility should include careful examination of all joints particularly the hips, knees, shoulders and temporomandibular joints. The active and passive ranges of movement should be measured and recorded.

ASSESSMENT OF RESPIRATORY FUNCTION

The costovertebral joints are affected at an early stage with a resultant effect on thoracic movement and respiratory function. Regular recordings of chest expansion are made at two levels: the xiphoid process (7th rib) and the nipple (4th rib). The measurements should be noted in full expiration and full inspiration, as well as the difference between them. Vital capacity (VC), peak flow and forced expiratory volume in one second (FEV_1) are taken regularly. As thoracic mobility is lost, more reliance is placed on diaphragmatic breathing and, in advanced cases when all other respiratory movement is lost, patients may be wholly dependent on this type of breathing.

Treatment

Although ankylosing spondylitis is a crippling disease with severe predictable deformity and loss of mobility, patients are able, with appropriate management, to retain a high level of functional independence. Physical treatment aims to retain spinal mobility, minimise spinal deformity when mobility is lost, relieve pain and improve endurance. This is achieved mainly through active exercise.

As already mentioned for the programme to succeed, the patient must know the purpose of each exercise and be committed to a daily routine which includes a considerable amount of activity. Hospital sessions are in *addition* to the home programme which must be taught carefully and checked frequently by the physiotherapists. Exercises for the home programme should be simple, specific and require little or no apparatus for their successful performance. They will include mobilising exercises for the spine, hips and thoracic cage, posture correction and activities designed to improve muscle endurance.

Attendance in the department enables the physiotherapist to check the patient's condition, assess the validity of the home programme and provide an additional range of treatment. Several patients may be treated together as they usually respond well to group work.

MAINTENANCE OF MOBILITY

Movement of affected joints will retard the rate of ankylosis, but will not prevent it occurring. It is most important that all joints are moved daily through their fullest possible range of movement to gain maximal delay of the ankylosing process. Maitland mobilisation techniques can be used when joints are in a state of exacerbation or quiescence to free movement within the existing range. Although these techniques can be used on any joint, they are particularly valuable in treating the facet joints of the spine and the costovertebral joints; the grade and type of mobilisation is determined by the degree of disease activity. Vigorous active exercises are performed wherever possible and it is advantageous to use a medium that supports body-weight thus allowing muscular effort to be devoted solely to producing movement. Support of the lower part of the body in axial suspension centred over the lumbar spine will allow flexion, extension or lateral flexion to be achieved by swinging to either side from a side-lying or lying position. Similarly hip extension and abduction can be encouraged.

Pool therapy is useful in encouraging joint mobility; the warmth of the water effectively reduces protective muscle guarding thereby enabling the patient to make full use of available joint ranges by formal exercise or free swimming. Swimming, particularly the breast stroke, is encouraged; this will not only improve endurance, but will also encourage extension of the spine and mobilisation of the hip and shoulder girdle. Bad Ragaz patterns for arms, legs and trunk are effective in restoring mobility.

Exercises to improve movements of the thoracic cage, and breathing exercises to improve the respiratory excursion will be required.

MINIMISING OF DEFORMITY

When ankylosis occurs the patient will be at a disadvantage if his spinal posture is markedly flexed. Early and continued attention to good positioning can reduce the tendency to assume a flexed position. Sleeping on a firm mattress should be encouraged, with the use of only one pillow to help retain the extended spinal position. Adjustment of the height of chairs and work surfaces will help to reduce the tendency to stoop. At all times the patient must actively retain an erect posture. A period of prone or supine lying each day will preserve hip extension, but the wearing of spinal supports or prolonged bed rest is discouraged as extensor muscles will weaken and the extended position will not be retained.

RELIEF OF PAIN

Pain is not a significant feature but it can be present when joints are in a phase of exacerbation. Relief of pain and associated protective muscle spasm can be achieved by applications of heat. Hot packs, radiant heat and short wave diathermy have been found effective, but short wave diathermy may aggravate symptoms when inflammation is present in the joints.

MAINTENANCE OF MUSCLE POWER AND IMPROVEMENT OF ENDURANCE

Although ankylosing spondylitis is an inflammatory disease of joints, muscle weakness is not a significant feature, therefore an increase of muscle power is not an essential part of the exercise programme.

Muscles will be strengthened by the increase in exercise taken by the patient and so this is an incidental benefit of the treatment programme. Muscle power is retained by working against maximal resistance for a short time, the resistance being offered manually or mechanically through springs, weights or water. Endurance is improved by working muscles against submaximal resistance for progressively longer times. Patients are best treated in groups in the gymnasium or hydrotherapy pool. Group treatments foster improved motivation and competition between patients, which, in turn, encourages more sustained effort. It is economical on time for the physiotherapist can effectively treat several patients simultaneously. Swimming is encouraged, particularly the breast stroke and the front crawl.

These patients are quite able to undertake a full day programme in the physiotherapy department which should include group activities, individual exercise against spring or other mechanical resistance, posture correction, games, circuits and pool therapy.

PSORIATIC ARTHRITIS

It is estimated that between 1 and 2 per cent of the population suffers from psoriasis, though this may be an underestimate, for psoriasis can be so mild that even the patient is unaware of it. Rheumatoid arthritis is also a common disease and both conditions may occur in the same patient. Apart from this, a sero-negative arthritis, differing from rheumatoid arthritis is also recognised in association with psoriasis.

Heredity is an important factor in psoriasis and in psoriatic arthritis. In at least a third of cases there is a family history of psoriasis. Certain HLA antigens other than B27 are frequent. When sacro-iliitis and spinal involvement occur as part of the arthritis, the HLA B27 is commonly found, but not quite as frequently as in ankylosing spondylitis.

Patients suffering from psoriasis may develop axial changes of mild ankylosing spondylitis. On the other hand there seems to be a relation between psoriasis and Reiter's syndrome, and indeed the pustular forms of psoriasis may be indistinguishable from the skin lesions of Reiter's. Even allowing for these associations there remain a group of psoriatic patients with an arthritis which would seem to be related to their psoriasis.

Clinical features

The following clinical groups can be distinguished:
1. Patients in whom distal interphalangeal joint involvement is a major feature. This is often associated with the nail changes of psoriasis (Fig. 17/7).
2. Patients with a severely deforming arthritis, sometimes known as arthritis mutilans, and giving rise to reabsorption of phalanges in hands and feet such that the soft tissues seem to telescope ('opera-glass' hands) This is a rare form.
3. A sero-negative polyarthritis difficult to distinguish from rheumatoid arthritis but usually less extensive and symmetrical, with a better prognosis, absence of rheumatoid factor and a tendency to more marked flexor tendon sheath involvement (e.g. 'sausage' fingers).
4. An oligo-articular (few joints) or even monarticular disease.
5. A spondylitic arthritis. This resembles, and may be indistinguishable from, ankylosing spondylitis. At the other end of the scale sacro-iliitis may be the only feature of axial involvement.

Features of one group may be present in the others.

The skin lesions of psoriasis may be mild or extensive and occur in different forms, the commonest being a dry scaly eruption often

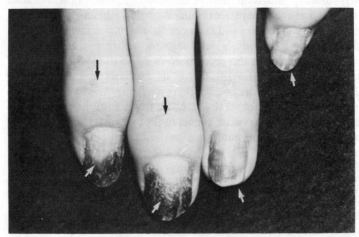

Fig. 17/7 Pitting and discolouration of the finger nails due to psoriasis. *Note* the distal interphalangeal arthropathy

beginning on the extensor aspects of the elbows and knees. Scalp lesions are common and may be dismissed as dandruff. They appear typically along the hair line and behind the ears. In the absence of obvious lesions a careful look in the navel and between the buttock cleft may reveal small patches of psoriasis. Skin changes usually precede arthritis but in about 20 per cent of cases the reverse is true and more rarely the two occur simultaneously.

Nail changes are much more closely related to the presence of arthritis than are the skin lesions and may occur without the latter. There is a greater tendency for them to be recognised either at the same time as, or following, the onset of arthritis. Pitting is a characteristic feature but is not specific (Fig. 17/7). Onycholysis (separation of the distal nail bed) often with a brownish discolouration just proximal to the region of lifting is more specific.

Apart from the uncommon mutilans group, the prognosis of the arthritis is usually good.

Investigations

There are changes in the non-specific indicators of inflammation (ESR etc). The rheumatoid factor test is negative. Tissue typing is not of sufficient value yet to use as a routine investigation. It has been said that the uric acid is sometimes raised due to the excessive cell turnover in the skin lesions but this seems not to be the rule.

The radiological changes are similar to those seen in rheumatoid arthritis with a few differences. Distal interphalangeal erosion is not seen in rheumatoid arthritis. In psoriatic arthritis, dissolution of the terminal phalanges may occur and there is often pencilling of the distal part of the middle phalanx such that it comes to a sharp point (Fig. 17/8). Periostitis is more common and the appearance of sacro-iliitis with or without spinal syndesmophytes is something not seen in rheumatoid arthritis. Paravertebral calcification may be found.

Treatment

The management of skin and joint changes are usually quite separate though a few approaches supposedly improve both.

SKIN
Topical therapy includes one or more of the following:
(1) coal tar derivatives; (2) dithranol; (3) corticosteroid preparations; (4) ultraviolet irradiation; and (5) salicylic acid.

Preparations of coal tar with or without salicylic acid are useful in

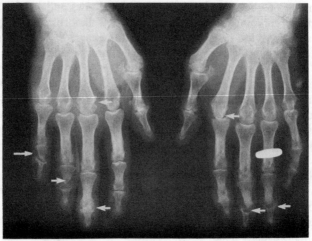

Fig. 17/8 Radiograph of hands affected by psoriatic arthritis

some cases and may be combined with the use of ultraviolet irradiation. If this is not successful, dithranol, (0.05% increasing to 2%) may be used but has to be applied carefully and exactly to the lesions as it is a skin irritant. It is better used for larger plaques on trunk and limbs, avoiding flexor creases. It may be combined with tar baths and ultraviolet irradiation for a three-week period, preferably with the patient in hospital. Corticosteroids may be used for smaller patches and for lesions around the face, ears and neck. Various shampoos are available for the scalp.

In severe cases, systemic therapy is required. Methotrexate can be given by mouth once a week but regular blood checks are required and there is a real danger of hepatic damage, especially if used long term. Methotrexate sometimes has a beneficial effect on the arthritis as well as the psoriasis. Other newer drugs (e.g. hydroxyurea and etretinate) are currently being assessed, and, of late, the use of long wave ultraviolet irradiation in conjunction with a psoralen drug has aroused much interest (see *Cash's Textbook of General Medical and Surgical Conditions for Physiotherapists*).

Nail disease is difficult to treat. Rarely radiotherapy has been used. The frequently associated distal interphalangeal joint involvement may respond to intra-articular corticosteroids.

JOINTS

Treatment resembles that used in rheumatoid arthritis. However, antimalarial drugs occasionally make the skin lesions worse and sudden change in systemic corticosteroid therapy can also result in an exacerbation. Despite the dangers of rash with gold therapy, it is not contra-indicated in psoriatic arthritis. Indeed, it is the most useful disease-modifying drug in this condition. Azathioprine has sometimes proved helpful. Unless there is infection, surgery is not contra-indicated. Psoriatic skin heals well.

REITER'S SYNDROME AND REACTIVE ARTHRITIS

Reiter's syndrome is a sero-negative asymmetrical arthritis with one or more of the following: urethritis, balanitis, skin lesions, (keratoderma blennorrhagica), oral ulceration and conjunctivitis. It is usually a sexually acquired disease though confusion arises when a similar picture occurs following bowel infections (*Yersinia, Salmonella, Shigella,* etc). Such a picture has been referred to as 'post-dysenteric Reiter's disease' and also 'reactive arthritis'. Features may be indistinguishable from Reiter's syndrome and although some patients may clearly fall into one or other group, others do not and a differentiation between Reiter's syndrome and reactive arthritis may be artificial. In both cases there is a strong association with the presence of HLA B27 or closely related antigens. It is estimated that there is a 1 in 5 chance of a B27-positive individual developing either ankylosing spondylitis or a reactive arthropathy. The situation is fascinating and highlights the relationship between disease, genetic make-up and environmental factors.

In the case of non-specific (i.e. non-gonococcal) urethritis, attempts to isolate an organism have not been uniformly successful but numerous authors claim to have isolated *Chlamydia* species. A further source of infection relating to the genito-urinary tract may be from the prostate.

Thus we are aware of a number of infections involving the genito-urinary tract and bowel which may, in susceptible individuals, be followed by Reiter's syndrome or reactive arthritis. The possibility of a similar sequence of events occurring in ankylosing spondylitis must be remembered.

Clinical features

Sexually acquired form: This is a relatively common disease particularly affecting young men. It is rare over the age of 50. The incidence in women is difficult to determine, for it is either under-diagnosed or much less common.

Urethritis and, after a latent period of a few weeks, arthritis are the commonest features occurring in over 90 per cent of patients. The urethritis may be minimal and easily forgotten, but usually there is a discharge, often with dysuria, which can persist for a long period. (In the female the urethritis and/or cervicitis is usually symptomless.)

The arthritis is often acute and usually involves the lower limb joints. It may be monarticular, involving knee or hind foot most frequently. If more than one joint is involved the arthritis, unlike rheumatoid arthritis, is asymmetrical. Plantar fasciitis and tendonitis, especially around the ankle and in the back are common causes of pain and tenderness. Dactylitis ('sausage toe') with diffuse swelling, redness and pain is a feature of the disease. The arthritis may settle but usually recurs weeks, months or even years later. In other cases it is persistent and chronic. As with other diseases related to HLA B27 positivity, sacro-iliitis can exist along with varying degrees of spondylitis. Although the back changes may mimic ankylosing spondylitis, there is perhaps a greater incidence of 'skip' lesions in Reiter's syndrome. About one-third of patients with the disease and positive tissue-typing will develop back changes and it especially occurs in those with severe and recurrent or persistent disease.

Conjunctivitis is present in approximately 60 per cent of cases. It can be very mild and transient. Occasionally a more severe uveitis leading to impaired vision is present in those patients with severe and recurrent arthritis.

Twenty-five per cent of patients demonstrate muco-cutaneous lesions with stomatitis, balanitis and keratoderma blennorrhagica. The oral ulcers occur on the palate, tongue, buccal mucosa and sometimes the lips. They settle spontaneously. Balanitis takes the form of small vesicles which rupture to form ulcerations of the glans penis. They may coalesce (circinate balanitis). If infection supervenes the changes can be persistent. Keratoderma is seen most frequently on the soles of the feet, although rarely can involve many areas of the body, especially flexor creases (Fig. 17/9). The initial lesions are vesicular but become hyperkeratotic, hard and sometimes horn-like. Clinically the changes may be impossible to distinguish from psoriasis. As with some other features of the disease the skin lesions usually settle but may be recurrent or persistent. Nail involvement is less common but again relates to the accumulation of hard keratotic material, this time under the nail which is thus lifted up. The nail itself takes on a dirty yellow colour and is thickened.

Several of the features of Reiter's syndrome are seen to be transient

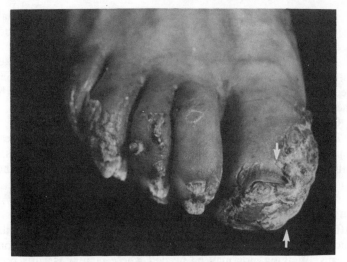

Fig. 17/9 Keratoderma blennorrhagica and nail changes in
Reiter's syndrome

but possibly recurrent. The most persistent feature which gives rise to long-term problems is the arthropathy. At one time it was thought that prognosis was good but it is now appreciated that for many this is not so and only in very few cases do all the manifestations of the disease settle. Even if they do, recurrence is always a possibility.

Laboratory investigations are not helpful in making a diagnosis. Radiographs are likely to be normal in the early stages. Periostitis is not uncommon. New bone formation in the form of a calcaneal spur at the origin of the plantar fascia is common but not specific for the disease. Eventually the changes of sacro-iliitis and spondylitis (usually not complete resulting in 'skip' lesions) can be demonstrated in about 30 per cent of cases.

Management

The arthritis of Reiter's syndrome is usually acute and severe, necessitating splintage and possibly bed rest. Non-steroidal anti-inflammatory drugs should be used but may not be sufficient to control the pain. In such circumstances a short reducing course of corticosteroids may be used and this is often the quickest way of controlling the symptoms. Long-term corticosteroid therapy is not recommended. Intra-articular corticosteroids can also be used. When the acute stage is over, mobilisation can begin.

The disease can be aggressive and severe, and in such cases trials, using methotrexate and azathioprine, are in progress indicating how severe the problem can be.

The urethritis is often treated with tetracycline. This is more likely to clear the sepsis associated with balanitis. Other antibiotics have been used (e.g. lincomycin) but there is no evidence to suggest that they have a role in treatment.

Ocular lesions may require the use of topical steroids.

Patients may be very sensitive about the nature of the disease especially when it is consequent upon extra-marital relationships. A full understanding is required and it can be difficult to gain their confidence.

PHYSIOTHERAPY

Affected joints are treated by free active exercise to maintain mobility and improve muscle power following pain relief by conventional means. Walking aids may be needed where plantar fasciitis poses problems of locomotion. Long-standing cases resemble ankylosing spondylitis and should be managed in the same way.

REACTIVE ARTHRITIS AND 'POST-DYSENTERIC REITER'S SYNDROME'

In this form the sex discrepancy is not so obvious and the age limits are much wider. Several members of the same family are sometimes affected. In many cases it is possible to isolate an organism. The management is as for Reiter's syndrome.

There is still confusion about terminology but it seems reasonable to consider this group with Reiter's syndrome. In practice these patients develop an *arthropathy* similar to that seen in Reiter's syndrome but the majority do not manifest the other changes.

ARTHRITIS ASSOCIATED WITH INFLAMMATORY BOWEL DISEASE (ENTEROPATHIC ARTHRITIS)

Ulcerative colitis and Crohn's disease (regional ileitis) are both inflammatory conditions of the bowel, and can be difficult to differentiate. Ulcerative colitis tends to be diffuse, whereas Crohn's disease is more of a granulomatous condition. Both are associated with bouts of severe diarrhoea, often with blood and mucus, anaemia, weight loss and general ill-health.

In ulcerative colitis the disease is confined to the large bowel whereas the lesions of Crohn's disease can occur anywhere in the gastro-intestinal tract.

There are two forms of arthritis which may be associated with these diseases. The first is a peripheral arthritis (often called enteropathic arthritis), and the second an axial arthritis resembling ankylosing spondylitis. The peripheral arthritis is often monarticular, and its activity relates closely to the activity of the bowel disease. The spondylitis will progress in a fashion totally unrelated to bowel disease activity. Thus treatment of the bowel lesion will improve the peripheral arthritis but not the spondylitis. The incidence of sacro-iliitis is 14 per cent and of spondylitis 6 per cent. The peripheral arthritis is sometimes self-limiting but obviously potentially recurrent.

Because of the extent of the lesions in Crohn's disease, surgery has a limited role. In ulcerative colitis, colectomy, which may be carried out to eliminate complications such as massive haemorrhage and the late development of malignancy, results in complete resolution of the peripheral joint problem (though the arthritis is *not* an indication for bowel surgery).

Treating the bowel lesion improves the enteropathic arthritis and the treatment used may also be helpful directly (e.g. corticosteroids, sulphasalazine). Apart from this, if required, non-steroidal anti-inflammatory drugs, local steroid injections and active exercises to avoid contractures can be used.

There is an increased frequency of HAL B27 in those patients with spondylitis and bowel disease but this is not as great as in ankylosing spondylitis, (approximately 70 per cent in ulcerative colitis and 50 per cent in Crohn's disease.)

BIBLIOGRAPHY

Goff, B. and Rose, G.K. (1964). The use of a modified spondylometer in the treatment of ankylosing spondylitis. *Rheumatism*, **20**, 3, 63–6.
See also Bibliography page 409.

Chapter 18

Miscellaneous Inflammatory Arthropathies

by D.J. WARD, MB, FRCP

and M.E. TIDSWELL, BA, MCSP, ONC, DipTP

Under this general heading may be considered the crystal arthropathies; diffuse connective tissue diseases; polymyalgia rheumatica; erythema nodosum; Sjögren's syndrome; haemophilic arthritis; and arthritis related to infection and malignancy. They are rare by comparison with rheumatoid arthritis and osteoarthritis, but physiotherapists may encounter patients with them and be asked to treat them.

CRYSTAL ARTHRITIS

This term relates to gout, pseudo-gout and hydroxyapatite arthropathy.

Gout

Gout is characterised by one or more of the following:
1. A rise in the serum level of uric acid.
2. Attacks of acute arthritis, tenosynovitis or bursitis related to the deposition of urate crystals.
3. The presence of tophi – deposits of urate occurring in the vicinity of peripheral joints and characteristically in the pinna of the ear. There may be an associated chronic arthritis.
4. Renal disease.
5. Renal calculi.

The sex ratio male/female is 6:1. Although the finding of a raised serum uric acid level is characteristic it is not always present. Uric acid levels vary even in gouty subjects and a normal value does not exclude the disease. It may be necessary to have serial estimations carried out if the diagnosis is suspected. Again, there are many factors which may influence the level of uric acid in the blood, e.g. age, sex, body bulk, diet, drugs (especially diuretics and low doses of aspirin), alcohol, other diseases (e.g. of the thyroid) and genetic. While it is far too simple just to relate gout to a raised uric acid level, there is no doubt that the disease is caused by an excess of urates either due to increased production or decreased excretion. There are rare forms related to enzymatic abnormalities (e.g. Lesch-Nyhan syndrome) and these conditions are usually associated with other clinical patterns such as neurological disease. Here, we are concerned with the common form of gout, not the exotic.

CLINICAL

Acute gout: This is a painful, acute condition. In over 70 per cent of cases the attack involves the metatarsophalangeal joint of the big toe, which becomes red, hot, swollen and exquisitely tender such that even bed clothes resting on it result in agony. Acute episodes may occur spontaneously or, in susceptible individuals, be precipitated by factors such as trauma, surgery, systemic illness, starvation diets, gourmandism, alcohol excess and drugs. Diuretics may commonly provoke an acute attack of gout and, ironically, so may the drugs used to treat the disease over a long-term period (e.g. uricosuric drugs and allopurinol). Other joints which may be involved in an acute attack include the ankle, knee, hands and wrists. The presentation may resemble septic arthritis. Such episodes are rare in the male before puberty or in the female before the menopause.

After a period of a few days the symptoms and signs usually settle with desquamation of the skin overlying the affected joint. Such episodes may or may not recur. If they do, then it may be at intervals of weeks, months or years and the frequency determines the need or otherwise for long-term drug treatment. Following recurrent attacks, there is the danger of chronic gout developing with loss of cartilage and bone and the deposition of urates (tophi). Considerable disability results and osteoarthritis is inevitably superimposed.

Acute gout may be confused with infection (commonly), trauma, episodic rheumatoid arthritis or another crystal arthropathy (e.g. due to pyrophosphate crystals – pseudo-gout).

Chronic gout: This is almost always the sequela of many acute attacks of gout but there can be problems in diagnosis. Chronic gout of the small joints of the hands or feet may masquerade as osteoarthritis especially in elderly women. Deposits of urate (tophi) have to be differentiated from those of fats (xanthomata) and occasionally the chronic tophaceous disease may resemble nodular rheumatoid arthritis. Rheumatoid arthritis and gout rarely occur together in the same patient.

Tophi are nodular thickenings commonly occurring in the vicinity of joints affected by recurrent attacks of acute gout (usually hands and feet) (Fig. 18/1). They may also occur in tendon sheaths, bursae and the cartilage of the ear. Sometimes they simulate infection and present as a discharging lesion.

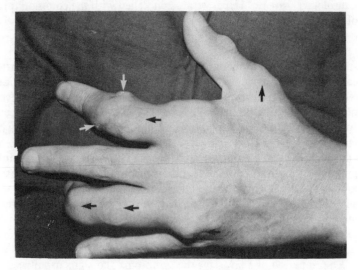

Fig. 18/1 Tophaceous gout. *Note* the sites of previous urate discharge

Renal disease is commonly present although it does not materially affect life expectancy. Renal calculi occur in approximately 10 per cent of patients.

DIAGNOSIS
The clinical picture is often typical with an acute attack involving the first metatarsophalangeal joint (podagra). If it is possible to obtain fluid from an affected joint the diagnosis can be confirmed by the finding of monosodium urate crystals in the fluid as determined by the use of polarising light microscopy. Similarly in chronic gout urates can be identified either from biopsy of a tophus or from the discharge which may result from one. It should be remembered that a raised serum uric acid (hyperuricaemia) can be present without any

symptoms and gout can occasionally occur even though the level is normal. If repetitive estimations are carried out, however, practically all gouty subjects can be shown to have an elevated uric acid level.

The history of acute attacks, the presence of tophi, a developing chronic arthritis and the finding of a raised uric acid level in the serum are the hallmarks of gout. Added to this list must be the occurrence of renal calculi in some 10 per cent of patients. Radiological examination may show characteristic changes if there are associated soft tissue changes due to tophi (Figs. 18/2, 18/3). Joint changes are, however, difficult to differentiate from those of rheumatoid arthritis.

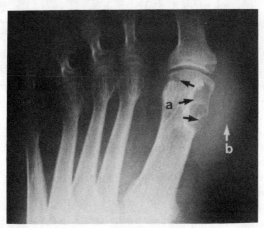

Fig. 18/2   Radiograph of a foot affected by gout. (a) Cystic and erosive change in the region of the first metatarsophalangeal joint. (b) Soft tissue swelling due to a tophus

There is a close relationship between gout, hyperuricaemia, obesity, liver dysfunction (? due to excess alcohol intake), hyperlipaemia (excessive fat levels in the blood), hypertensive and ischaemic heart disease and diabetes mellitus.

TREATMENT
Acute attack: One of the non-steroidal anti-inflammatory drugs described in Chapter 16 should be used. Indomethacin (by mouth or by suppository), diclofenac (by mouth or by injection) or azapropazone are commonly used. Colchicine is an alternative, though diarrhoea is common if treatment is to be effective. Rarely, corticosteroids (systemic or intra-articular) have been used but are seldom necessary. Rest will usually be insisted upon by the patient.

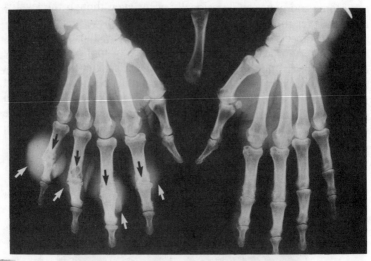

Fig. 18/3 Radiograph of hands affected with gout. *Note* soft tissue lesions (tophi) as well as those in bone and joint

Long-term management: As this is life-long there must be well-defined indications. These are:
1. Recurrent attacks of acute gout (more than two a year).
2. Chronic tophaceous gout.
3. Renal disease.
4. A persistently high uric acid level especially if there is a family history of hypertension.

Allopurinol (Zyloric) is the drug of choice, but should not be started until an acute attack has subsided. It should be used with caution in the presence of severe renal or hepatic disease. It should not be used intermittently for the treatment of acute gouty arthritis. Once started, it should be continued. Paradoxically, it can even precipitate acute gout so that when started, it should be covered by the use of a non-steroidal anti-inflammatory drug for several weeks. Occasionally allopurinol may give rise to a hypersensitivity reaction with rash and, should this occur, the older uricosuric drugs such as probenecid (Benemid) or sulphinpyrazone (Anturan) may be used, though they are usually less effective, especially when renal disease is present.

Pseudo-gout

This is very similar to gout but is due to the deposition of calcium pyrophosphate crystals. It tends to occur in an older age-group than gout and commonly affects knees and wrists. It has to be considered as a possibility if a patient, especially with osteoarthritis, has an acute attack of pain at these sites, and if there is radiological evidence of calcification of the cartilage (chondrocalcinosis) (Fig. 18/4). It can be polyarticular leading to chronic synovitis and gives rise to both acute and chronic arthritis.

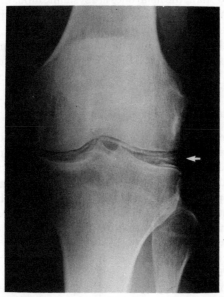

Fig. 18/4 Radiograph of left knee joint showing chondrocalcinosis in pseudo-gout

There are several different forms of the disease: hereditary (especially in Czechoslovaks, Chileans and Dutch); idiopathic (but possibly familial); and associated with various metabolic diseases (hyperparathyroidism, haemochromatosis, and possibly hypothyroidism and diabetes mellitus).

Treatment is similar to that for gout but a search must be made for underlying metabolic disease, and management may well include treatment of osteoarthritis.

Hydroxyapatite crystals are probably related to joint disease more often than is realised, especially osteoarthritis. The crystals can only be recognised by electron microscopy and as yet their role in the development of arthritis has to be determined.

Finally, a crystal arthritis may occasionally result from the injection of microcrystalline corticosteroids.

DIFFUSE CONNECTIVE TISSUE DISEASE

This heading encompasses a number of disorders which often have considerable overlap; the main ones are systemic lupus erythematosus (SLE), systemic sclerosis (scleroderma), dermatomyositis and poly-arteritis nodosum. Syndromes either representing an intermediate disease or with features similar to one of the above include mixed connective tissue disease (MCTD), Wegener's granulomatosis, and polymyositis.

Systemic lupus erythematosus (SLE)

This is a disease of younger women (female to male ratio 10:1). Mild cases may be common but there is a real danger of the condition being incorrectly/over-diagnosed on the basis of laboratory tests. There is a marked immunological response and several different antibodies make their appearance, the commonest being anti-nuclear antibody (ANA) and anti-DNA (deoxyribonucleic acid) antibody. The disease can be drug-induced (e.g. hydralazine).

CLINICAL FEATURES
1. A rash is common. Typically it is the so-called 'butterfly' rash on the face. Skin lesions can be widespread and include alopecia.
2. Arthralgia/arthritis. Erosive change is not common, but deformities can occur and mimic rheumatoid arthritis.
3. Raynaud's phenomenon.
4. Central nervous system disease.
5. Renal disease, which can either be relatively benign or life-threatening.
6. Other lesions affecting the lungs, pleura, etc, and there may be various haematological changes apart from the development of numerous antibodies. These include anaemia related to the disease, sometimes a haemolytic anaemia, low platelet and white cell counts and a raised ESR.

Clinical management tends to be more conservative than it used to be, but non-steroidal anti-inflammatory drugs, corticosteroids and cytotoxic drugs may be indicated. Antimalarial drugs are useful for the skin and joint lesions. Various less well-tried procedures include plasma exchange, bolus high dose intravenous steroid therapy and lymphatic drainage, and are reserved for severe cases.

PHYSIOTHERAPY
The majority of patients with this disease display joint symptoms similar to those present in rheumatoid arthritis with episodes of joint effusion, pain and loss of function. Bone and cartilage destruction is rare, so patients have little residual deformity. Involvement of the flexor tendons of the fingers produces transitory triggering. The physiotherapist should teach the patient how to manage joint symptoms during acute episodes, concentrating on relief of pain, reduction of swelling and improvement of muscle strength.

Generalised muscle tenderness with associated reduction in power and endurance is observed and probably contributes to the lassitude and reluctance to move that is noted in patients early in the disease or during acute exacerbations. A general programme of exercise geared to improving muscle strength and endurance will relieve symptoms.

Education of the patient is essential to enable a normal life to be led, and the patient should recognise the fluctuations of the disease, avoid over fatigue and prolonged physical and mental stresses. Patients should also be aware that the disease is exacerbated by ultraviolet irradiation, with alopecia and the development of butterfly distribution facial skin rashes being superimposed on joint exacerbations. Many systems may be involved with pleurisy, pericarditis and progressive lung shrinkage being common signs; they must be considered when the overall management of the patient is being discussed. Low doses of steroids such as prednisolone, additional analgesics and anti-inflammatory drugs during acute episodes, combined with a sensible lifestyle, have substantially improved the prognosis of these patients who can expect to survive a normal life span.

Systemic sclerosis (scleroderma)

Raynaud's phenomenon is common in the early stages and is accompanied by swelling of the fingers. The skin becomes tethered to underlying structures such that it cannot be pinched up on the dorsum of the finger (sclerodactyly) (Figs. 18/5, 18/6). Apart from the skin involvement of the hands, the face is often affected resulting in diminished oral aperture and tightening around the nose and the eyes. Eventually calcification occurs and forms nodular excrescences which sometimes discharge. Calcification is part of a variant of systemic sclerosis known as the CRST syndrome (Calcification; Raynaud's

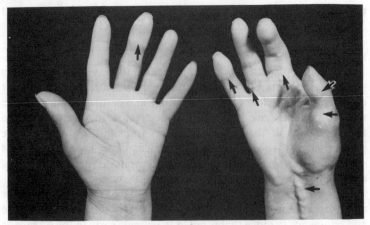

Fig. 18/5   Systemic sclerosis with multiple calcific deposits

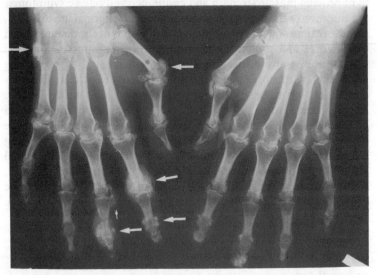

Fig. 18/6   Radiograph showing calcification in hands affected by
systemic sclerosis

phenomenon; Sclerodactyly; Telangiectasia, e.g. of the lips). In this
syndrome there may also be diminished motility of the lower third of
the oesphagus but no other systemic involvement, whereas in
systemic sclerosis itself, other viscera are eventually involved such as
the kidneys. Renal involvement leads to progressive hypertension late
in the disease.

Drug management is disappointing, though penicillamine, with or without colchicine, may help, especially the skin changes. Hypertension may require treatment with a beta-blocker drug.

PHYSIOTHERAPY

The disease produces overt and covert features in many of the body systems. The progressive thickening and tethering of the skin of the fingers is the most likely aspect to require physiotherapy. As the skin becomes shiny, tight and loses hair and sweat glands, joint movement is inhibited and muscle power is reduced.

Loss of function due to the skin changes is an early and disabling feature of the disease, and physiotherapy is directed to preserving mobility, delaying the development of predictable contractures, and preserving muscle power by any suitable method(s). Massage, passive stretching and active exercises all have their place. Progression of the disease is not affected by physiotherapy, but the patient's life can be made more tolerable by such attempts to delay the inevitable loss of function.

Dermatomyositis: polymyositis

In this condition inflammatory changes occur in skin and muscle. Some times the latter only is present (polymyositis). It can present either in the child or the adult and in the latter there is a significant chance of underlying neoplasm being present.

The skin changes may come before or after muscle weakness. A facial rash may resemble that seen in SLE but there is often a violaceous (heliotrope) colouration, especially on the eyelids and sometimes associated with peri-orbital oedema. Elsewhere, the rash tends to occur on extensor aspects; over the knuckles it forms thin erythematous lesions (collodion patches). Erythema of the nail-fold is common.

Muscle weakness in the limbs is more obvious in proximal muscles. If respiratory muscles are involved (usually severe cases), regular vital capacity measurements are required.

Calcification in muscle planes may be apparent on the radiograph and nodular calcific lesions can occur in skin and elsewhere, even in the tongue and brain.

The prognosis is usually, but not always, better in the child. Muscle enzymes, especially creatinine phosphokinase (CPK) are elevated and sequential levels indicate the response to treatment. Corticosteroids (e.g. prednisolone) should be used when muscle weakness is pronounced, especially early in the disease, or if skin ulcers develop.

They should be withdrawn slowly when clinical and laboratory indices improve but re-introduced if, as is not infrequently the case, relapse occurs. Occasionally, azathioprine or methotrexate may be required.

PHYSIOTHERAPY
As both these diseases are characterised by progressive weakness of all voluntary muscles the physiotherapist will be involved in management of the patient over the stages of deteriorating function and, hopefully, recovering power. During acute phases of the disease, the patient is confined to bed when careful monitoring of posture ensures maintenance of muscles and other soft tissue length. Pillows may be required to be placed strategically to retain the lumbar and neck curves. Fracture boards and the use of resting splints to retain functional positions of knees and ankles are indicated.

During the recovery phase, physiotherapy aims to maintain adequate ventilation, improve muscle power and prevent contractures developing. Careful monitoring of the patient's progress is required at all stages of the disease with accurate assessment and recording.

Mixed connective tissue disease (MCTD)

This is an example of an overlap syndrome and is a composite of SLE, systemic sclerosis and dermatomyositis. In all these conditions, arthritis or arthralgia may constitute a real or apparent clinical situation requiring differentiation from the inflammatory arthropathies.

Polyarteritis nodosum (PAN)

Arteritis is the basis of this disease and the causes, as well as the manifestations, are protean. Inflammation of blood vessels with resultant ischaemia of the end-organ will give rise to a clinical picture dependent upon the extent and distribution of the vessels involved. It is a multi-system disease, but purpura, vasculitic skin lesions, abdominal pain and renal disease leading to hypertension are prominent features.

In its acute stage corticosteroids are essential. If response is poor, cytotoxic drugs, plasma exchange or pulse therapy may be required.

Wegener's granulomatosis is similar to polyarteritis nodosum, but upper respiratory (sinusitis, nasal ulceration) and pulmonary lesions are more common, whereas hypertension is less so.

POLYMYALGIA RHEUMATICA

When symptoms referable to the shoulder girdle in particular, and to the pelvic girdle less often, were not able to be fitted into a well-defined diagnosis the term polymyalgia rheumatica tended to be used. Clearly defined features have now established this disease in its own right as part of a vasculitic (arteritic) abnormality.

The onset is usually after the age of 60, and may be acute or insidious. General ill-health is often a prominent feature but all too often the patient presents with neck and shoulder-girdle pain which is often dismissed by the observer as hysterical in origin. Pain and stiffness occur in the early morning. There is tenderness of musculature without wasting. The ESR is high. Liver function tests are frequently abnormal. Synovitis may occur in the hands and knees. Corticosteroid therapy is very effective and should be continued for a period extending up to two years. This is one of the few conditions in which treatment should be tailored to the level of the ESR.

Although there is usually remission occurring within a two-year period there is an important association with the disease. This is a giant cell arteritis manifested especially by temporal arteritis. Frontal headache is then a common feature. The temporal arteries become tender, thickened and often non-pulsatile, and there is a real danger of blindness; the use of corticosteroids becomes essential.

ERYTHEMA NODOSUM

It is difficult to relate this disease to others in this section. Nonetheless, it can be associated with joint disease. The lesions of erythema nodosum occur typically on the front of the shins. They are red, raised, blotchy areas initially up to the size of a 10-pence piece, or slightly larger. There may be pain and the lesions often become confluent such that the picture resembles, and is often misdiagnosed as, cellulitis.

Precipitating diseases include streptococcal infection (e.g. sore throat), sarcoidosis (with hilar lymphadenopathy on radiological examination) as well as less common ones. In the practice of rheumatology the most frequent association is that of erythema nodosum, hilar lymphadenopathy and joint symptoms, that is sarcoidosis. This can involve many organs of the body but in the form associated with erythema nodosum, the disease is self-limiting in over 90 per cent of patients. The leg lesions, radiographic changes and arthritis/arthralgia usually settle without residua thus differing from other forms of sarcoidosis. Occasionally corticosteroid therapy may be indicated to shorten the duration of symptoms.

Arthritis related to inflammation of the bowel (ulcerative colitis and regional ileitis) has been mentioned previously, and can be associated with erythema nodosum (see p. 368).

SJÖGRENS SYNDROME

Dry eyes, (keratoconjunctivitis sicca), dry mouth (xerostomia) and a peripheral arthropathy occurring together are called *Sjögrens syndrome*. Dry eyes and dry mouth occurring together are referred to as the *sicca syndrome*.

Approximately half the patients suffering from Sjögrens syndrome will have rheumatoid arthritis and in the remaining half, other connective tissue diseases, thyroid, hepatic and renal diseases are common. Rarely, a malignant lymphoreticular disease may develop. Sicca syndrome may be present in 25 per cent of patients with rheumatoid arthritis usually presenting as keratoconjunctivitis. The patient complains of a gritty feeling in the eye. Redness and superficial ulceration may occur. Tests for tear secretion will confirm the diagnosis. Artificial tears can do much to alleviate the symptoms in most cases but may have to be used at very frequent intervals. Dry mouth is less common but extremely distressing and difficult to treat. Various mouthwashes containing hypromellose can be tried but if the condition is severe they may be of little help. Severe dental caries may result.

PHYSIOTHERAPY
Joint symptoms are treated as affected joints in rheumatoid arthritis and where there is involvement of the upper respiratory tract, chest physiotherapy will be required.

SEPTIC ARTHRITIS (see Chapter 5)

VIRAL ARTHRITIS

Several different viruses throughout the world may be associated with arthralgia or arthritis. Rubella (German measles) and hepatitis B arthritis are good examples and deserve special mention. The arthritis may be related either to the disease or, less often, to vaccination. Various articular complaints may also accompany most of the common viral infections but are usually minimal, transient and occur as a late manifestation.

ARTHRITIS ASSOCIATED WITH MALIGNANCY

Although direct involvement of a joint by local primary or secondary bone malignancy can occur, neoplastic polyarthritis is practically never seen. Acute leukaemia in childhood can result in asymmetrical polyarthritis (differential diagnosis of juvenile polyarthritis). Hypertrophic pulmonary osteoarthropathy (due to carcinoma of the lung) in the adult includes non-inflammatory joint effusions and peri-articular bone pain.

HAEMOPHILIC ARTHRITIS

This is a disease of males transmitted by females and is due to a deficiency of Factor VIII. Haemarthrosis is common and acute, particularly involving knees, elbows and ankles. There may be premonitory symptoms of aching or pricking and this is very important since the situation must be treated as early as possible. Pain, swelling and loss of movement develop rapidly and the patient may seem ill and have pyrexia.

Treatment must be prompt and consists of the replacement of Factor VIII (anti-haemophilic globulin) either by transfusing fresh frozen plasma or, preferably, freeze-dried concentrate of Factor VIII. Some families have even been trained to start this at home, so urgent is the replacement required. Additional measures include immobilisation, and the administration of analgesics. In rare cases elevation and ice packs may be used. Fortunately most cases respond to replacement therapy, immobilisation and analgesics; joint aspiration – a dangerous procedure – is infrequently required. Following the acute episode, rehabilitation is necessary.

PHYSIOTHERAPY

Rest of the affected joint is essential to prevent further trauma and further bleeding. Splintage is the best method as movement is prevented and protective muscle guarding will be reduced. When all danger of further bleeding is past, a programme of mobilisation and muscle strengthening is followed. Progress is slow as rapid increase in activity can cause further bleeding. Joints frequently affected may require permanent splintage to protect the joint from trauma.

BIBLIOGRAPHY

See page 409.

Chapter 19

Osteoarthritis

by D.J. WARD, MB, FRCP
and M.E. TIDSWELL, BA, MCSP, ONC, DipTP

This is the commonest single form of arthritis and dates back to ancient times. Examples may be found in many different species apart from man. It is the end result of a series of changes which may be triggered by many different mechanisms, and several of these are now recognised. The arthritis is designated as *primary* or *secondary* depending upon whether a precipitating factor is known. As more causes are found, the incidence of the primary type diminishes.

Osteoarthritis is often regarded as a progressive process associated with getting older. There is, however, little evidence to support either an ageing or 'wear and tear' phenomenon. It should be regarded as the end result of abnormal mechanical, inflammatory, metabolic, physiological or pathological factors. There is no doubt that the incidence of the disease is higher in the elderly, but the clinical presentation may not be apparent for many years after the abnormal factors pertain and thus there can be a long interval during which the changes take place. During this time there is even the chance of reversibility if the initiating factors are corrected. It becomes obvious that recognition of these factors and their correction should reduce the incidence of osteoarthritis since there is very little change in articular cartilage during the human life-span under normal conditions.

Terminology is confusing. Because the disease does not display such intense inflammatory changes as are seen in rheumatoid arthritis there has been a tendency to call it 'osteoarthrosis'. Although mild, and probably secondary, inflammation is present however, and there seems little point in changing from osteoarthritis. Degenerative joint disease is unsuitable as is also hypertrophic arthritis (a reference to the new bone formation – osteophytes – seen in the disease) and none of these terms adequately describes the true nature of the process. *Osteoarthritis* is the term used in this chapter.

EPIDEMIOLOGY

Radiological evidence is much commoner than clinically recognisable disease. Symptoms may be present only in some 15 per cent of those with radiological change, but after the age of 60 over 80 per cent of the population will have some radiological evidence of osteoarthritis. Factors triggering the disease may be present at birth or in early childhood, and even at the age of 20 there is a 10 per cent incidence of radiographic abnormality.

It is equally as common in men as in women overall but under the age of 50 there are more men, and over the age of 50 more women, affected.

The disease occurs throughout the world. There is no climatic, geographic or racial factor involved. Differing prevalence for osteoarthritis of various joints is more likely to be related to cultural and industrial variations. For example, the squatting position more favoured by Asian communities may in some way protect the head of the femur and explain the lower incidence of osteoarthritis of the hip in Orientals.

It has been implied that osteoarthritis is responsible for much time lost from work. This is not entirely correct since many patients are at, or beyond, retirement age, especially since early retirement and redundancies are becoming increasingly evident.

AETIOLOGY AND PATHOGENESIS

As already mentioned, classification of osteoarthritis is based on the concept of primary and secondary disease. This may not be a valid classification in that all cases could be regarded as secondary. Some authors would prefer to differentiate between multiple site involvement and the occurrence of osteoarthritis in only one or two joints. For now, however, we will retain the concept of primary and secondary though it must be appreciated that this situation will probably change.

Primary osteoarthritis

This includes:
1. *Primary generalised osteoarthritis.* This occurs particularly in post-menopausal women and may be regarded as a hereditable form of the disease. Proximal and distal interphalangeal joints in

the hands, the carpometacarpal joint at the base of the thumb, cervical and lumbar spine, knees and great toes are most commonly involved. Primary generalised osteoarthritis affects women more than men (ratio 10:1) and is typified by more severe symptoms at the onset. During the acute onset the joints look inflamed and are red and tender. The acute phase may last for several months but gradually osteophyte formation and deformity develop. Symptoms may be episodic and the patient sometimes has a mild generalised illness. In this disease, osteophyte formation is a pronounced feature. Heberden's nodes occur at the distal interphalangeal joints in the hands and Bouchard's nodes at proximal interphalangeal joints (Fig. 19/1).

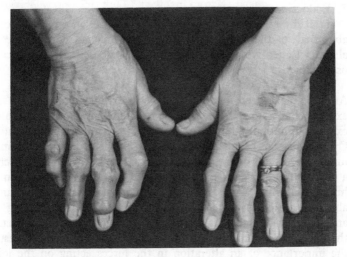

Fig. 19/1 Heberden's and Bouchard's nodes in osteoarthritic hands

2. *Erosive interphalangeal osteoarthritis.* Again with involvement of proximal and distal interphalangeal joints but with a different clinical and radiological pattern. The joints are subjected to attacks of inflammation with redness, tenderness and pain. Radiological changes include an erosive element and can mimic those seen in rheumatoid arthritis.
3. *Idiopathic.* In many such cases, especially with hip involvement, there is probably an underlying cause which it may not be possible to identify as yet.

Secondary osteoarthritis

This may be initiated by a number of factors including:
1. Developmental, e.g. hip dysplasia, slipped upper femoral epiphyses, osteochondritis dissecans, unequal leg lengths, etc.
2. Inflammatory, e.g. rheumatoid arthritis and the spondyloarthropathies.
3. Infective, e.g. septic arthritis.
4. Metabolic, e.g. gout, pseudo-gout, haemochromatosis, hydroxyapatite crystal arthropathy (with chondrocalcinosis), Paget's disease.
5. Traumatic, e.g. articular surface fracture, occupational (miners, sportsmen), hypermobility syndrome.
6. Neuropathic.
7. Endocrine, e.g. acromegaly.

In all these secondary cases either the stress on a joint becomes abnormal, or the ability of the joint to withstand normal stress is altered. Repetitive normal use of a normal joint does not cause osteoarthritis.

Attempts have been made to study osteoarthritis by inducing it in experimental animals. The results are interesting though difficult to explain. Immobilisation in plaster leads to cartilage degeneration. Overuse has not been shown to be associated with cartilage damage unless there is considerable overloading as well. Altered forces across a joint will induce cartilage degeneration and this is reflected in the human following various injuries to joints. Instability leads to changes almost identical to osteoarthritis – for example after cutting the anterior cruciate ligament of the knee, though this does not occur if the knee is immobilised in flexion postoperatively, again suggesting the importance of an alteration in the forces acting on the joint. Patellectomy can be shown to be followed by cartilage change and in the human the adverse effect of this procedure is well known. In these experimental models, the forces and stresses acting on a joint are altered. If the joint itself is rendered abnormal, then it loses its ability to absorb even normal stresses.

CONGENITAL OR DEVELOPMENTAL FACTORS

In the case of hip dysplasias, epiphyseal abnormalities, osteochondritis dissecans, etc, the joint is abnormal and there is an imbalance between the stresses on the joint and the ability to absorb those stresses. Scoliosis and inequality of leg length, however, alter the normality of forces acting on hip and knee. In both circumstances osteoarthritis ensues. In congenital hip dysplasia there is a shallow acetabulum facing anteriorly and laterally and providing a poor cover for the femoral head.

INFLAMMATORY FACTORS

After years of involvement by inflammatory disease such as rheumatoid arthritis or one of the spondyloarthropathies, it is common to find that a joint develops more the changes of osteoarthritis with little or no excess of synovial fluid and no synovitis, but marked crepitus and sometimes osteophyte formation. Instability and lack of alignment are additional factors.

Septic arthritis can also cause sufficient damage to lead to osteoarthritis.

METABOLIC FACTORS

There are a number of so-called deposition diseases in which various substances may be deposited in cartilage. Haemochromatosis is often associated with chondrocalcinosis. Ochromosis is a rare disease in which homogentisic acid is deposited. In gout, urate crystals are deposited in the joint and in pseudo-gout whether with or without general underlying disease, pyrophosphate crystals are identified. (There are several different conditions which may be associated with pyrophosphate crystal deposition, such as haemochromatosis, hyper-parathyroidism, and many cases which are idiopathic.) In the 1970s it was realised that a number of patients diagnosed as primary osteoarthritis had hydroxyapatite crystals in their joints and although the role of these crystals has been the subject of much debate, it is possible that they are related to the development of osteoarthritis. Of course, in a number of the above situations, osteoarthritis may be due either to a post-inflammatory factor or a deposition factor – or even both.

TRAUMATIC FACTORS

Articular and peri-articular structures respond well to regular exercise and this has no part to play in the onset of osteoarthritis providing the joint mechanics are not altered. Obviously, correction of mechanical faults and proper rehabilitation after injury are very necessary; there is no doubt that minor injuries beset athletes and sports people more frequently than those with more sedentary habits and as a result there is a higher incidence of osteoarthritis. Again it is stressed that it is only in the case of trauma or biomechanical fault that this happens and not in the case of regular exercise.

Unusual activity (repeatedly) is known to lead to osteoarthritis (e.g.

in the knees of coal miners). In the hypermobility syndrome, abnormal stresses are caused by the joint laxity allowing an excess of movement and this results in premature osteoarthritis.

Trauma, if it gives rise to micro-fractures in subchondral bone, if it causes a major fracture through the joint or if it results in dislocation, may in this direct fashion alter both the forces exerted on the joint and the ability of the joint to resist them.

NEUROPATHIC
In the case of neuropathic joints there is sensory loss from articular and peri-articular tissues with removal of impulses necessary for the reflex activity required to maintain a joint's stability. The joint becomes relatively unstable and thus prone to osteoarthritis. Syphilis, syringomyelia and diabetes mellitus are some of the conditions associated.

ENDOCRINE FACTORS
Certainly acromegaly is associated with joint changes. In this condition there is an increase in growth hormone which results in changes in the cartilage and eventual osteoarthritis.

Diabetes mellitus and hypothyroidism have been said to carry an increased tendency to develop the disease but evidence is not very great. In both cases, however, there are possible ways in which cartilage may be altered. Sex hormones may also have an influence.

Osteoporosis reduces the chances of developing osteoarthritis, the bone being more compliant and more effective as a shock absorber.

Finally one has to consider the role of obesity. It seemingly has little part to play unless a malalignment of hip or knee is caused by the sheer excess of tissue in the thighs. Other than this, however, it may well accelerate osteoarthritis of hip and knee arising from other causes and especially if there is instability. The knee joint is the one most related to obesity.

Pathology

There are two obvious pathological processes. The first is the progressive destruction of articular cartilage, and the second is the formation of new bone at the margins of the joint (ostephytes). The relationship between these processes is still not clear. It is a generally held view that the primary change occurs in articular cartilage and here the main biochemical change is a decrease in proteoglycans. The latter and collagen are the two most important substances necessary for the integrity and normal function of cartilage. The loss of proteoglycans and the consequences of a diminished amount in cartilage are essential steps in the development of osteoarthritis. There is a loss of stiffness and elasticity altering the effects of mechanical forces. The loss of proteoglycans also adversely affects cartilage lubrication. There is also a change in water content and the ability to absorb water. This latter fact may cause diffusion of degradative enzymes from synovial fluid. Histological studies show localised areas of softening in which the cartilage becomes irregular (fibrillation). Clefts develop and in time extend down to, and penetrate, subchondral bone with the formation of cysts. A continuing process of degradation results in fragments of cartilage being flaked off into the synovial cavity. These are phagocytosed and a mild inflammatory reaction is triggered. Eventually, bone may be completely denuded of cartilage and the bone-end become very smooth (eburnation). Until the final stages of the disease, reparative processes are taking place and in the early stages some, if not all, of the changes may be reversible.

New bone formation starts at the beginning of the disease though the largest osteophytes are usually seen in those patients who have long-standing and slowly progressive disease. They may not be directly related to the cartilage destruction and could be dependent upon vascular changes. They may be responsible for some of the pain and restriction of movement experienced by the patient. Other sources of pain are the thickened fibrotic capsule, the synovium and sometimes subchondral bone (e.g. due to increased venous pressure caused by cysts) but not the cartilage itself. Pain arises where there are nerve endings.

The changes seen are common to all forms of osteoarthritis.

Clinical features

Patients complain of pain, stiffness, deformity and loss of function. The symptoms do not always correlate with radiological findings, e.g. there may be few symptoms even in the presence of marked radiological changes. The reverse is also true, and pain may be severe despite minimal clinical and radiological findings. Usually there are increasing complaints over a number of years but occasionally the history can be relatively short, a matter of a few months only, despite extensive radiological disease.

PAIN

This is usually related to the joint involved but in the case of the hip may be referred to the knee or to the thigh. With a combination of lumbar spine and hip disease, it can be difficult to isolate the site giving rise to most pain.

The pain is described as dull and aching, but in erosive interphalangeal osteoarthritis it can be more acute. Acute pain occurring in a knee joint should always make one think of chondrocalcinosis, pseudo-gout or gout as underlying factors in patients with osteoarthritis.

Pain is made worse by movement and, in the lower limbs, by weight-bearing and walking. Initially it is relieved by rest, but later in the disease rest pain can be severe and ultimately lead to disturbance of sleep.

Pain arises in structures possessing nerve endings and may result from micro-fractures in subchondral bone, increased venous pressure in subchondral bone and osteophytes, synovitis, capsular thickening and subluxation. With cartilage damage alone, there is no pain, since articular cartilage does not contain nerve endings. This is the reason why the disease may be obvious radiologically long before symptoms appear. After osteotomy it is said that pain relief may be due to lowering of the venous pressure and/or the severing of nerve endings.

STIFFNESS

After resting, stiffness is a feature lasting for about 15 minutes. It is never as marked a feature as in rheumatoid arthritis but may occur in the morning after a night's sleep or after any prolonged disuse through the day. Patients learn to use their joints little, but often.

DEFORMITY

This is commonly observed in the hands and can be unsightly. In the lower limbs, flexion contracture of hip and/or knee is due to protective muscle spasm and varus deformity is common at the knee (Fig. 19/2). Due to the deformity and limitation of one joint, secondary change may occur in an unaffected joint (e.g. flexion deformity and limitation of the hip secondary to long-standing knee disease with flexion).

In time, peri-articular structures thicken, varying degrees of subluxation may occur, loss of congruity of the joint surfaces will limit movement and this may be further limited by the presence of large osteophytes.

The signs found in osteoarthritis depend to a certain extent on the site

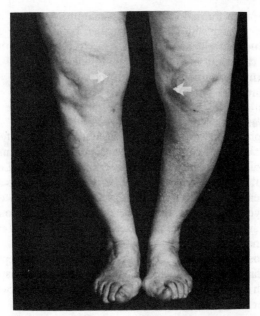

Fig. 19/2 Obesity and osteoarthritis of the knees showing a varus deformity

of the disease. In easily accessible joints, bony thickening, sometimes with tenderness, may be evident, as may deformity, subluxation, instability, and limitation. Crepitus may be felt and heard when moving a joint and is a fine or coarse creaking noise occasioned by irregular surfaces. Especially in the hip, a loud 'clunk' may be heard on movement, usually when there is a bone on bone situation. This sound can be heard from yards away, and a patient's approach may be heralded before he enters the room.

Investigations

RADIOLOGY
In the initial stages the radiological appearance may be normal. Subsequently the changes which are seen include:
1. Joint space narrowing. This reflects the gradual disappearance of cartilage.
2. Sclerosis (increased density) of bone beneath the cartilage as the process of eburnation takes place.

3. Osteophyte formation at the joint margins.
4. Cystic changes in the peri-articular bone. These are seen as translucent areas of varying size in close proximity to the joint. They can result in local collapse of bone.
5. Deformity resulting from subluxation.
6. The presence of loose bodies.
7. Irregularity of bone surfaces. This may be made even more obvious by the collapse of bone cysts.

Osteophyte formation is a curious event. Although osteophytes are typical of osteoarthritis their presence *alone* does not imply that the other radiological changes will necessarily develop. Loss of joint space, subchondral sclerosis and the presence of cysts are perhaps more reliable indices of progressive cartilage destruction. Osteophytes related to the hip can occur in numerous different patterns and it is an interesting exercise to relate the differing sites of formation around the hip with clinical presentation.

Ankylosis is unusual and erosions are not seen except in erosive interphalangeal osteoarthritis. Changes of osteoarthritis are uncommon at the metacarpophalangeal joints unless secondary to previous trauma or inflammation.

LABORATORY TESTS
There are no specific laboratory abnormalities in osteoarthritis except in some cases of secondary disease in which there may be specific tests for the primary disease. The haemoglobin, white cell count, platelet count and ESR are normal (except perhaps for a slight rise in the ESR during the acute phase of primary generalised osteoarthritis).

Tests for rheumatoid factor are negative or only slightly positive in the same manner as is found in the general population. Serum proteins are normal.

Synovial fluid retains its viscosity and has a glairy mucous consistency. The protein content is rarely above 3g/100ml and the white count usually below 5.0×10^9/litre (often even less).

Medical management

From what has been said already it would seem that the most important approach should be a prophylactic one. Unfortunately we are not yet able to achieve this goal but continuing research into the mechanical stresses acting on a joint, the biochemistry of joint structures and the question of lubrication may radically alter the approach to osteoarthritis in the future. Situations which place abnormal stress on the affected joint must be avoided and this may include obesity. Attention must be given to conditions at work and in the home. Another approach to the question of prophylaxis is to identify the primary disease or condition leading to osteoarthritis and to apply effective treatment as early as possible.

Many patients will require no more than reassurance. The word 'arthritis' conjures up a picture of crippledom, and the fear of this must be dispelled. Fortunately, progression of the disease is usually slow and much of the patient's discomfort and disability can be relieved even though the pathological changes remain.

Rest relieves pain in the early stages but induces stiffness. Too much rest is not a good thing, neither is too much exercise. A suitable balance between the two must be established and varies from patient to patient. How much rest/activity and what kind will vary according to the joint involved. Immobilisation is not as necessary as may occasionally be the case in rheumatoid arthritis.

Drugs are frequently used but constitute only one aspect of the treatment of osteoarthritis. The object is to use general measures and hopefully avoid the need for drugs, but sometimes the latter are needed for symptomatic relief and to facilitate other approaches to treatment. Side-effects from drugs are frequently encountered and their use should be kept to a minimum. Pain and stiffness may be severe enough to justify the use of analgesics (paracetamol, salicylate, dihydrocodeine, etc), and it is common practice to use non-steroidal anti-inflammatory drugs as well (see p. 325). Systemic corticosteroid therapy has *no* place in the treatment of osteoarthritis but intra-articular or soft tissue injections may have a limited role. At least the latter may render the task of the physiotherapist easier. Other forms of medical therapy have been employed but are of doubtful value and may be dangerous. This applies to irradiation therapy, various attempts at improving lubrication (e.g. intra-articular silicones) and intramuscular injections of extracts of cartilage. There is no single curative medication available. The use of drugs combined with physiotherapy and general measures related to the correction of abnormal stresses, and the treatment of primary disorders should be satisfactory in the management of most patients. Reassurance is always required.

The disability created by osteoarthritis must be assessed as well as symptoms such as pain or stiffness, and, as with rheumatoid arthritis, assessments must take into account the total environment of the patient. This should be easier than in rheumatoid arthritis since change in the osteoarthritis is not as marked a feature and fewer joints are involved.

PHYSIOTHERAPY

Patients present to physiotherapy departments with varying distribution and degrees of deterioration in the affected joints and are treated according to the stage of the degenerative process. For treatment to be effective, the basic principles of assessment, planning, implementation, evaluation and modification, followed by reassessment are essential.

Assessment

A systematic approach is required in order to ensure that all relevant aspects of the patient's condition are considered. Careful recording of the findings of the assessment, treatment given and the patient's response is necessary. A great deal of information can be gained from the patient's notes, and the physiotherapy assessment should concentrate on those aspects of the patient's condition which concern the physiotherapist; these include pain, loss of function and joint stiffness.

PAIN

The level of pain experienced by the patient indicates the degree of joint irritability but not necessarily the amount of joint deterioration. Information concerning the pain can be elicited by careful questioning of the following points:
1. Site and distribution of the pain.
2. Quality: burning, aching, throbbing, searing.
3. Duration: permanent, persistent or intermittent.
4. Triggering factors: weight-bearing, jarring, sustained stress; specific movement, rest, posture, weather, emotional state; no recognisable trigger.
5. Relieving factors: rest, movement, postural adjustment, temporal adjustment; physiotherapeutic procedures, e.g. traction, application of external heat or cold, massage, manipulative procedures, resisted movement; analgesia.

LOSS OF FUNCTION

Damage to a single joint such as a hip or knee will have a significant effect on the patient's function. Although the patient may remain ambulant, he may have difficulty in negotiating stairs, bathing or certain aspects of self-care activities. Difficulties may be encountered negotiating transport, as he may be unable to get on or off a bus or train and may have difficulty driving. If the patient is working, restricted mobility may cause problems. If the joints of the upper limb are affected, this may be disabling to the housewife or office worker who requires precision movements and to be able to handle separate pieces of paper. The patient will be able to identify specific problems and treatment should be orientated towards their relief.

JOINT STIFFNESS

All affected joints display restriction of movement, and careful examination is required of the active and passive ranges so that deficiencies may be noted. The quality of movement, point of pain limitation or muscle guarding should be noted and recorded. Movement must be localised to the joint under examination and care taken to prevent movement in adjacent joints augmenting that present in the affected joint.

Large joints are examined effectively using a goniometer to record ranges of motion, but small joints, e.g. of the fingers, can be measured by applying a malleable wire to the extensor aspect of the fingers, bending it to maintain contact with the skin through the range of motion and then transferring to graph paper the trace of the wire.

When examining joint movement, the physiotherapist must also check accessory movements at the joints involved. These movements are an essential part of normal movement and cannot be performed voluntarily in isolation. Restriction of accessory movements due to mechanical disruption of the joint surfaces will give rise to pain on movement and will preclude normal range or smooth quality of movement within the existing range.

Assessment is completed by noting the posture, identifying any deformity or asymmetry of limb lengths and testing the strength of muscles around the affected joints using the MRC scale.

Treatment

Once the patient's problem(s) has been identified, treatment is directed towards improving function within the limits imposed both by the state of the affected joint(s) and the requirements of the person's lifestyle. As always, successful management rests upon the co-operation and understanding of the person. Instruction in posture improvement, adequate rest in suitable positions, a programme of graded exercises, selection and use of appropriate walking aids, and dietary advice if obesity is present, will all contribute to an easier way of life.

AIMS OF TREATMENT
1. To control pain.
2. To prevent further strain or damage to affected joints.
3. To improve movements.
4. To improve muscle power.
5. To maintain or improve functional independence.

TO CONTROL PAIN
Pain may be caused by (1) destruction of cartilage leaving subchondral bone exposed and vulnerable; (2) osteophytes tearing synovial lining of the joint capsule or breaking off and forming loose bodies in the joint; or (3) jarring of the joint or subjecting it to unacceptable stress such as weight-bearing or exercise.

Various physiotherapeutic techniques can be used to help relieve pain. (These are in addition to any analgesics which may be prescribed.)

Traction: Distraction of joint surfaces, either manually or mechanically; either intermittently or prolonged, will reduce pain by relieving pressure on sensitive intra-articular structures. Protective muscle guarding is reduced and this will also ease the pain.

Heat: Superficial or deep heat will relieve discomfort by reducing the protective muscle spasm. Hot packs, radiant heat, paraffin wax or short wave diathermy are all beneficial.

Cold: The application of cold is often more effective than heat. Ice packs or ice-towelling techniques are useful.

Ultrasound: This is indicated when pain is centred on peri-articular soft tissues.

Interferential: This is used for its analgesic and circulatory effects. It is able to be used in the presence of metal implants. Currents between 0–10Hz are used to provide muscle stimulation by a current which is more comfortable than faradism. Care must be taken not to reduce pain and protective muscle guarding to the point where the patient will further damage affected joints by overactivity.

Hydrotherapy: The warmth of the water and its buoyancy are helpful in relieving pain particularly when weight-bearing joints are affected.

TO PREVENT FURTHER STRAIN OR DAMAGE TO AFFECTED JOINTS

The identification of activities which produce strain followed by reduction or elimination of them is obviously the best method. Improvement of posture, the selection of an appropriate walking aid or correction of leg length inequality by a shoe-raise may also be required. A period of rest in the corrected position during the day will ease strain and should be encouraged.

TO IMPROVE MOVEMENTS

As there is no systemic involvement in osteoarthritis, vigorous techniques can be used to improve joint movement once the protective muscle spasm has been reduced (see above). Mobilisation may be active or passive.

Active: Methods include the use of suspension therapy for the larger limb joints and lumbar spine. Pool therapy is beneficial for the lower limb joints, as are PNF techniques such as hold-relax and slow reversal hold-relax used in appropriate patterns.

Passive: These techniques are used where mechanical dysfunction or alteration of the length of peri-articular soft tissues are limiting movement. (See Chapters 10 and 11.)

TO IMPROVE MUSCLE POWER

Muscle power can only be improved by active exercise. At each attendance the physiotherapist will select the appropriate starting positions, type and quality of resistance so that the patient works to the limit of his capabilities in order to hypertrophy muscle. Endurance will be increased by working muscles for a longer time against a submaximal resistance.

TO MAINTAIN OR IMPROVE FUNCTIONAL INDEPENDENCE

By relieving pain and muscle guarding the patient's level of functional independence may improve; if problems remain the solution may lie in the use of an alternative method or, where this cannot be achieved, by supplying an aid, for example a stocking gutter, elasticated shoe laces or a half-step.

When joint deterioration coupled with increasing pain become intolerable surgery will be considered (see Chapters 20 and 21).

INDIVIDUAL JOINTS

Spine (see Chapter 12)

Shoulder

Osteoarthritis of the glenohumeral joint is uncommon as a primary event but may occur secondarily after trauma or other joint diseases, such as rheumatoid arthritis. Extra-articular disease of soft tissues is by comparison very common (e.g. adhesive capsulitis, rotator cuff syndrome and tendinitis with or without calcific deposits) and other causes of shoulder pain must be considered before accepting a diagnosis of osteoarthritis (e.g. inflammatory arthritis, neurological and vascular lesions, referred pain, etc). Osteoarthritis of the acromioclavicular joint is a rare cause of pain.

Elbow

This is an uncommon site for osteoarthritis except after trauma.

Hand

The distal interphalangeal joints are the most frequently affected in the hand, with the clinically characteristic Heberden's nodes. These relate to osteophytes formed at the joint margin and are seen as prominences around the joint. Bouchard's nodes are similarly formed around the proximal interphalangeal joints but occur less frequently (Fig. 19/1). The osteophytic outgrowth may occur in one or two fingers, especially after injury, or simultaneously and spontaneously in all fingers. They are much more common in women and one must remember that activities requiring 'pinch' are more often undertaken by women. The loading set up by pinch is surprisingly severe. In the case of women, one parent usually has had similar lesions, whereas in men, both parents will have been affected. Nodes tend to make their appearance, without symptoms initially, especially after the age of 45. Pain frequently ensues and may persist for a number of years; both pain and osteophyte formation will inhibit function. It is interesting that nodes are more severe in the dominant hand and either do not appear, or regress, in paralysed limbs. Eventually, pain will decrease though the unsightly swelling remains.

Lateral deviation and flexion of the distal phalanx may be noted.

Occasionally cystic swellings will develop in association with the nodes (especially Heberden's nodes). They contain gelatinous material, can be painful and may burst. Treatment is not very satisfactory but wax baths and intra-articular steroids may help. Minor surgery is of benefit if painful cystic lesions develop; in some cases these are acute, hot and tender and will settle spontaneously. The diagnosis is usually easy but the possibility of gout has to be considered.

Almost as common in the female is osteoarthritis of the carpometacarpal joint of the thumb (trapezio-metacarpal joint). The trapezium-scaphoid joint is also involved. This results in a squared appearance of the thumb. Patients find it very difficult to grasp objects and any function involving the thumb becomes painful and difficult. Excision of the trapezium or a silastic implant will give considerable relief though it may take up to six months for power to return.

Erosive interphalangeal osteoarthritis gives rise to intermittent, apparently inflammatory, bouts of pain. Ankylosis is more common than is the case with Heberden's and Bouchard's nodes and cartilage destruction is even more severe. Radiologically erosions are present but this would seem to be a distinct entity and differs from both rheumatoid arthritis and classical osteoarthritis.

Let us consider the metacarpophalangeal joints. It has been taught that osteoarthritis involves the distal and proximal interphalangeal joints but not the metacarpophalangeal joints. Additionally, rheumatoid arthritis involves the metacarpophalangeal and proximal interphalangeal joints but not the distal interphalangeal joints. These are good guidelines. Occasionally, however, radiographs will show evidence of osteoarthritis in the metacarpophalangeal joints. Is this primary, post-traumatic or post-inflammatory? The answer has not been resolved, but poses the question – are some typical osteoarthritic changes secondary to a mild unrecognised inflammatory arthritis? In other words, do we really know the true clinical spectrum of rheumatoid (or other) arthritis?

Calcification in the triangular ligament of the wrist sometimes associated with calcification in the articular cartilage of the knee may represent a different form of osteoarthritis, related to the deposition of hydroxyapatite crystals.

Finally, osteoarthritis in the hand may occur without other joint involvement or as part of a more generalised disorder. You must consider the hand as part of the whole. You must assess the disability, including the psychological as well as the painful distress. You must also realise that the discomfort and aesthetic displeasure are nought in comparison with the disastrous consequences resultant upon the effect of rheumatoid arthritis involving the hand. The pain will diminish in time. The ugliness will not. The function will remain better than that in rheumatoid arthritis. Surgical treatment for the thumb can be very effective.

PHYSIOTHERAPY ASSESSMENT

In addition to assessing the joint range and muscle power, it is important also to assess sensation and the functional use of the hand.

Range of movement: Individual joint movement can be measured by moulding wire to the extensor aspect of the finger. Contact is maintained as the finger joints are flexed fully: a trace is taken of the position and transferred to graph paper. This is then repeated while the joints are extended.

Muscle power: The intrinsic and extrinsic hand muscles should be tested individually, and graded using the MRC scale.

Sensation: This tends to be diminished over the finger tips and is a contributory cause of hand clumsiness.

TREATMENT

Paraffin wax gloves will provide all-round warmth and is the most beneficial form of heat. The oiliness of the wax also lubricates the skin. Some patients may prefer immersion of their hands in a 50:50 mixture of crushed ice and water. Either form should be followed by mobilisation of the joints using traction, passive and active assisted movements.

Re-education of function requires particular attention to all grasping activities, gripping and precision movements. The needs of each patient must be known so that a rational treatment may be offered. For example, a postmistress or a banker who has to handle separate pieces of paper will be more affected by deterioration in hand function than a person who has a job not requiring manual dexterity.

Hip

Osteoarthritis of the hip can be bilateral but it is more usual for just one hip to be involved. In over 75 per cent of cases it is the consequence of congenital or developmental abnormality. Congenital dysplasia of the hip accounts for 25 per cent or more of cases. Slipped capital femoral epiphysis is also a common cause and avascular necrosis (Legg-Calvé-Perthes' disease) may be responsible. Not to be forgotten is the possibility of a previous inflammatory arthritis, especially Reiter's syndrome or an atypical spondyloarthropathy. If severe enough, congenital abnormalities may present with symptoms in childhood, but a significant number may not and in these cases, osteoarthritis of the hip will present as a disease of middle-age.

Congenital hip dysplasia in a child results in a limp as early as two or three years of age. If the diagnosis is missed and there is only partial subluxation, the teenager will present with pain. In even less severe cases osteoarthritis in middle-age will be the presenting feature. The same sequence of events takes place in other congenital or developmental abnormalities. In some cases symptoms related to the abnormality will start early, in mild form, and continue into adult life merging into the symptoms of osteoarthritis.

Congenital hip dysplasia is more common in females and a slipped upper femoral epiphysis is found more often in males.

Pain arising from the hip may be felt in the groin, lateral buttock or thigh and is not uncommonly referred to the knee. Internal rotation is the first movement to be impaired but subsequently extension, abduction and flexion become restricted. Increasing adduction deformity leads to relative and then absolute shortening of the limb. The gait becomes antalgic (i.e. the body leans to the affected side during the stance phase of walking.) The patient stands with the affected side elevated but this can only be possible as a result of lumbar scoliosis developing and the heel will not meet the ground unless there is flexion of the knee on the unaffected side. A Trendelenburg gait is the result.

Trendelenburg's sign: This is an indication of the gluteal muscles' potential to abduct the hip when weight-bearing, and is positive if abduction is not possible.

To elicit the sign instruct the patient to stand on the affected leg and raise the other knee as in marking time. Normally the buttock of the raised leg rises higher than that of the standing leg. If the sign is positive, the buttock of the raised leg droops below the other.

Leg-length shortening may be apparent, as measured from the umbilicus (or xiphisternum) to the medial malleolus. True shortening is ascertained by measuring the distance from the anterior superior iliac spine to the medial malleolus on both sides.

It must be obvious that changes in the lumbo-sacral spine are a frequent consequence of hip disease. Scoliosis, changes in lumbar lordosis and osteoarthritis (e.g. of the facet joints) result from altered mechanical stress on the spine. It can be difficult to differentiate between pain arising from the hip and that from lumbo-sacral spine disease, whether the latter be primary or secondary to the hip disease. This is an important aspect to take into account when considering hip surgery. Often pain is due to both conditions.

The contralateral knee is sometimes placed under undue stress and this will encourage the development of osteoarthritis here, again as a secondary phenomenon.

Paget's disease of bone is quite common in the pelvis, and may be unilateral. In such a situation it is often associated with osteoarthritis of the hip and the questions are posed – which condition is giving rise to the pain or is it due to both? Which condition should be dealt with first? Generally speaking, the osteoarthritis is more likely to be the source of most pain in this combination but as surgery carries a danger because of the increased vascularity of bone in Paget's disease, the latter should be treated first (either by calcitonin, disodium etidronate or a combination of these).

Having regard for the above problems, osteoarthritis of the hip is usually a good condition to treat. Total hip replacement gives excellent results (see Chapter 21). Before surgery is considered, simple measures should be tried. These include weight loss (if obesity is evident), the use of a stick in the contralateral hand, local steroid infiltration of the trochanteric bursa, analgesia, traction and physiotherapy.

PHYSIOTHERAPY ASSESSMENT
Gait, general appearance and posture can be observed as the patient enters the department for treatment. See page 197 for assessment details.

TREATMENT
Relief of pain: During an acute inflammatory episode, complete bed rest for a few days with traction may be indicated but usually less radical approaches will provide considerable ease. Application of ice packs to the joint, or iced towels placed along the length of muscle fibres around the joint will reduce muscle spasm, and so reduce pain. Intermittent traction distracts joint surfaces releasing trapped synovia. Short wave diathermy is the deepest form of penetrating heat available in a physiotherapy department; while a significant number of patients will gain relief from its application, some find the pain exaggerated by it and will gain more benefit from radiant heat irradiation. Ultrasound, immersion in a treatment pool or repetitive exercise in a weight-relieved position may all help reduce protective muscle guarding and thus reduce pain.

Mobilisation of joints and prevention of deformity: Once pain and protective muscle guarding have been reduced, mobilisation commences by passive or active means. It is advisable for the patient to spend some time during the day in a corrected position; prone is ideal, but this will be precluded in advanced cases by hip flexion deformity, and then the patient should lie supine with the hip extended as far as possible.

Manipulation under general anaesthesia may be recommended to be followed by active exercise to maintain the range of movement regained. Maitland mobilising techniques of low grades when the hip is irritable, progressing to higher grades as irritability subsides, produce good results. Traction is also an effective passive measure.

Active extension and abduction of the hip can be encouraged using suspension apparatus to support the weight of the leg. Deep water exercises in the treatment pool and proprioceptive neuromuscular facilitation techniques are beneficial, particularly hold-relax and slow-reversal hold-relax in the extension, abduction and medial rotation pattern.

Strengthening of muscles: Muscle contractions against a graded resistance offered by gravity, manually or by mechanical means using water, springs, pulley circuits or weights are effective in strengthening muscle groups weakened by disuse or pain. Exercises may be performed in lying, side lying, prone lying, sitting or standing.

Gait re-education and posture correction: A temporary raise may be required on the shoe of the adducted leg to equalise leg lengths and eliminate toe walking on that side or walking with a flexed knee on the contralateral side. Pace length, timing and the correct sequence of heel strike, weight transference and push-off should all be considered. Re-education may be started in the pool and progress to dry land with support from elbow crutches or walking sticks. A single walking stick in the contralateral hand will provide some weight relief. Patients who do not use sticks are encouraged to carry heavy loads such as a shopping bag or a suitcase in the opposite hand as this relieves strain on the affected hip.

A minimum of 45 degrees of active hip flexion is required to climb stairs and as many patients cannot achieve this they should be taught to trail the affected leg in ascent and lead with it in descent. The non-affected leg will then take the strain of raising or lowering the body-weight.

The patient should be reminded continually about his posture and any deviation corrected.

Functional independence: Patients with an OA hip may require training in changing position from lying to sitting, moving in bed, getting into and out of bed and from standing to sitting. They may need to be shown how to get in and out of a car and they should be advised about car seating. Not only should they be taught how to climb house stairs but also how to negotiate the high step on and off a bus or train.

In later stages of the disease, home adaptations may be needed to facilitate self-care, and the occupational therapist may be asked to advise about aids which will compensate for the lack of movement in the hip. These include a pincer-grip extension hand for picking up small objects from the floor; elasticated shoe laces; sock or stocking gutters; or a half-step to aid climbing.

Knee

Osteoarthritis may occur in the patello-femoral joint or in the medial or lateral compartments of the knee. Patello-femoral arthritis can occur on its own or following disease in the knee joint, and typically gives rise to pain anteriorly.

Initiating factors in osteoarthritis of the knee include fractures involving the tibial plateaux and/or femoral condyles, instability (e.g. after ligamentous damage) and severe lateral deformities, and post-inflammatory states. Special instances include the development of arthritis after patellectomy, following a torn meniscus and in association with chondromalacia patellae. The incidence of change after meniscectomy is high and although a damaged meniscus interfering with joint function has to be removed, care must be taken to ensure that the procedure really is essential. *Chondromalacia patellae* occurs in a younger age-group (15–30) than patello-femoral osteoarthritis. There is pain with activity. Descending a flight of stairs or getting up quickly from a crouching position typically induce symptoms, which can be elicited also by passively depressing the patella in the femoral groove as a patient contracts the quadriceps. Symptoms tend to come and go but can be severe. Eventually osteoarthritis may supervene and the symptoms generally become more severe at this stage.

In the case of osteoarthritis of the knee, pain is more marked with weight-bearing and, initially at least, is relieved by rest. Transfers, kneeling and climbing stairs are especially likely to bring on symptoms. Muscle wasting, especially quadriceps, is apparent. There is little or no evidence of soft tissue swelling but small effusions are common. The fluid is less inflammatory than that in rheumatoid arthritis, being more viscous and having a lower protein content and white cell count. There may be instability in both lateral and antero-posterior planes. Flexion becomes limited and it is common to develop lack of full extension. A varus deformity is more common than valgus and may be passively reversible only to reappear with weight-bearing. If the degree of varus deformity is less than 15 degrees then appropriate splintage (especially using a telescopic valgus-varus support (TVS)) might prevent progression in the degree of varus and in reversible cases perhaps improve mechanical forces with the hope of slowing down the arthritic process (Fig. 19/3(a) and (b)).

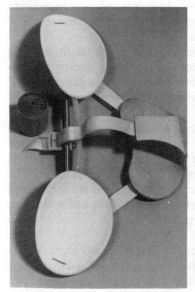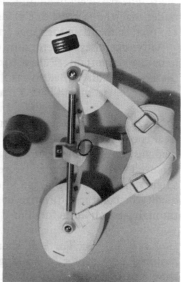

Fig. 19/3   TVS brace: (a) inner surface; (b) outer aspect

Crepitus is very commonly elicited. Locking or an acute exacerbation of pain may be caused by a loose body or a damaged meniscus.

PHYSIOTHERAPY ASSESSMENT

Gait, general appearance and posture can be observed as the patient walks into the department for treatment. See page 198 for assessment details.

TREATMENT

Relief of pain: Radiant heat, short wave diathermy, interferential or ice packs encircling the joint may be used beneficially. Local areas of persistent pain may be treated by counter-irritant doses of ultraviolet irradiation. Where there is nipping of the synovial membrane, traction will be of benefit.

Maintenance of movement and improvement of range: Patellar movements (distal, proximal and oblique) should be maintained by moving the patella passively in all directions. In severe lesions manipulation under anaesthesia may be necessary after which active exercise will be required to maintain the range gained.

Active exercises concentrating on establishing full extension of the joint are important. Pulley circuits, suspension therapy, hydrotherapy particularly Bad Ragaz flexion and extension patterns, PNF techniques, etc will all have a relevant part in the programme.

Strengthening of muscles: Although all the leg muscles may be weakened, it is the quadriceps muscles, and particularly vastus medialis, on which strengthening will be concentrated. This can be achieved by using progressive resistance on land or in water. The single most useful technique to employ is PNF for it can improve quality of contraction, range of movement, power and endurance through being used in functional patterns.

Gait re-education: The gait should be analysed and corrected as required (see Chapter 2). Walking aids may be needed and the patient should be trained in their correct use. If both knees are affected two sticks will be needed and the patient taught to use them as a normal four-point gait pattern; if only one knee is affected then a single stick used in the opposite hand is sufficient.

Gait re-education includes management of stairs, slopes, standing to sitting and bed to chair transfers. Postural awareness needs to be stimulated and the patient encouraged to assume a more efficient posture.

In severe cases it may be necessary to provide some form of orthosis (see Chapter 1). If external splintage is used particular attention must be paid to the maintenance of the quadriceps muscle strength.

Feet

Involvement of the hind foot is rare and is usually the result of injury. Conversely the incidence of osteoarthritis of the first metatarso-phalangeal joint (with or without hallux valgus deformity) is high. The joint becomes restricted and take-off during gait can be very painful. This state, progressing to hallux rigidus, can be alleviated by wearing thick, stiff-soled shoes or inserting a steel bar into the medial sole of the shoe. Osteophytes form and bursitis adds to the pain. Especially with hallux valgus, footwear becomes a problem and patients are happier in old shoes or slippers which have adapted to the deformed foot.

Temporomandibular joint

The cause of osteoarthritis at this site is uncertain although occlusional abnormalities and other repetitive insults relating to mastication have been variously blamed. It may be the end result of long-standing pain and imbalance related to tendons, muscles and soft tissue. Crepitus is common and there is pain and tenderness.

Sacro-iliac joints

Symptoms include low back pain, tenderness over the sacro-iliac joint and stiffness after rest. There seems to be no active inflammation present and it is frequently unilateral with radiological changes differentiating it from true sacro-iliitis.

BIBLIOGRAPHY

Davies, B.C. (1967). A technique of re-education in the treatment pool. *Physiotherapy*, 53, 2.

Hollis, M. (1981). *Practical Exercise Therapy*, 2nd edition. Blackwell Scientific Publications Limited, Oxford.

Hollis, M. and Roper, M.H.S. (1965). *Suspension Therapy*. Baillière Tindall and Cassell, London. (Now out of print but will be found in libraries.)

Hyde, S.A. et al (1980). *Physiotherapy in Rheumatology*. Blackwell Scientific Publications Limited, Oxford.

OSTEOARTHRITIS

Knott, M. and Voss, D. (1968). *Proprioceptive Neuromuscular Facilitation–Patterns and Techniques*, 2nd edition. Harper and Row, London.

Powell, M. (1981). *Orthopaedic Nursing and Rehabilitation*, 8th edition. Churchill Livingstone, Edinburgh.

Savage, B. (1984). *Interferential Therapy*. Faber and Faber, London.

Skinner, A.T. and Thomson, A.M. (eds) (1983). *Duffield's Exercise in Water*, 3rd edition. Baillière Tindall, London.

Wynn Parry, C.B. (1982). *Rehabilitation of the Hand*, 4th edition. Butterworths, London.

Equipment note

The TVS brace is manufactured by Northern Scientific Equipment Ltd (Medical Division), Bridge Road Works, Lymington SO4 9BZ, from whom an illustrated brochure may be obtained giving full instructions in its use and application.

Chapter 20

Osteotomy, Arthrodesis and Girdlestone Arthroplasty

by G.J. BENKE, FRCS, FRCS(Ed)

OSTEOTOMY

This term describes an operation which achieves its effect by division of a bone. It may be used to correct deformity or relieve pain.

The operation is carried out in three stages:

1. The bone is divided as near to the deformity or painful joint as possible. This may be done as a single cut, generally transverse or oblique. Sometimes two cuts are made so that a triangular wedge of bone is removed.
2. The deformity is then corrected. This correction must be complete if recurrence of the deformity is to be avoided. Following this the bone ends should lie in close apposition (Fig. 20/1).
3. The part is then splinted. A plaster of Paris cast may be sufficient if the areas of bone in contact are large. Alternatively, some form of

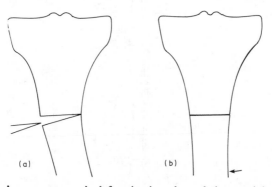

(a)   (b)

Fig. 20/1 An osteotomy. A deformity in a bone being straightened by removal of a wedge

internal fixation or an external fixator is used. It is important that the correction is maintained until the osteotomy has united.

Indications for use

There are many situations where this procedure may be applicable. In general the following objectives may be achieved.

(a) *Improved function*: For example, if a shoulder has become fixed in adduction and internal rotation because of disease, an osteotomy may be used to correct this and so improve function in the arm as a whole.

A malunited Colles' fracture may occasionally give rise to significant disturbance of wrist function. Correction by distal radius osteotomy may considerably improve this.

(b) *Correction of a cosmetic defect*: Osteotomy is rarely indicated for this alone.

(c) *Relief of abnormal stresses on joints which may precipitate early degenerative changes*. For example, in standing the load axis of the leg runs from the centre of rotation of the femoral head through the knee near its mid-point to the mid-point of the ankle. Normally this means that the two halves of the knee joint are loaded equally (Fig. 20/2). This axis may be altered in its relation

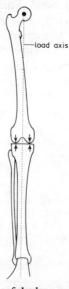

load axis

Fig. 20/2   The normal load axis of the leg passes near the centre of the knee equally loading both compartments

to the knee and ankle by deformities in the femur or tibia which may arise as a result of mal-union of a fracture or bending due to pathological change such as in rickets or Paget's disease. The axis may also be altered by intertrochanteric osteotomy if the femoral shaft is not shifted appropriately (see Fig. 20/6). The overall effect of this may be to produce overloading of one or other side of the knee joint and this may precipitate degenerative changes on that side.

An appropriate osteotomy will restore the correct alignment and loading of the joints.

(d) *Increase in apparent length of a leg which may be apparently shortened by a fixed adduction or flexion deformity at the hip* (Fig. 20/3). These deformities may be corrected by an appropriate intertrochanteric osteotomy (Fig. 20/4). If the deformities are combined, they may both be corrected by removal of appropriate wedges of bone in both planes. This means the femoral shaft, and therefore the leg, is realigned under the hip obviating the need to tilt the pelvis in order to stand with the legs parallel.

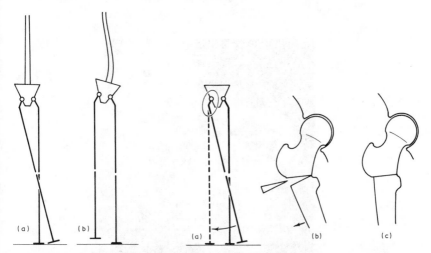

Fig. 20/3 (*Left*) Fixed adduction deformity of the hip. (a) The position of the adducted limb with the level pelvis. (b) The pelvis tilted to bring the affected limb parallel to the other limb. This is achieved by abducting the unaffected hip. *Note* the compensatory curve in the lumbar spine

Fig. 20/4 (*Right*) Correction of the adduction deformity by an intertrochanteric osteotomy. (a) The corrected position of the adducted limb. (b and c) The intertrochanteric osteotomy which corrects this deformity in the circled area of (a)

(e) *Treatment of osteoarthritis by relief of pressure within a joint*: Osteotomy may be indicated in the treatment of this condition in either the hip or knee joints. The objective of the osteotomy is to decrease the pressure in the joint by increasing the surface area being loaded and to decrease the tension in the muscles surrounding the joint.

Either a varus or valgus osteotomy may be performed according to which will restore the greatest congruous load-bearing area in the joint. This is based upon the principle that the greater the surface area of a structure that is being loaded, the smaller will be the pressure on each square unit of that area. For example, if a load of 200kg is put across an area of $2cm^2$, the pressure on the surface will be 100kg per cm^2. If the area being loaded is increased to $5cm^2$, the pressure will be 40kg per cm^2.

Many surgeons still have strong reservations about using joint replacement in younger patients, particularly if the problem is osteoarthritis. Osteotomy may provide a reasonable alternative method of treatment in this situation.

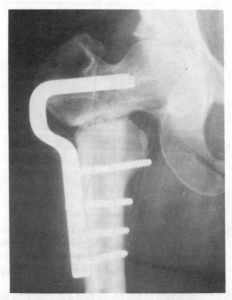

Fig. 20/5   A radiograph showing an osteotomy which has been performed for osteoarthritis of the hip. The osteotomy is fixed under compression with a right-angled blade plate

Hip osteotomy

At the hip a varus osteotomy decreases the angle between the femoral shaft and neck so rotating the femoral head further into the acetabulum. A valgus osteotomy increases this angle rotating the femoral head in the opposite direction. The osteotomy is carried out at the intertrochanteric level and is generally secured under compression by a blade plate (Fig. 20/5).

Bearing in mind the load axis in the normal anatomical situation (Fig. 20/2), it will be noticed that by simply decreasing or increasing the neck-shaft angle of the femur, this axis will be moved respectively medially or laterally in relation to the centre of the knee (Fig. 20/6a and b). By simply shifting the shaft medially without altering the neck-shaft angle, as in the original McMurray osteotomy, the load axis

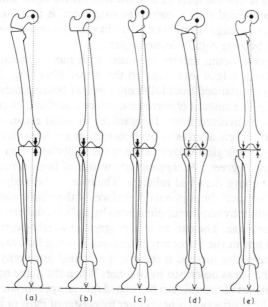

(a)   (b)   (c)   (d)   (e)

Fig. 20/6 Intertrochanteric osteotomy: variations in load axis produced by different femoral neck-shaft relationships. (a) Simple varus osteotomy shifts the axis medially overloading the medial knee compartment. (b) Simple medialisation of the femoral shaft (McMurray osteotomy) shifts the axis laterally overloading the lateral knee compartment. (c) Simple valgus osteotomy shifts the axis laterally with the same result as (b). (d) Varus osteotomy with medialisation of the shaft restores the normal relationship of the axis to the knee as does valgus osteotomy with lateralisation of the shaft (e)

will be moved laterally in relation to the centre of the knee (Fig. 20/6c). In order to keep the load axis in its normal relationship to the knee, a varus or valgus osteotomy must be combined respectively with some medial or lateral displacement of the shaft (Fig. 20/6d and e).

To the basic intertrochanteric varus or valgus osteotomy may be added elements of rotation, flexion or extension as appropriate.

The pressure across the joint is also decreased by lessening the tension in the muscles surrounding the joint. This is brought about by the alteration in the neck-shaft angle or by supplementary tenotomies.

Knee osteotomy

At the knee, genu varum and genu valgum deformities may result from osteoarthritis which predominantly involves respectively the medial or lateral compartment of the joint. If the other compartment is well preserved then a corrective osteotomy is indicated. This is designed to realign the tibia or femur in such a way that both sides of the joint become equally loaded again.

The genu varum deformity is met with more commonly and is treated by a valgus osteotomy in the upper tibia (Fig. 20/7). The procedure is planned from full-length weight-bearing radiographs of both legs. The amount of correction can be calculated by comparison with the uninvolved limb. In practice, to avoid recurrence of the deformity, a few degrees of over-correction are introduced (i.e. the normal physiological valgus between the femur and tibia is restored plus a few degrees). An appropriate wedge of bone is removed at a level just above the tibial tubercle. The base of the wedge is lateral. After its removal the adjacent cut surfaces of the tibia are apposed and held together by staples supplemented by a plaster of Paris cylinder or by plaster alone. The patient may progress to weight-bearing early as the final line of the osteotomy is transverse to the load axis.

An alternative method is the use of a domed osteotomy above the tibial tubercle as described by Maquet. When the dome has been cut the distal part of the tibia can be rotated into an appropriate amount of valgus. The correction is held either by plaster of Paris or by external fixation (Fig. 20/8). To allow appropriate movement of the tibia, the fibula must be divided. This is done obliquely about 7.5cm below the neck of the fibula to avoid damage to the peroneal nerve.

For the genu valgum deformity an upper tibial varus osteotomy may be used. However, the results for this are not so good as a femoral supracondylar osteotomy. The appropriate correction is again determined from weight-bearing radiographs of both legs.

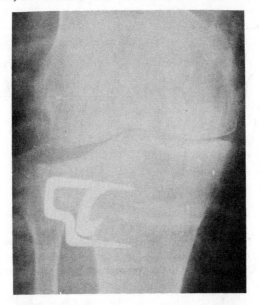

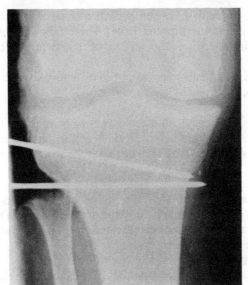

Fig. 20/7 (*Upper*)   Radiograph of a high tibial valgus osteotomy for genu varum. Here the deformity is secondary to osteoarthritis predominantly affecting the medial knee compartment. Fixation is by two staples. (*Lower*) The intra-operative radiograph illustrating how the wedge of bone to be removed can be determined with the help of two guide wires

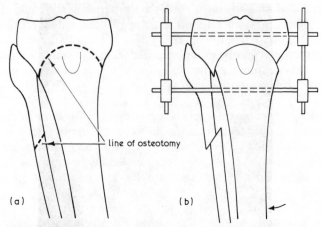

line of osteotomy

(a)   (b)

Fig. 20/8 High tibial dome osteotomy of Maquet. (a) The line of the tibial and fibular osteotomies. (b) The correction achieved by rotating the distal fragment. Correction held under compression by an external fixation device

Particular emphasis has been laid on osteotomies as they apply to osteoarthritis of the hip and knee. There follows a brief regional survey indicating where this method of treatment may be applied.

Scapula: Glenoid osteotomy described by Stamm in the treatment of a painful arc syndrome of the shoulder.

Humerus: Occasionally an osteotomy may be required in the upper part if the shoulder has become fixed in adduction or internal rotation as a result of disease. This is done to put the arm in a more functional position.

Elbow: Varus deformity of the elbow may occur as a result of mal-union of a supracondylar fracture of the humerus. This is an ugly deformity and may be corrected by removal of a wedge of bone on the lateral side of the humerus just above the elbow.

Occasionally severe residual backward angulation following this fracture may lead to a significant loss of flexion in the elbow joint. A corrective osteotomy inserting a wedge of bone into the lower humerus from behind will restore this.

Forearm and wrist: Mal-union of a Colles' fracture may occasionally require a corrective distal radius osteotomy.

Spine: Ankylosing spondylitis leads to a progressive stiffening of the spine. Sometimes, when fusion in the spine occurs in severe flexion the patient may not be able to see in front of him. To correct this an angular lordosis may be produced in the lumbar region by excising a wedge of bone from the adjacent bodies of two vertebrae having first removed their posterior elements.

Hip: A variety of hip disorders may be treated by osteotomy either of the pelvis (Salter, Pemberton, Chiari) or the upper femur in the intertrochanteric or subtrochanteric region. The following are the principal indications with the type of osteotomy bracketed.

(a) Congenital dislocation of the hip. (Pelvic or femoral osteotomy or both.)
(b) Congenital subluxation of the hip. (Pelvic or femoral.)
(c) Tuberculosis. (Femoral to correct fixed deformities following ankylosis.)
(d) Perthes' disease. (Femoral or pelvic.)
(e) Slipped upper femoral epiphysis – chronic type. (Dunn cervical osteotomy of the femoral head or intertrochanteric tri-plane osteotomy. The former is done if the epiphyseal plate is still open, the latter if it has fused with the epiphysis in the slipped position.)
(f) Osteoarthritis. (Femoral.)
(g) Un-united subcapital fracture. (Femoral.)

Femoral shaft: Occasionally this is necessary for congenital deformities; those which arise as a complication of diseases such as rickets or fibrous dysplasia; or as a result of mal-union of a fracture.

Supracondylar region of femur: For genu valgum or a fixed flexion deformity of the knee. Occasionally an osteotomy may be carried out in this region for a genu recurvatum deformity.

Upper tibia: Angulatory or rotatory deformities may be corrected by osteotomy in the upper tibia. Osteotomy for genu varum has already been discussed. Internal tibial torsion may be corrected by a rotational osteotomy just below the tibial tubercle in the upper part of the tibial shaft.

Shaft of tibia: Osteotomy may be used to correct a rickets' deformity or in painful Paget's disease with bow legs.

Lower tibia: A mal-united ankle fracture may lead to secondary degenerative arthritis. This may be prevented by an osteotomy just above the ankle joint. This is planned so that the ankle joint will be brought horizontal.

Foot: Osteotomies may be used in a number of deformities including talipes equino varus and claw foot. They may be carried out in the calcaneus, mid-tarsal and tarso-metatarsal regions.

Great toe: Osteotomy of the first metatarsal may be carried out to correct hallux valgus deformity. This is applicable in a younger person where the deformity is often based on a pre-existing primary metatarsus varus deformity and degenerative changes have not occurred in the first metatarsophalangeal joint.

ARTHRODESIS

The term arthrodesis refers to surgical fusion of a joint. The indications for this are pain and instability in a joint and, in some situations, following the failure of joint replacement. With the increase and improvements in the field of joint replacement arthrodesis is now carried out much less frequently.

In the lower limb, because of the larger stresses brought about by weight-bearing, arthrodesis as a primary procedure should only be used if adjacent joints and the joints of the other leg are sound. This applies to a much lesser degree in the upper limb where, for example, arthrodesis of a painful, unstable wrist in rheumatoid arthritis may in fact considerably improve the function of involved fingers and thumb.

A successful arthrodesis is a sure way of permanently relieving pain but it is bought at the price of stiffness. However, this may be a small price to pay in some situations.

Ideally arthrodesis is carried out as an intra-articular procedure. All articular cartilage is removed from both surfaces of the joint and the bone ends shaped to fit in the required position. They are held there either by internal fixation, an external fixation device or external splintage (e.g. plaster of Paris) or a combination of these methods, until the fusion is sound. Where possible compression is applied to the bone ends to promote fusion. Occasionally extra-articular arthrodesis is carried out. This usually applies to the hip and shoulder joints. Here the joint surfaces are not disturbed and fusion is achieved by bridging the joint by a bone graft adjacent to it, e.g. from the femur to the ischium.

Fixation positions

The optimum positions for arthrodesis in different joints are as follows.

Shoulder: In such a position that the hand can comfortably reach the mouth.

Elbow: Ninety degrees of flexion in clerical workers. Slightly straighter in labourers.

Wrist: A few degrees of extension unless both wrists are arthrodesed, in which case one should be fused in some flexion to permit the carrying out of certain toilet functions.

Thumb: Metacarpophalangeal joint in 20 degrees of flexion. Interphalangeal joint in slight flexion.

Fingers: Metacarpophalangeal joints in 20–30 degrees of flexion. (These joints are rarely fused.)
   Proximal interphalangeal joints in 40–50 degrees of flexion (less in middle and index fingers).
   Distal interphalangeal joints in 15–20 degrees of flexion.

Hip: In 15–20 degrees of flexion (to permit comfortable sitting); 10 degrees of abduction; and 5 degrees of external rotation.

Knee: Straight.

Ankle: Ninety degrees; (a little equinus in women who wear high heels).

Subtalar: Neutral (i.e. no varus or valgus).

Great toe: Metatarsophalangeal joint in a few degrees extension and slight valgus. (A little more extension for women who wear high heels.) Interphalangeal joint straight.

Lesser toes: Straight.

Arthrodesis is indicated in some painful arthritic joints especially if there is associated instability, or in joints which have become flail due to paralysis (e.g. in poliomyelitis). The indications in arthritic joints are becoming less and less with the advent of more and more joint replacements. However, certain joints still lend themselves to arthrodesis as a primary form of treatment. This particularly applies to the knee, ankle and wrist.

In osteoarthritis of the knee arthrodesis should be considered if this is the only joint involved, particularly in the younger patient.

The ankle joint replacement is not so reliable as those for the hip and knee joints and its only indication is in rheumatoid patients with joints of the foot involved as well. Otherwise arthrodesis is the treatment of choice for a painful arthritic ankle.

The wrist joint may be replaced. However, although movement is preserved power in the hand is less than that produced by an arthrodesis. If both wrists are involved, it is usual to replace one and arthrodese the other.

Arthrodesis of the shoulder joint is usually reserved for a flail joint as may follow a brachial plexus injury. Stabilisation of this joint may lead to improvement in the remaining distal function of the arm.

Tuberculosis may lead to destruction of a joint and fibrous ankylosis (Chapter 5). This may be painful. If this is the case, arthrodesis may be indicated. It is one of the few remaining indications for arthrodesing a hip joint.

Sometimes a joint may remain very painful following trauma. To relieve this arthrodesis may be required. This particularly applies to the subtalar joint following a serious fracture of the calcaneus. Such an arthrodesis is usually carried out after the passage of an adequate amount of time has allowed for spontaneous settling of pain. Occasionally the fracture is so severe that the subtalar joint is completely disrupted and arthrodesis may be necessary as an immediate form of treatment.

As indicated in Chapter 21 joint replacements are subject to complications which may include mechanical failure and infection. If this occurs following replacement of the knee, ankle or wrist, arthrodesis may become necessary as a salvage procedure.

If a hip joint replacement fails it may not be possible to revise it. If this is the case arthrodesis is not carried out but the joint components and cement are removed and the patient is left with a Girdlestone arthroplasty.

GIRDLESTONE ARTHROPLASTY

Girdlestone described this operation as treatment of a tuberculous hip which had become secondarily infected. The operation he described involved a very radical excision of tissue. This included excision of the upper half of the greater trochanter and the whole of the femoral neck and head. The acetabulum was curetted to remove all necrotic and infected bone; enough bone was removed from the acetabulum and ilium to allow free drainage of an intrapelvic abscess. Any involved soft tissue was also excised.

This procedure is considered by many to be very radical but occasionally may be required if there is extensive involvement of the joint and surrounding tissues. Earlier diagnosis and the availability of more effective antibiotic therapy have reduced the need to carry out this procedure for tuberculosis.

Now the principal use of this operation is as a salvage procedure for a failed hip joint replacement. The procedure is less radical than that initially described by Girdlestone. The greater trochanter is preserved. After removal of the joint components and all cement, necrotic soft and bony tissue is completely excised. Any remaining femoral neck is then trimmed off.

After operation the patient is rested in bed with the leg on skeletal traction for up to six weeks. Movement of the hip can be started in traction as pain settles. The patient is then mobilised with crutches and if possible should remain non-weight-bearing on the affected side for a few months to allow good fibrosis to establish in the old joint space. If weight-bearing is commenced too early there will be a tendency to increase the inevitable shortening of the leg which follows this procedure. If the patient is elderly and frail it may be best to accept this and allow weight to be taken earlier. Attempts to make such patients non-weight-bear may produce two undesirable effects. First, excessive demands may be put on their limited energy reserves and second, locomotion may become very unstable leading to an increased risk of falling.

Previously a weight-relieving caliper was employed for several months. Opinions are divided on this and many surgeons now would not advocate its use but rather would accept the inevitable shortening and compensate this by an adequate shoe-raise. Very few patients with a Girdlestone arthroplasty will walk without an aid. The minimum aid required by most is two walking sticks.

BIBLIOGRAPHY

Pauwels, F. (1976). *Biomechanics of the Normal and Diseased Hip. Theoretical Foundation, Technique and Results of Treatment.* Springer-Verlag, New York.

Chapter 21

Joint Replacement

by G.J. BENKE, FRCS, FRCS(Ed)

Over the last 25 years, joint replacements have become established in the practice of orthopaedic surgery. Although for several years preceding this surgeons used many materials in the attempt to achieve this purpose, it was not until Sir John Charnley developed the concept of metal articulating with plastic (high density polyethylene) that the real breakthrough was achieved. At the same time as Charnley was developing the earlier version of his arthroplasty, McKee developed a hip joint in which both components were metal. Although many of these did reasonably well, the articulation of metal on metal did not prove satisfactory because of the higher frictional forces involved which led to a high incidence of loosening. On the other hand, metal articulating on high density polyethylene produces much less friction, hence the name given to the Charnley hip prosthesis – low friction hip arthroplasty (Fig. 21/1).

Early attempts at joint replacements not only failed because of the inadequate properties of the materials, but also because of the difficulties in obtaining a secure and reliable fixation to the bone. This was overcome by the introduction of methylmethacrylate cement as this provided a more secure fixation. This cement is not an adhesive. It achieves its supportive function by being tightly packed around the prosthetic component and interlocking into the cancellous bone immediately adjacent to the cortex. This interlocking is sometimes supplemented by keying holes such as those that are drilled into the floor and roof of the acetabulum. Although the use of cement has revolutionised the insertion of a joint replacement, it is by no means the perfect answer. In fact, the bone-cement interface remains the potentially weak link in the system and the part most susceptible to mechanical failure, a fact highlighted by the current strenuous research to develop uncemented prostheses.

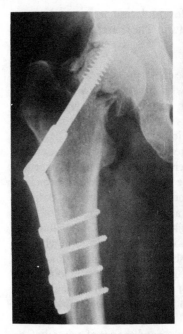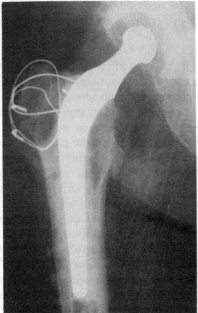

Fig. 21/1 Charnley low friction hip arthroplasty. It has been carried out following failure of fixation of a subcapital fracture (*Left*). *Note* the greater trochanter has been reattached by wires

Other materials are used for joint replacements, the chief of which is silastic. Its use will be referred to in consideration of the replacement of smaller joints such as the metacarpophalangeal joints of the hand.

INDICATIONS

Before considering some of the joints in more detail, we must be clear about the indications for carrying out these procedures. It must be stressed that a joint replacement is not the panacea of all joint problems and that some clearly defined objectives must be kept in mind when it is being considered. In making this decision the surgeon must take into account the potential complications of a joint replacement. The whole team must also be aware of these. They will be considered in more detail at the end of the chapter.

In determining the indications for replacing a joint we must consider the objectives of this procedure. These are:
1. To relieve pain
2. To improve function.

Of these, the first will always be the most pressing as, apart from causing distress, pain will interfere with function. Few patients are referred for consideration of such procedures simply for the improvement of function when pain is not a significant feature. Many patients perform well with a stiff joint providing there is not a significant element of pain associated with it, as is seen with a successful arthrodesis (see Chapter 20). However, in certain situations, joint replacement may be indicated when the principal problem is stiffness. An example of this would be in a patient, particularly a female, who has fixed adduction contractures of both hips. This will not only make walking difficult, but will cause problems relating to toilet functions. Sometimes a stiff joint which is pain-free may lead to abnormal stresses in adjacent joints which may cause them to become painful. Mobilisation of the stiff joint by a replacement may improve the pain, or prevent it from worsening. An example of this is backache related to fixed flexion deformities of the hip.

In summary, a patient can be offered a good chance of pain relief, as high as complete relief in 90 per cent of hip replacements, but he should be cautioned that although movement in a stiff joint can usually be improved, this is unlikely to be as dramatic as the degree of pain relief.

Bearing in mind these objectives, we can understand in what conditions the use of a joint replacement is most applicable. The great majority are carried out in patients with rheumatoid arthritis and similar inflammatory joint diseases such as ankylosing spondylitis, or osteoarthritis, both primary and secondary.

More rarely, a joint replacement may be used in the treatment of pathological bone near a joint. For example, a total hip replacement may be used to replace the femoral neck if it is involved by a malignant tumour.

Sometimes they are used in the primary treatment of fractures. For example, some surgeons consider that a displaced subcapital fracture of the femur should be treated by a total hip replacement, rather than a hemi-arthroplasty such as a Thompson or Austin Moore prosthesis. These are also a form of joint replacement. They are stemmed prostheses which replace the neck and head of the femur. The former is designed to be used with cement, whereas the latter is not. Of the two, the Thompson prosthesis is used more commonly. Here the new articulation is between a metal femoral head and the patient's acetabulum.

INDIVIDUAL JOINTS

Keeping in mind the preceding general comments, the replacement of specific joints will be considered in an order which will reflect the frequency with which the joint is replaced and, to a point, the degree of success achieved with it.

In Chapter 22, emphasis will be placed on treatment as it relates to physiotherapists. Ideally any postoperative programme should be outlined to the patient before his operation. In this way, those involved can establish a good rapport with the patient and can teach him what will be expected of him in the early postoperative period when pain can prove to be a distraction to learning new things. It will help to secure in the patient's mind the aims he is trying to achieve and the rate of progress he is likely to make.

Hip joint

Replacement of the hip joint is the most commonly performed arthroplasty and there is no doubt that it achieves the highest success rate of all the artificial joints. There is evidence to show that they will survive for at least 15–20 years. In spite of this it must be remembered that many surgeons still have strong reservations about using this procedure in younger patients who will generally put greater demands on the replacement. This will lead to greater mechanical stresses on the joint which, in turn, will make the outcome less certain in the longer term. However, if there is some form of inherent brake on the activity level of the patient their younger age will not hold quite the same significance. This is well shown in those with rheumatoid arthritis, where the general level of activity is frequently reduced by multiple joint involvement and also by the systemic nature of this disease. This is a very different situation from that of the young patient, whose only problem is osteoarthritis of one hip joint. This concern applies to all joint replacements, but more particularly to the weight-bearing joints.

The hip replacements that are used at the present time are basically of two types:

The first are referred to as *conventional* arthroplasties. These are composed of a plastic acetabular cup and a stemmed femoral component which is fixed into the medullary cavity of the upper end of the femur. The Charnley arthroplasty is the forerunner of many others which show various modifications. Mostly these joints are anchored by cement. However, some are being developed where the parts, particularly the femoral component, are not dependent on cement for their fixation.

The second type are *resurfacing* procedures. In these a thinner, larger diameter plastic cup is used in the acetabulum, and the femoral head is prepared in such a way as to accept a thin metal cup to cover its surface. The femoral neck is entirely preserved and no cement is passed into the intramedullary cavity. Of the types available the ICLH, Tharies and Wagner arthroplasties are the most commonly used.

The surgical approach to the hip joint may be antero-lateral, lateral or posterior. Some surgeons prefer to detach the greater trochanter to facilitate access to the joint. This is particularly useful if any technical difficulties are anticipated. The trochanter is reattached at the close of the operation, generally by a wiring technique (see Fig. 21/1).

Assuming correct placement of the components, when the antero-lateral and lateral approaches are used, in most cases the joint tends to be more stable in flexion and internal rotation, i.e. with the patient sitting. However, the hip is more stable in external rotation and extension, i.e. with the patient lying flat, when the joint is inserted through the posterior approach. For a few days after operation the patient will frequently be nursed with a wedge pillow between the legs. Such a pillow encourages abduction of the hips, a position which gives good stability. Apart from these points, the general principles of postoperative management are the same whichever approach is used.

Knee joint

Replacement of the knee joint may be partial or total.

Examples of partial replacements are the McIntosh and Sledge prostheses. In the former, a part of one or both of the tibial condyles is removed and replaced by a metal disc. The femoral condyles articulate with the upper surface of the disc. The latter type involves replacement of either the medial or lateral compartment of the tibio-femoral articulation. This is achieved by inserting a metal runner on the appropriate femoral condyle which glides on a polyethylene component on the adjacent tibial condyle. The components are secured by bone cement. This concept is useful in advanced osteoarthritis involving one compartment only, seen in valgus and varus knee deformities, and can be considered when it is judged that the condition is beyond the scope of treatment by osteotomy. The third compartment of the knee, namely the patello-femoral articulation, may be the only part significantly affected by osteoarthritis. Resurfacing of the patella and adjacent femoral intercondylar areas with plastic and metal liners have produced replacement for this joint also. The results of these procedures are still under evaluation.

Total knee replacement, which in fact does not routinely involve resurfacing of the patella, has also become an established procedure. Although the results of this procedure may be very good, overall the outcome is less satisfactory and more uncertain than for hip replacement. There are two principal reasons for this. First, the superficial nature of the joint tends to give more problems relating to wound complications. Secondly, the very complexity of the normal knee joint biomechanics presents difficulties. Unless design of the prosthesis permits gliding and rotational movements as well as hingeing, torsional forces will be produced which will tend to produce loosening of the components.

It is with these features in mind that the concepts of knee joint replacement have evolved. It is beyond the scope of this book to consider this in detail. It will therefore be simpler to consider the types of joint under three headings.

CONSTRAINED JOINTS
These represent the simple hinge (e.g. Waldius, Shiers, McKee and Stanmore types) in which the femoral and tibial components are stemmed, and also linked together to allow only hingeing movements. Their major advantage is the inherent stability produced, leaving no dependence on the knee ligaments to achieve this. However, they have two disadvantages. First, they are exposed to torsional forces which will tend to promote loosening; and secondly, they require excision of larger amounts of bone for their insertion, which may make arthrodesis difficult as a salvage procedure.

UNCONSTRAINED JOINTS
Here the surfaces of the tibia and femur are covered with polyethylene and metal respectively with no linkage of the components. These have the advantage of introducing an element of rotation and gliding which will decrease the torsional forces which tend to promote loosening. They also involve excision of much less bone and, in the event of failure, may be salvaged more easily by either a hinged prosthesis or arthrodesis.

They do, however, depend on proper tension in the collateral ligaments to provide good stability. Examples of these joints are the ICLH and Geomedic types.

SEMI-CONSTRAINED JOINTS

These have been designed to incorporate as many advantages of the first two types as possible. Examples of these are the Sheehan and Attenborough prostheses (Fig. 21/2). They comprise two components with a linkage system. This is not rigid like a simple hinge. Thus, features of a hinge joint have been produced giving greater inherent stability while maintaining some freedom of rotation and gliding to minimise torsional stresses.

The joints are inserted through an anterior mid-line, or parapatellar skin incision. The capsule of the knee is opened by a medial parapatellar incision. The components are introduced in such a manner as to produce a stable knee with correction of valgus or varus

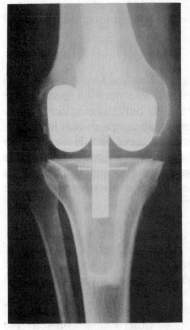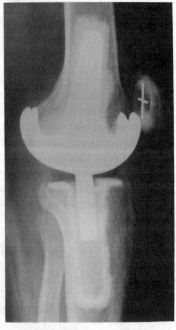

Fig. 21/2 An Attenborough total knee replacement for a rheumatoid knee joint (AP and lateral views)

deformities while leaving no fixed flexion. The ultimate range of flexion is unlikely to be much beyond 90 degrees in most cases.

The hip and knee joint replacements have been considered in detail as they are by far the most commonly replaced joints. Most joints in the upper and lower limbs now have replacements, but all are much less frequently used. Therefore, they will only briefly be referred to by way of description.

Finger joints

Small silastic joints are used in rheumatoid arthritic patients, particularly in metacarpophalangeal joints which have subluxed anteriorly and in an ulnar direction. Function may be considerably improved by correcting these deformities. Similar replacements may be used in the proximal interphalangeal joints.

One basic point must be stressed when considering such treatment in the rheumatoid hand. The overall function of the hand must be assessed. Even with marked deformities, adapted function may be so effective as to obviate the indication of a joint replacement, which may only achieve an improved cosmetic effect while diminishing the functional efficiency of the hand as a whole.

Wrist joint

Arthrodesis (Chapter 20) has produced excellent functional results when used to treat a painful wrist. However, replacements have been introduced which are most effectively employed in rheumatoid arthritis. An example of such a joint is the silastic replacement designed by Swanson, particularly used in the destroyed, anteriorly subluxed wrist. It allows for stabilisation with realignment while maintaining some movement.

Shoulder joint

These are basically designed on a ball and socket principle. In order to retain any possibility of functional movement, the integrity of the tuberosities with their muscle attachments must be preserved. They are perhaps most effective in pain relief in rheumatoid arthritis. Whereas this is generally good, improvement in the range of movement is not usually comparable.

Elbow joint

Various designs have been produced either involving a hinged joint or a resurfacing type of procedure. They are mostly used in rheumatoid arthritis. Osteoarthritis is relatively uncommon in this joint and rarely requires such treatment.

Ankle joints

Replacements have been designed, but at the present time are rarely carried out. Arthrodesis of the ankle is very effective if the joints of the foot are normal. However, preservation of some ankle movement by joint replacement may be most helpful to a patient where this is not the case. Again these are more commonly used in rheumatoid patients.

Silastic joints have been designed for treatment of hallux valgus and hallux rigidus. Here the implant is basically acting as a spacer to fill the gap left by excision of bone.

COMPLICATIONS

Many of the patients undergoing joint replacements are elderly, in some there may be medical problems, others have rheumatoid arthritis, of whom some may be on steroid therapy. As a consequence, the general complication rate is by no means insignificant.

Appropriate physiotherapy can help in avoiding three of these complications in particular. The first is deep venous thrombosis, the prevention of which can be considerably helped by promotion of good circulation in the lower extremities. The second is postoperative chest infection. Patients with underlying pulmonary problems, e.g. bronchitis, will be particularly at risk. Good pre-operative and postoperative breathing exercise regimes will help to avoid this. The third is avoidance of skin pressure problems by appropriate care to vulnerable areas both before and after operation. Ideally there will be a reciprocal integration of these aspects of management involving the whole team. However, the principal burden of avoiding these complications will fall on the nursing and physiotherapy staff.

As indicated at the outset of this chapter, joint replacements must not be looked upon as the panacea of all joint problems. There may be some serious local complications namely, dislocation, infection, loosening or component failure. Some of these may be amenable to appropriate treatment often involving one or more further major operations.

The final outcome, particularly with infection, may be removal of the joint and salvage by arthrodesis or excision arthroplasty (e.g. Girdlestone arthroplasty of the hip (p. 422)).

However, for the patient with severe pain and limitation of function, the successful replacement of one or more involved joints, together with good rehabilitation, may so transform his life that these risks may quite justifiably be taken.

BIBLIOGRAPHY

Charnley, J. (1979). *Low Friction Arthroplasty of the Hip. Theory and Practice.* Springer-Verlag, New York.

See also end of Chapter 23.

Chapter 22

Physiotherapy Following Joint Replacement, etc

by J.A. BENTLEY, MCSP, ONC

Patients admitted to hospital for total joint replacement may have had severe, disabling pain in one or more joints for many years. The operation is performed primarily to relieve pain, increase range of movement and improve function. The patients are closely involved in the rehabilitation programme and the procedures preceding and following surgery should be carefully explained. They should know what to expect, what is expected of them, and understand that *their* motivation and perseverance are essential factors to *their* successful rehabilitation. A successful rehabilitation programme also depends upon communication and co-operation between medical, nursing, physiotherapy and occupational therapy staff working closely together to form, with the patient, a positive and progressive team.

The patient is admitted two to three days prior to surgery to enable investigations, including radiographic examination, to be carried out and assessments made; it is the latter which particularly concerns the physiotherapist.

Assessment enables a rapport to be established between the physiotherapist and the patient; hopes and expectations can be discussed and a realistic approach taken to the outcome of the operation. A functional assessment to establish the ability to run a household, perhaps hold down a job or do the shopping, get into and out of a car or travel on public transport will give an idea of the pre-operative independence. The difficulties he experiences in the simple everyday activities of dressing, bathing, sitting and rising from an armchair, negotiating stairs and thresholds will also indicate the aids and adaptations which may be needed when the patient returns home. The help and support that is received from family and friends may be an important factor when they are discharged from hospital, and where problems exist the social worker should be asked to see the patient.

A single joint cannot be treated in isolation; the physiotherapist must bear in mind the interdependence of one joint or limb with another, and support or exercise as appropriate those joints not immediately affected. The following routine maintenance exercises to assist venous return, prevent deep venous thrombosis and chest complications should be taught, and the importance of practising them assiduously after operation should be stressed.
1. Deep breathing exercises.
2. Bilateral foot exercises.
3. Isometric quadriceps and gluteal exercises.
4. Active exercises for the sound limb.
5. General arm exercises.

TOTAL HIP REPLACEMENT

Treatment is determined by the type of operation and the surgical approach which is used. With the Charnley total hip replacement, because the great trochanter with its muscle attachment is detached and then wired back to the femoral shaft, abduction must be maintained and adduction avoided until sound healing in the tissues around the joint and great trochanter has occurred. Partial weight-bearing is permitted after the wound drainage tubes have been removed, but full weight-bearing is delayed for six weeks.

When the posterior approach is used hip flexion must be carefully controlled to avoid the danger of dislocation. This may occur if undue stress is put on the structures around the posterior aspect of the joint which have been incised and, until the tissues are healed, flexion is restricted to 45 degrees. Sitting out in an armchair may be delayed for a few days and the patient should not sit bolt upright – but lean back in the chair – to minimise hip flexion. Full weight-bearing within the patient's tolerance is allowed.

Pre-operative

Prior to surgery the postoperative management should be explained, a functional assessment made and the routine maintenance exercises taught. In the physical assessment the following should be observed and recorded.
(a) The type of gait and walking aid used.

(b) The range of active and passive movement in both hips – and whether the limiting factor is pain or stiffness.
(c) The degree of muscle wasting present through the limb.
(d) The mobility of the lumbar spine and any increase in the normal lumbar curve.
(e) The presence of pain whether at rest or on weight-bearing.
(f) The presence of deformity.
(g) The inequality of leg lengths.
(h) The amount of intercondylar and intermalleolar separation.

LEG MEASUREMENT
To measure leg length the patient should lie supine with the pelvis level and the feet a little apart: for *true* length measure from the anterior superior iliac spine to the tip of the medial malleolus; for *apparent* length from the umbilicus to the tip of the medial malleolus.

Postoperative

DAY 1–5
Following surgery the patient is nursed in the supine position for the first 24 hours, after which he is raised to a semi-recumbent position. The lower limbs are held in abduction by means of a Charnley wedge, or a firm pillow placed between the malleoli.

Active and active-assisted hip and knee flexion and abduction exercises in a small range are given in addition to the routine maintenance exercises already described. After 48 hours, the wound drainage tubes are removed, and if the patient's general condition is satisfactory, weight-bearing commences. The patient moves to the edge of the bed, to the same side as the affected limb which is supported and maintained in abduction by the physiotherapist. The patient rests on the side of the bed, both feet on the floor, and with minimal flexion of the affected hip and knee. With the help of the physiotherapist and the support of a walking frame, the patient stands up taking partial weight on the affected leg. After practising weight transference and balance exercises, a few steps may be taken, and the patient then returns to bed.

DAY 5–7
Active and active-assisted movements to the affected hip are gradually increased in range and the patient encouraged to practise them frequently. A sliding board may be used for active hip flexion and abduction exercises but care must be taken to ensure that correct movements are occurring at the hip and that the limb does not rotate

laterally. General posture in bed must be observed and corrected as necessary. The patient may be allowed to sit out in an armchair for short periods during the day at the discretion of the surgeon. Weight-bearing with the aid of elbow crutches, and re-education in walking progresses and the walking distance is increased each day. At this stage the patient may walk with the affected limb in some abduction giving the impression of inequality in leg length, this disappears as the limb adopts a more normal or neutral position.

The physiotherapist must observe any circulatory disturbance and report to the nurse in charge of the ward the presence of pain or discomfort in the calf muscles, any restriction in dorsiflexion of the ankle or swelling of the limb.

DAY 7–12

By this time the patient is up for most of the day, dressed and wearing comfortable shoes, able to sit and rise from an armchair of appropriate height, get into or out of bed unaided, walk to the bathroom and negotiate stairs.

Stair drill: to ascend: Hold the banister rail with one hand, an elbow crutch in the other hand while carrying the second elbow crutch horizontally in this hand. Place the sound limb up on to the step and bring the affected limb up to it.

Stair drill: to descend: Hold the banister rail with one hand. Place the elbow crutch and the affected limb on to the step below and bring the sound limb down to it. Negotiating stairs with alternate steps may not be achieved for three months.

The patient should rest in the supine or prone position for an hour during the day to prevent any tendency to a flexion deformity recurring. To turn into the prone position the patient should roll on to the sound side with the operated limb supported in abduction during the turn.

Isometric exercises for the quadriceps and gluteal muscles, mobilising and strengthening exercises for both limbs, including bilateral abduction exercises, continue. The affected hip is not allowed to flex beyond 90 degrees until the structures around the joint are soundly healed, and maximal range of movement is not achieved for some months. Inequality in leg length must be adjusted by raising the appropriate shoe. Balance exercises and gait training are practised in front of a mirror so that the patient can see and feel the correct pattern of walking.

The patient must be warned to avoid bending and rotating the hip, as in reaching forward to fasten a shoe, because of the risk of dislocation. If necessary the occupational therapist will teach the patient how to dress and use the various aids which are available and will also assess the need for aids and adaptations in the home.

When the wound is soundly healed the sutures are removed and by day 12–14, if all is well, the patient is discharged. The majority of patients do not require outpatient physiotherapy. They are advised:

(a) To use common sense and treat the new hip with care.
(b) To rest for an hour in the supine or prone position every day for the first few weeks.
(c) To walk little and often taking equal strides with each step.
(d) To use aids for picking up objects from the floor.
(e) To avoid adduction as in crossing one knee over the other.
(f) To avoid maximal flexion of the hip for the first few months.

The surgeon will see the patient four to six weeks post-surgery when elbow crutches may be replaced by walking sticks. These are retained for three months, or for as long as the patient's needs dictate.

TOTAL KNEE REPLACEMENT

Total knee replacement is indicated where there is severe disabling pain with associated instability and deformity of the joint resulting from advanced osteoarthritis or rheumatoid arthritis.

Total knee prostheses may be classified into three basic groups (see p. 429).

Physical assessment

The following should be observed and recorded.

(a) Type of gait and the walking aid used.
(b) The presence of deformity and instability on weight-bearing and non-weight-bearing.
(c) The active and passive range of movement in both knees.
(d) The quality of quadriceps contraction.
(e) The quality and power of movement through the range.
(f) The presence of muscle wasting throughout the limb.
(g) The mobility of the patella and presence of effusion.
(h) The impairment of other joints.
(i) The presence of pain at rest, on weight-bearing.

The patient is instructed in the routine maintenance exercises already described with particular emphasis on teaching bilateral isometric quadriceps exercises.

Postoperative

DAY 1–5

Following surgery the limb is supported in a pressure bandage and back splint and the foot of the bed is elevated to assist venous return and minimise swelling. Vigorous bilateral foot exercises, isometric quadriceps exercises with concurrent dorsiflexion of the ankle to reinforce the contraction, and routine maintenance exercises are commenced at once, and the patient encouraged to practise them frequently throughout the day. When the wound drainage tubes have been removed and the patient can straight leg raise (SLR) with a good quadriceps contraction, weight-bearing is allowed within the tolerance of the patient. A walking frame may be necessary at first but the patient progresses quickly to elbow crutches or walking sticks.

DAY 5–12

At the discretion of the surgeon the pressure bandage is reduced and the back splint removed for knee mobilising exercises. Some surgeons restrict flexion to 30–40 degrees until wound healing has occurred. Active knee flexion and extension exercises, initially with the heel supported on the bed, commence with emphasis on obtaining full extension of the knee with a good quadriceps contraction. A small wedge or firm pillow which is gradually increased in height, can be placed under the thigh to enable the patient to exercise the knee actively against gravity. As control and strength improve knee exercises are given over the side of the bed or plinth. The foot should be supported on a stool or by the physiotherapist at the maximum point of flexion, to minimise pain and inhibition of movement until the patient can control the movement through the range. The range of movement should be measured and recorded each day.

Active, active-assisted and resisted exercises, hold/relax and facilitatory techniques to gain range and restore strength and stability are gradually included, with particular emphasis on active extension of the knee. When the control of movement through the range is satisfactory, weight-bearing exercises may be given. Isometric exercises, rhythmical stabilisations and weight transferences may be practised in standing but the splint is retained for walking until 70–90 degrees of flexion has been achieved. When the wound has healed the sutures are removed and the patient attends for hydrotherapy.

As soon as the back splint is discarded re-education of walking is added to the physiotherapy programme. A mirror may be used at first so that the patient can see and feel the correct pattern of walking. As confidence and ability improve the patient progresses to walking up slopes, over uneven ground and up and down stairs; the ability to climb stairs with alternate steps may not be possible for some weeks. At this time the patient may visit the occupational therapy department for advice on aids and adaptations which are available.

Progress varies with each patient; some attaining 90 degrees of flexion, full extension of the knee and good control through the range with ease, while others have difficulty in gaining range and control of movement and, despite all efforts, develop an extensor lag. It is the latter group who particularly need encouragement, skilled handling and expertise. Where progress has been slow, a manipulation under anaesthetic may be necessary to increase the range of flexion. Treatment is commenced immediately after manipulation – ice packs are applied over the quadriceps muscle to relieve pain, reduce swelling and facilitate movement, and are followed by mobilising exercises to maintain the degree of flexion and restore rhythmical movement through the range. Depending upon progress the patient is discharged three to four weeks after operation. Treatment should continue until a painless rhythmical range of movement with stability has been achieved.

McIntosh knee prosthesis: hemiarthroplasty: bicompartmental tibio-femoral replacement

This type of replacement may be indicated when the patient complains of pain in the knee related particularly to the lateral or medial aspect of the joint, and when tibio-femoral arthritis has been found predominantly in one or other compartment.

Pre- and postoperative treatment closely follows the regime for total joint replacement, but re-education progresses rather more quickly. Following surgery the limb is supported in a pressure bandage and back splint. As soon as the patient can straight leg raise with a good quadriceps contraction weight-bearing is allowed with the aid of elbow crutches or walking sticks. On the fifth postoperative day the pressure bandage is reduced and knee mobilising exercises commence. The back splint is retained for walking until the patient has good control of movement through the range, full active extension and 70–90 degrees of knee flexion. Re-education of walking, knee mobilising and strengthening exercises continue and when the wound is healed the sutures are removed. Treatment is continued until satisfactory movement has been achieved.

TOTAL ANKLE REPLACEMENT

Physical assessment

The following should be observed and recorded.
(a) Gait pattern.
(b) The range of movement of the ankle and subtalar joints.
(c) Muscle power and degree of ligamentous stability around the ankle.
(d) Muscle wasting present throughout the limb.

The patient is instructed in the routine maintenance exercises with particular attention to teaching bilateral dorsiflexion and plantar flexion exercises.

Postoperative

After surgery the foot is supported in a pressure bandage with the foot of the bed elevated to minimise swelling. Routine maintenance exercises and toe flexion and extension exercises of the affected extremity commence on the first day after surgery. When the drainage tubes have been removed, the patient is allowed to sit out in a chair, care being taken to ensure that the limb is not allowed to assume a dependent position or take any weight. On the fifth day some surgeons reduce the pressure bandage and, if the wound is satisfactory, permit active dorsiflexion and plantar flexion of the ankle. Other surgeons continue immobilisation and restrict movement until the sutures are removed, at about 10–12 days.

Graduated active movements of the foot and ankle are practised with particular emphasis on dorsiflexion and plantar flexion exercises; but care must be taken to avoid stretching the scar and tissues surrounding the joint until sound wound healing has occurred. Partial weight-bearing on the affected limb commences at the discretion of the surgeon, gradually progressing – within the tolerance of the patient – to full weight-bearing using one stick. As the range of movement in the ankle increases and gait improves, the patient progresses to walking up and down slopes and over uneven ground.

The patient is discharged two to three weeks after surgery and should continue to practise the specific exercises for the affected ankle and gradually resume normal activities.

UPPER EXTREMITY JOINT REPLACEMENT

Joint replacement in the upper extremity, although still in the early stages of development, may be indicated in a small group of patients who have severe and persistent pain, limitation of movement and loss of function in one or more joints. These symptoms may be caused by advanced rheumatoid arthritis, post-traumatic arthritis or primary osteoarthritis. The operation is primarily performed to relieve pain which may then lead to an increased range of movement and improved function.

The patient's co-operation is an important factor in rehabilitation after operation and an explanation of the pre- and postoperative treatment should be given so that the patient understands the regime to be followed.

Functional and physical assessment

These particularly complement each other in the upper limb and should be made prior to surgery. The following should be observed and recorded:

The ability to take the hand to the mouth.

The ability to take the hand to the head and comb the hair.

The ability to dress and to attend to personal toilet with or without aids.

The ability to carry out normal activities or occupation (Lettin et al, 1982).

The active and passive range of movement.

The presence of pain on movement/at rest.

Muscle power throughout the limb.

The impairment of other joints.

SHOULDER ARTHROPLASTY

The prostheses at present in use have been discussed in Chapter 21.

Physiotherapy will vary, to some extent, with the type of prosthesis, the surgical approach and the condition of structures surrounding the joint. When the rotator cuff is intact, less protection of the joint will be required; whereas when there is a tear in the rotator cuff requiring repair or reconstruction, the shoulder will be protected and treatment delayed until healing has occurred. The following is an outline of treatment following interposition silastic cup arthroplasty (Varian, 1982. Personal communication).

The cup is made from high performance silastic and is a full hemisphere with an internal diameter of 44mm; larger or smaller sizes are also available. Interposition arthroplasty, which may be defined as the insertion of material into a joint without significant bone resection, is feasible only in patients suffering from rheumatoid arthritis. In rheumatoid arthritis the ligaments around the shoulder joint remain slack as the cartilage and bone are eroded, so leaving room for a prosthesis. In osteoarthritis the ligaments tend to remain tight which makes insertion of the prosthesis difficult. A simple anterior approach with a shoulder strap incision is used, the deltoid and pectoralis major muscles are parted; coracobrachialis is retracted medially; subscapularis is divided; the joint is opened up; and the cup is inserted over the head of the humerus. After surgery the arm is immobilised in a Velpeau-type bandage, or in a sling worn under the clothes, for three weeks, during which time hand, wrist and finger movements are encouraged. A sling is then worn, outside the clothes, for a further three weeks. All movements of the shoulder joint, except lateral rotation, commence. Shoulder shrugging and pendular exercises, and, with the patient in the supine position, active and active-assisted movements to the shoulder and elbow are started. Facilitatory techniques to gain range and strength are added to the programme and exercises in the sitting position are gradually introduced. By the sixth week lateral rotation is allowed and the patient may attend for hydrotherapy. Treatment continues for three months and the patient is then encouraged to practise simple functional exercises at home and resume normal activities.

TOTAL ELBOW REPLACEMENT

The increasing knowledge of biomechanics and kinematics of the elbow, and of biomaterials has produced a significant transition since the early days of elbow joint arthroplasty. New implants and techniques continue to be developed but elbow joint arthroplasty still remains a salvage procedure (Coonrad, 1982). It is indicated for patients with advanced rheumatoid arthritis where joint destruction precludes procedures such as synovectomy or excision of the head of the radius; traumatic arthrosis due to persistent subluxation or dislocation of the joint; or bone stock loss from trauma or tumour; or for those patients who have bilateral elbow ankylosis. The operation is primarily performed to relieve pain, restore or maintain mobility and improve stability. It is contra-indicated if the shoulder on the same side is ankylosed, if there is infection or if the limb has to perform tasks involving weight being taken through the joint.

After surgery the arm is supported in a pressure bandage and posterior shell and the limb elevated. The degree of flexion is determined by the type of prosthesis and the surgical technique. Mobilisation of the elbow commences when the swelling and postoperative oedema has subsided, any time between five and fourteen days after operation. The splint is removed for active flexion exercises, gentle passive extension and active pronation and supination exercises. The splint is replaced after exercising and is retained for four weeks until the triceps is secure and the tissues around the joint are healed. Graduated mobilisation continues until satisfactory functional movement has been achieved, and the patient has a stable, painless joint for sedentary use. The patient must be advised against overloading the elbow joint by lifting or carrying awkward or heavy objects, or by using the arm for weight-bearing (as when using elbow crutches or a walking stick).

TOTAL WRIST ARTHROPLASTY

The aims of wrist arthroplasty are to provide a pain-free, stable but mobile, joint in patients who require some pain-free movement at the wrist because of occupational or recreational needs. A few degrees of wrist movement can increase the reach of the fingers by several centimetres and so improve potential function.

Following operation, the hand and wrist are supported in a voluminous dressing and plaster splint, and the arm is elevated to minimise swelling. After three to five days a plaster of Paris cast with the wrist in a neutral position is applied and is worn for approximately two to four weeks to allow soft tissue healing to occur. The patient is encouraged to actively exercise the shoulder, elbow and fingers on the affected side in as full a range as possible. When the cast has been removed, active and active-assisted movements are given to gain range of flexion and extension and to improve muscle power. Normal activities within the ability of the patient are resumed as soon as possible.

SILASTIC IMPLANT OF THE
METACARPOPHALANGEAL JOINT

Joint replacement of the metacarpophalangeal joints is indicated for patients who have severe and persistent pain due to destruction of the joint surfaces, and subluxation or dislocation of the joints usually caused by rheumatoid arthritis. In some cases quite gross dislocation may be associated with good function and little or no pain, therefore, deformity in itself is not necessarily an indication for surgery, which may improve the cosmetic appearance of the hand but do little or nothing to improve the function. The operation is performed to provide a stable joint, improve mobility but primarily to relieve pain.

Following resection of bone the implant maintains the joint space and alignment and provides an internal mould for the development of a functional joint capsule. This capsule can be adapted by forces applied to it in the early stages so it is important that alternating flexion and extension movements are given in order to achieve the desired range of movement. The co-operation and involvement of the patient in the rehabilitation programme has already been mentioned and it is particularly essential after surgery to the hand. No joint can be treated in isolation and the range of movement in the shoulder, elbow and wrist must be maintained to prevent any tendency for a shoulder-hand syndrome to develop.

After surgery the hand is supported in a pressure dressing with the arm elevated to minimise swelling. Postoperative treatment will vary according to the wishes of the individual surgeon as well as with the facilities available. Wynn Parry (1981) advocates resting the hand in a plaster cast until the extensor expansion has healed, restricting flexion at the metacarpophalangeal joints to 30 degrees but permitting movement at the interphalangeal joints. The patient is readmitted to hospital after three weeks for a daily intensive rehabilitation programme; dynamic bracing is not then used. Madden et al (1977), when the postoperative swelling has subsided, usually five days after surgery, apply a dorsal splint with the wrist held in 15–20 degrees of extension, which incorporates a rod outrigger with rubber bands and finger loops, and recommend early passive movement and prolonged dynamic splinting (Fig. 22/1). The Swanson regime allows protective movements when the postoperative swelling has subsided three to five days after surgery (Swanson et al, 1982).

A dynamic brace is then applied over a light dressing and this is worn continuously day and night for three weeks (Figs. 22/2 and 22/3). The rubber band slings placed over the proximal phalanges

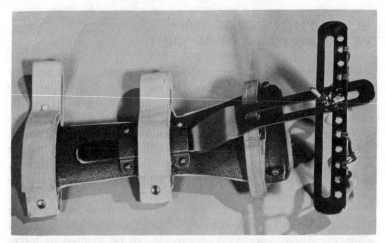

Fig. 22/1 Dynamic brace. *Note* the adjustable transverse bar with holes along its length, through which rubber bands with finger loops are threaded. By loosening the wing nut, this bar can be moved up or down the longitudinal bar, adjusted sideways and/or rotated. Out-rigger bars can be fitted to the splint as required

guide the alignment of the digits into the correct position to prevent the recurrence of ulnar deviation. The tension of the rubber bands must be tight enough to support the finger and yet loose or flexible enough to allow 70 degrees of flexion at the metacarpophalangeal joints.

Specific exercise periods to gain range of movement and increase the strength of the flexors and intrinsic muscles of the hand commence at this time. If at all possible 70 degrees of flexion should be achieved by the end of the third week, because the reconstructed joints start tightening up during the second postoperative week and will be quite tight by the end of the third week. If flexion is restricted at the metacarpophalangeal joints, and movement is found to be occurring at the interphalangeal joints, small aluminium splints taped on to each finger to immobilise these joints will help to localise flexion at the metacarpophalangeal joints; or the rubber bands may be lengthened to decrease the extensor force and facilitate flexion; or, if necessary, a flexion cuff may be worn for periods during the day to flex the metacarpophalangeal joints passively.

After three weeks, if progress is satisfactory, the extensor part of the splint is discarded during the day and is worn only at night for a

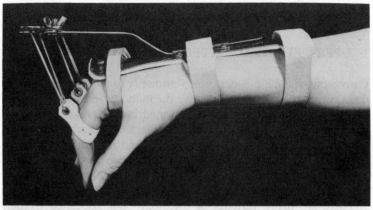

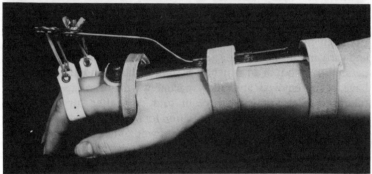

Fig. 22/2 and Fig. 22/3 Application of the dynamic brace shown on a model. It may be applied over a light dressing, or a felt pad, to prevent pressure following surgery

further three weeks. Active physiotherapy and occupational therapy to gain range, increase muscle strength and improve function continue at specific times during the day. The patient is encouraged to practise the exercises frequently. If, however, there is a persistent extension lag; or a tendency to flexion contracture; or if there is ulnar deviation of the fingers, the dynamic brace should be retained and active treatment continued for several more weeks or months. Active treatment is usually continued for about three months or until there is adequate flexion to permit the patient to grasp small objects and to use the hand for careful normal activities.

OSTEOTOMY OF THE HIP:

1. UPPER FEMORAL OSTEOTOMY

Osteotomy of the hip is performed primarily to relieve pain, correct deformity and maintain or improve the mobility and stability of the affected limb. The operation is indicated in early cases of primary degenerative arthritis, where the patient has severe disabling pain but before the hip joint is severely damaged and movements seriously restricted. The patients therefore are younger in age than those requiring a total joint replacement and do not usually have the added problems of other stiff and painful joints.

There are many varieties of osteotomy and associated fixation devices, and postoperative treatment will vary to some extent according to the technique used and the wishes of the surgeon. Complete immobilisation of the affected limb is not usually practised and early mobilisation is the general rule. Some surgeons permit their patients to sit out in an armchair as soon as the wound drainage tubes have been removed and allow partial weight-bearing, within the tolerance of the patient, three or four days after surgery. Other surgeons prefer to restrict mobilisation for seven to ten days, keeping their patients non-weight-bearing until wound healing has occurred, and the tissues and muscles of the thigh are less painful.

In the immediate postoperative period the patient practises the routine maintenance exercises already described, paying particular attention to bilateral isometric quadriceps and gluteal exercises. No specific exercise programme is given for the affected hip but the patient is encouraged to move around in the bed as much as possible and actively to mobilise the knee. Straight leg raising as an exercise is avoided until healing of the structures around the hip joint has occurred. Undue strain or stress on the limb may delay union and the patient should be taught how to support the limb when getting out of, and into, bed, and how to sit down and rise from a chair. Partial weight-bearing with the aid of elbow crutches of 10–15kg commences at the surgeon's discretion and continues for four to six months. The patient is taught to walk up and down slopes, over uneven ground and how to negotiate stairs and thresholds, before being discharged 12–14 days after surgery.

The patient may attend as an outpatient for a course of hydrotherapy if the facilities are available. When union has been achieved, walking sticks replace the elbow crutches and the patient gradually progresses to full weight-bearing and normal activities.

2. TIBIAL/LOWER FEMORAL OSTEOTOMY

An osteotomy may be carried out around the knee to relieve pain and correct deformity of the joint. Commonly this is performed in the region of the proximal tibia or distal femur, but it may be carried out at both levels at the same time (Benjamin, 1969). The deformity may be due to changes in the bone and associated soft tissue contractures. This degeneration in the medial part of the joint with loss of cartilage and erosion of the subchondral bone will lead to a varus deformity of the knee and a similar process in the lateral compartment to a valgus deformity. A pure varus or valgus deformity of the knee may also be associated with a flexion deformity and not infrequently there may also be a rotational element to the tibial position. Surgery attempts to correct the deformity and at the same time realign the limb so that the forces then passing through the knee joint will not predispose to a re-occurrence of the deformity (see Chapter 20).

The ultimate goal is a solid bony union at the site of the osteotomy leaving the leg in the corrected position and with maximum mobility at the knee joint. After having performed the osteotomy some surgeons fix the two bone fragments with staples or a compression clamp across the osteotomy site, whereas others do not fix the bone but simply immobilise the leg in a plaster of Paris cylinder. Clearly the need to obtain union at the osteotomy site, which to some extent is related to the technique of fixation of the osteotomy, dictates the speed with which the knee may be mobilised postoperatively. Certain of the regimes related to the techniques of fixation of the osteotomy are outlined below.

Following surgery the knee is immobilised in a pressure bandage and back splint. Routine maintenance and isometric quadriceps exercises are practised immediately. When the patient can straight leg raise with a good quadriceps contraction, weight-bearing with elbow crutches, within the tolerance of the patient, may be permitted. The pressure bandage is removed between the eighth and tenth day after operation and a plaster of Paris cast is applied. Immobilisation continues for six weeks, the patient continuing to weight-bear with elbow crutches. The plaster cast is bivalved when bony union has occurred, the posterior half being retained for walking until 70–90 degrees of knee flexion has been obtained. Knee mobilising and strengthening exercises are given, but in the initial stages care must be taken to avoid excessive leverage when giving resisted exercises.

Treatment continues until there is a satisfactory range of flexion, full knee extension and good control of movement through the range.

At the discretion of the surgeon, and as the patient's ability dictates, walking sticks replace the elbow crutches which are then gradually discarded and the patient resumes normal activities.

An alternative method of immobilisation is the application of a cast brace after the pressure bandage has been reduced at two weeks. This permits early mobilisation of the knee; it is retained for six to eight weeks until union has occurred.

Another method is the use of compression clamps which are applied at operation and retained for six to eight weeks. This allows knee mobilisation to commence immediately after surgery, and weight-bearing with elbow crutches after eight to ten days. When the pins are removed a plaster cast is applied for two weeks for support until the pin tracks through the bone have healed.

REFERENCES

Benjamin, A. (1969). Double osteotomy for the painful knee in rheumatoid arthritis and osteoarthritis. *Journal of Bone and Joint Surgery*, **51B**, 694–9.

Coonrad, R.W. (1982). *Seven Year Follow-up of Coonrad Total Elbow Replacement*. Included in *Symposium on Total Joint Replacement of the Upper Extremity*, (ed Inglis, A.E.). C.V. Mosby Co, St Louis.

Lettin, A.W.F., Copeland, S.A. and Scales, J.T. (1982). The Stanmore total shoulder replacement. *Journal of Bone and Joint Surgery*, **64B**, 1.

Madden, J.W., de Vore, G. and Aren, A.J. (1977). A rational postoperative programme for metacarpophalangeal implant arthroplasty. *Journal of Hand Surgery*, 2(5), 358.

Swanson, A.B., de Groot Swanson, G. and Leonard, J. (1982). *Postoperative Rehabilitation Programme in Flexible Implant Arthroplasty of the Fingers*. Included in *Symposium on Total Joint Replacement of the Upper Extremity*, (ed Inglis, A.E.). C.V. Mosby Co, St Louis.

Wynn Parry, C.B. (1981). *The Rheumatoid Hand*. Included in *Rehabilitation of the Hand*, 4th edition. Butterworths, London.

BIBLIOGRAPHY

Inglis, A.E. (ed) (1982). *Symposium on Total Joint Replacement of the Upper Extremity*. American Academy of Orthopedic Surgeons. C.V. Mosby Co, St Louis.

Laskin, R.S. (1979). Symposium on disorders of the knee joint. *Orthopedic Clinics of North America*, **10**, 1.

Bayley, J.I. and Kessel, L. (1982). *Shoulder Surgery*. Springer-Verlag, New York.

Chapter 23

Fractures – 1. Clinical

by E.R.S. ROSS, FRCS, FRACS

A fracture is a break in the continuity of a bone accompanied by soft tissue damage. Figure 23/1 illustrates the importance of the soft tissues.

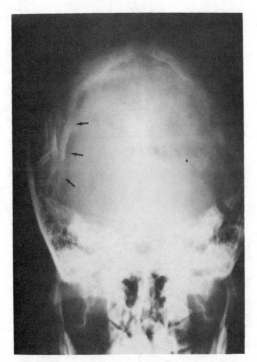

Fig. 23/1 Depressed fracture of the skull. Treatment of the fracture relates more to underlying brain damage, possible extradural haematoma due to torn meningeal vessels and to the care of an unconscious patient

MECHANISM OF INJURY

Bone is broken by direct or indirect violence. A motor car bumper hitting the tibia of a pedestrian is an example of direct injury (Fig. 23/2). A skier, whose foot is trapped in the ski as he falls, will sustain an indirect twisting injury to the tibia (Fig. 23/3). Bone does not break randomly. Patterns of fractures occur in bones as a result of the type of injury. The pedestrian will sustain a transverse fracture, the skier a spiral fracture (Fig. 23/4). Study of the pattern of fracture gives a clue to the mechanism of injury which indicates how much energy was expended in creating the fracture and hence the likely soft tissue damage. A fracture is reduced by reversing the direction of the force which caused the injury.

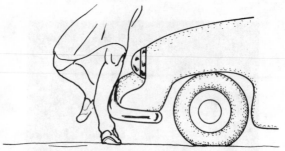

Fig. 23/2   Direct injury

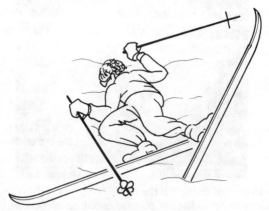

Fig. 23/3   Indirect injury

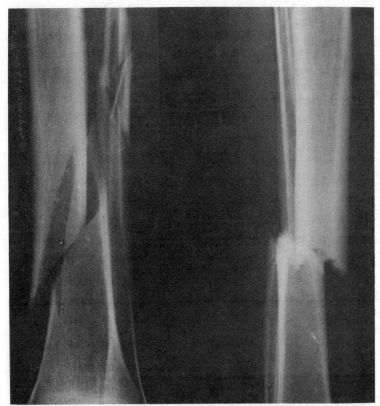

Fig. 23/4   The result of a twisting injury on the left (spiral), and a direct blow on the right (transverse)

DIAGNOSIS

The history: This explains how an injury occurred and thus the likely fractures for which to look, e.g. a fall on the outstretched hand could result in a scaphoid fracture; a fracture of the distal radius (Colles' fracture); fractures of the shafts of the radius or ulna; a fracture of the radial head; a supracondylar fracture of the humerus; a fracture of the shaft or neck of the humerus; or a fracture of the clavicle!

Symptoms: Pain pin-points the site of injury. (Pain should be relieved at the earliest opportunity by simple splintage, analgesics, local anaesthetics or Entonox.)

Signs: Deformity (Figs. 23/5, 23/6): this may be obvious or it may be hidden in bulky muscle or by haematoma or swelling. In all fractures blood vessels are torn inside the bone, in the surrounding periosteum or in muscle. This causes immediate swelling. Over the next few hours inflammation increases or sustains the swelling. There is vasodilatation and more fluid, proteins and blood cells of various types are released into the area. Local increase of temperature occurs. Crepitus (which is a grating sensation in the examining fingers) should not be deliberately elicited because it causes more pain.

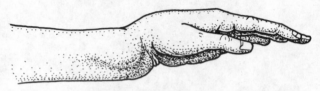

Fig. 23/5   The dinner fork deformity of Colles' fracture

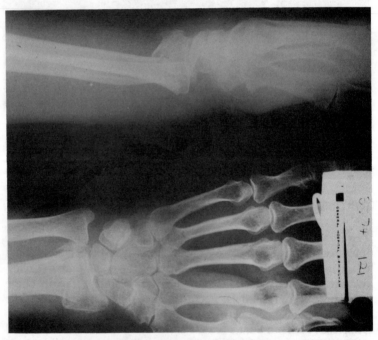

Fig. 23/6   Radiographic appearance of a Colles' fracture: antero-posterior and lateral views

Radiographs: These should be considered an integral part of the examination. However, if they are used to confirm fractures and delineate the nature of a fracture rather than 'to look for a fracture', more information is gained.

Special techniques: Computerised axial tomography (CAT), tomography, cineradiography, radionuclide bone scanning, radiculography, and arteriography all have a place in fracture management.

FRACTURE HEALING

Bone is a unique tissue in that it does not heal by a scar but by the actual reconstitution of the injured tissue, i.e. bone heals by forming new bone. Although phases of healing are described there is marked overlap.

The inflammatory phase

Torn blood vessels, medullary, periosteal and soft tissue produce a haematoma in and around the fragments. Then follows vasodilatation with release of proteins and cells into the area; polymorphonuclear leucocytes, histiocytes and mast cells begin to clear up the debris.

It is fundamental to realise that the bone ends are dead. Even if cell death has occurred over only a distance of a few millimetres, its presence precludes direct healing between the bone ends except under exceptional circumstances which will be described under primary bone healing, page 458.

The phase of cellular proliferation (Fig. 23/7)

It is in this phase that callus is formed. This tissue bridges the gap from living bone on one side of the fracture to living bone on the other side. The bone which is laid down rapidly may well be a product of cells which are derived from dormant cells of the periosteum. These latter produce collagen and ground substance which is mineralised, thus bridging and stabilising the fracture. In some areas of this surrounding collar of proliferating tissue, cartilage is formed. Possibly where proliferating cells outstrip their blood supply they become cartilage-forming cells rather than bone-forming cells. Cartilage can temporarily fill the gap but is less demanding on oxygen for its formation and will be replaced by a process of endochondral ossification. This type of bone formation is found in normal bone growth at the epiphyses and in that situation produces an increase in

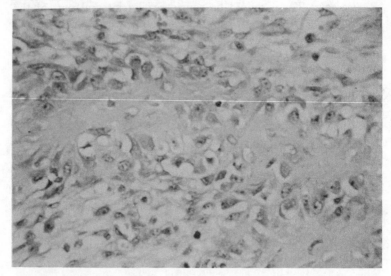

Fig. 23/7 The cellular phase. A central seam of osteoid is surrounded by osteoblasts

length of the bone. Here it adds to the woven bone of the callus. This process of external callus formation is seen in the diaphysis of a long bone (Fig. 23/8).

A similar activity is going on in the tubular cavity (the medulla). This is a relatively slow process and contributes little to stability in shaft fractures, unless the external callus response fails. In cancellous bone there is an excellent blood supply and a huge surface area, and medullary callus formation is the principal means of healing. In a markedly offset fracture the external and medullary callus may meet and unite the fracture.

Phase of remodelling

Once the fracture has united, the callus mass must be adapted to the requirements of function. In the normal skeleton the process of removal and replacement of bone are continuously at work. Osteoclasts remove bone and osteoblasts lay it down again. In cancellous bone, blood vessels are never far away and so the process occurs on the surface of the trabeculae, sometimes called *creeping substitution*. In the cortical bone of the shafts of long bones the cells

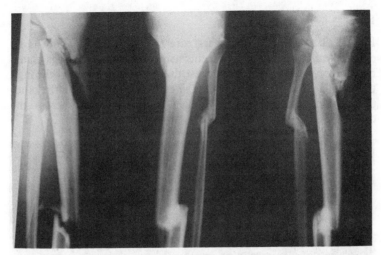

Fig. 23/8 *Left*: A comminuted fracture of the tibia, and fracture of the fibula. *Centre*: The lower tibial fracture and the fibular fracture have healed by external callus bridges. *Right*: The upper tibial fracture runs into the cancellous area, and not much external callus is seen. The fracture is, nevertheless, united. *Note* how the separate fragment has joined proximally but not distally at this stage

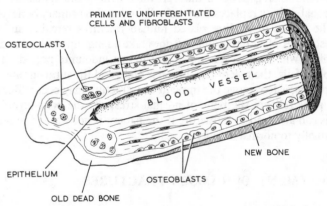

Fig. 23/9 An osteon. *Note* the multinucleate osteoclasts which form the 'cutter head'

need to take a blood supply with them. Thus a unit called an osteon is formed (Fig. 23/9). This mechanism remodels bone throughout life, and fractures as required.

Primary bone union

Figure 23/10 shows a plated fracture at eight weeks. There is no external callus visible. Experiments using osteotomies in dogs plated by compression techniques suggest that osteons can tunnel through the small area of dead bone on one side directly into that on the other thus creating new living Haversian systems directly across the osteotomy.

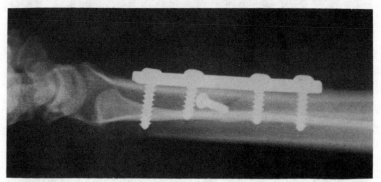

Fig. 23/10   A plated fracture of the radius showing no external callus

Where small gaps occur these are filled with medullary callus, then osteonal activity replaces the whole. Whether this primary bone union is the means of healing plated human fractures remains an open question. A plated human bone does take a long time to heal and the implant will need to remain in situ for an indefinite period. If the implant fails, the risk of non-union is high, and the surgeon must not be too eager to remove the implant or refracture may occur. Because the plate relieves the bone of normal stressing, the bone atrophies. This can also lead to refracture if the patient is not warned to return gradually to normal activity.

TREATMENT OF CLOSED FRACTURES

'It is appropriate to remember that fractures are capable of healing in the natural state without any human assistance. When contemplating the effects of a specific treatment it is wise to bear this mechanism in mind so that modifications imposed upon it by the particular treatment can be fully appreciated' (McKibbon, 1978).

Fractures may be accompanied by other general problems: airway obstruction, shock from blood loss, visceral injuries, loss of consciousness. Discussion of these is beyond the scope of this chapter but the treatment of a fracture may be dictated by the nature and extent of concomitant injury as much as by the particular nature of the fracture itself.

All trauma is accompanied by profound metabolic changes. Sodium and water are retained while potassium is lost over the first 10 days. Protein is broken down and this is principally at the expense of muscle. A relative glucose intolerance arises from major changes in hormone secretion as a response to stress. Little if anything is known on how these factors influence rehabilitation programmes.

Guidelines to fracture care (Fig. 23/11)

REDUCE THE FRACTURE IF REDUCTION IS REQUIRED

Restoration of function is the aim of all fracture care. Bearing this in mind reduction of a fracture will aim to restore (a) axial alignment, (b) length and (c) joint surfaces or relationships of one joint to another. Reduction may be by a closed method, e.g. manipulation. There are

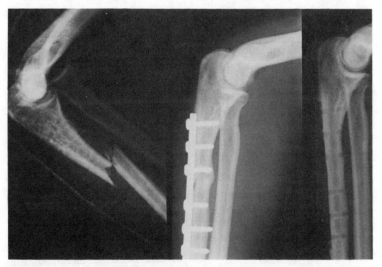

Fig. 23/11 A Monteggia fracture-dislocation. *Left*: A closed reduction has been attempted. The radial head remains dislocated, the ulnar fracture is not reduced and is shortened. *Centre*: Open reduction has been performed. *Note* that the radial head is now reduced. The ulnar fracture is held by a plate. *Right*: The appearance after plate removal

occasions when closed reduction fails and open reduction is then performed.

HOLD THE REDUCTION

If no reduction has been attempted clearly there is no need to hold it. However, rest of the part may be offered by simple splintage, e.g. a sling for a fractured clavicle or a plaster of Paris back-slab for a greenstick fracture of the radius. Holding a reduction does not necessarily immobilise the fracture. It has been shown by cine-radiography that a fractured tibia in a functional brace may shorten by a centimetre on weight-bearing. This does not result in non-union. The important factor then is not relative movement at a fracture but the elimination of shear stress (see Chapter 2).

A reduced fracture can be held by:
1. Traction.
2. Plaster splintage of conventional type.
3. Functional braces.
4. Internal fixation.
5. External fixation.

Traction: See Chapter 6.

Plaster of Paris (POP): The widespread use of POP attests to its ease of use, general application, low cost and acceptability to patient and surgeon alike. Analysis of most POP casts will show that they work on the principle of three-point fixation (see Chapter 1).

In the early phase of acute inflammation swelling occurs. This swelling inside a rigid POP may embarrass the circulation or produce pressure effects on nerves. This must be carefully looked for in the first 24 hours. Using incomplete plasters or splitting ALL coverings down to the skin is safer. The main disadvantage of traditional POP casts is that joints are prevented from moving, and oedema cannot easily be dissipated. Both factors contribute to rehabilitation problems later. Delayed splintage or conversion to a functional brace at an early stage can overcome this. If the fracture can be stabilised on traction while oedema and swelling are vigorously treated, and joint movement restored before a plaster is applied, little fear of 'fracture disease' need arise.

Functional bracing: This is as much a philosophy of fracture management as a technique. At its heart are the ideas that rehabilitation of the soft tissues and joints, by function of the part during the phase of fracture healing, may enhance fracture healing and certainly restore the patient to normal function at the earliest opportunity. A brace can be made from many different materials and individual bones have their own particular type of brace (Fig. 23/12).

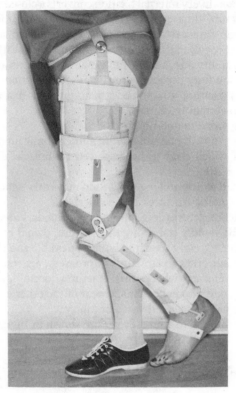

Fig. 23/12   A femoral functional brace

It is important that the brace fits snugly round the injured part. Soft tissue support is thought to contribute to fracture support and this means careful adjustment of the brace throughout the period of treatment. Braces are not applied straight away but usually when swelling and pain are no longer present. There is some evidence that a femoral fracture may be braced when the fracture is still deformable but not displaceable. This is a clinical decision but occurs at about six weeks. Tibial fractures may be braced a little earlier. A transverse fracture which has been reduced will be very stable to axial forces and thus ideal for bracing at two to three weeks. Sarmiento (1981) has shown that oblique fractures will not shorten more than at the time of initial injury. This may be unacceptable and thus bracing will be delayed while length is maintained by some other method until the fracture is more stable.

Internal fixation: Every internal fixation converts a closed fracture into an open fracture thus creating an entry route for infection. The advantages of internal fixation must be weighed against this background. Providing the patient's condition is right, the surgeon's training and ability adequate, a full range of implants are available, theatre staff are fully capable with the instrumentation, and aseptic facilities and routine guaranteed, then internal fixation may be considered in certain fractures.

1. Fractures prone to non-union.
2. Fractures prone to mal-union which might limit function.
3. Fractures which tend to be displaced by muscle action, e.g. a patella fracture.
4. Fractures in which prolonged traction may carry added risks, e.g. intertrochanteric fractures in the elderly.
5. Pathological fractures, e.g. through a secondary deposit from a tumour. By rapidly stabilising the fracture, pain is eased, nursing care facilitated, early return to home is possible and the limb may be used while other treatment is in progress, e.g. radiotherapy.
6. Multiple injuries – where two fractures occur in one limb, stabilising one can make management of the other easier.
7. Fractures with associated vascular injury.

Examples of internal fixation devices are shown in Figure 23/13.

TREATMENT OF OPEN FRACTURES

An open or compound fracture is one in which the skin is broken allowing access to bacteria or bacterial spores. Regardless of the size of the wound, whether bone has penetrated the skin from inside or there is severe soft tissue loss, contamination is assumed.

The limb should be splinted initially and the wound covered with a sterile dressing. Appropriate antitetanus therapy is given. Penicillin may be used as an adjunct to surgery but is never a substitute. The wound must then be thoroughly cleaned. This is performed under general anaesthesia without a tourniquet. All dead tissue is removed. The soft tissues inevitably swell and there is usually difficulty in trying to close wounds. Therefore, wounds should be left open so that more skin will not die; this allows any exudate to drain freely and does not form a nidus for bacteria to multiply, and the danger of precipitating a *compartment syndrome* is reduced. Compartment syndromes are so

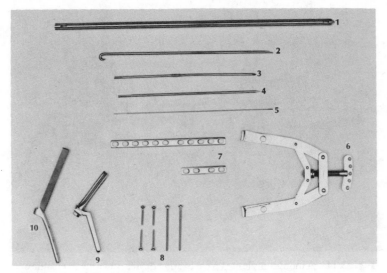

Fig. 23/13   (A) Fixation devices: 1. Küntscher nail; 2. Rush nail; 7. A-O dynamic compression plates; 8. A-O cortical screws; 9. McGlaughlan plate; 10. Capener nail-plate. (B) Instruments for skeletal traction: 3. Denham pin (*note* the central thread); 4. Steinmann pin; 5. Kirschner wire; 6. Wire tightener

called because muscles are grouped together and surrounded by fascial envelopes: as the tissues swell from injury the pressure within those tissues rises. Fascia does not stretch much and consequently the pressure rises. At 10–30mmHg below diastolic pressure blood flow to muscle ceases. An infarct or death then occurs in the muscle. To prevent this happening the fascia is split and the skin is left wide open. Compartment syndromes also occur in closed injuries.

The fractures must be stabilised. The methods already outlined may be applicable, but where severe soft tissue damage has occurred the use of an *external fixator* may be considered (Fig. 23/14): pins are placed in the bone away from the damaged area and a frame constructed to hold them. The advantages of such a system are:

1. The bone is stabilised thus giving the soft tissues the best chance to heal.
2. Wounds can easily be inspected and dressed.
3. Split skin grafts or other plastic procedures can be performed easily.
4. The limb can easily be elevated.

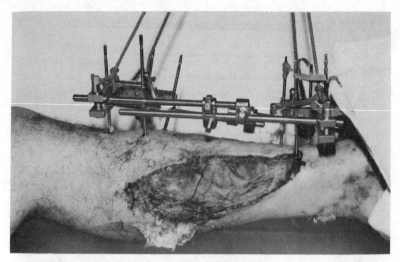

Fig. 23/14 A more complex external fixation device, but a very versatile one. *Note* the ease with which a split skin graft can be applied and managed

Bone healing may be a problem with this technique. Several factors contribute: bone may be devascularised at the time of injury; bone may actually be lost at the time of injury or subsequently; infection occurs despite meticulous attempts to prevent it; and possibly some fixation systems are so rigid that this has an adverse effect on healing. An interesting development from using external fixation devices is the plotting of healing curves. By applying strain gauges to the bars of the device the increasing stiffness of a fracture can be plotted. Where the stiffness plateaus or decreases decisions can be made as to the subsequent management of the fracture.

CHILDREN'S FRACTURES

The general principles outlined above apply but there are important differences. Usually union is not a problem in children's fractures and the capacity for remodelling is very great. Thus a deformity which may be unacceptable in an adult is not necessarily so in a child. Shortening of a femoral fracture in an adult for instance is permanent and is avoided. In the child overgrowth of the fractured side occurs and can compensate for up to one inch of shortening depending on the age of the child. As skeletal maturity is reached the capacity to remodel decreases.

Figure 23/15 shows the growth plate of a long bone in a child. Injuries of the growth plate can occur, and the importance of the Salter Harris classification is that it indicates how the injury may progress. Types I and II heal well. Types III and IV are intra-articular injuries and may need operation and fixation to ensure joint surface integrity, and to accurately reposition the growth plate so that growth plate tethers are reduced. Type V injuries are serious in that they may be difficult to recognise initially and only present when they begin to cause a problem: unequal growth of the epiphysis because part of it has fused, or unequal growth in a two-bone system like the radius and ulna when one epiphysis of one bone is completely arrested. All epiphyseal injuries should be followed up till no growth arrest is assured.

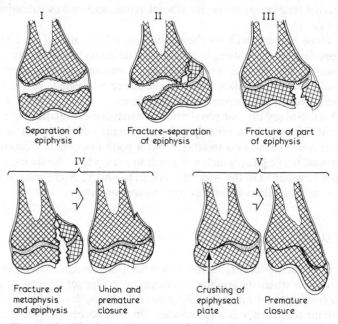

I · Separation of epiphysis

II · Fracture-separation of epiphysis

III · Fracture of part of epiphysis

IV · Fracture of metaphysis and epiphysis · Union and premature closure

V · Crushing of epiphyseal plate · Premature closure

Fig. 23/15   The Salter Harris classification of epiphyseal injuries

The majority of fractures in children will be treated by closed methods. Joint stiffness is rarely a problem since the length of time to healing is usually less than three months. In general physiotherapy has little part to play except perhaps for patients treated on traction for femoral fractures.

FRACTURES WITH ASSOCIATED INJURIES

Nerves and blood vessels may be damaged when a bone is fractured, e.g. the radial nerve in a humeral fracture or the femoral artery in a low femoral fracture. Potential damage of this kind is always carefully looked for on presentation, but the physiotherapist should look for any developing problems subsequently.

Arterial damage produces a pulseless, pale, cold distal extremity which may also have altered sensation as a result of the ischaemia. Reduction of a fracture or dislocation will sometimes unkink or relieve pressure on a vessel. If, in a closed injury, simple manipulation does not restore the circulation, exploration of the vessel is indicated. Arteriography can be of help but the site of arterial damage is frequently self-evident. Stabilisation of the fracture by internal or external fixation protects the arterial repair and makes subsequent care easier.

Nerve damage will be shown by loss of sensation (not always appreciated by the patient immediately after injury) and loss of muscle power. If the nerve is simply squeezed a neuropraxia results which should recover spontaneously. If the nerve is divided, primary or delayed repair will depend on many factors.

Suffice to say that the physiotherapist may have to adapt treatment in the light of these other problems. Details will be found in the appropriate section on treatment but a good example is a common peroneal nerve palsy which will result in a drop foot. Ankle mobility must be retained in the hope of eventual recovery. Night splintage to prevent an equinus deformity may be appropriate.

DISLOCATIONS

In this context only traumatic dislocations are considered. A joint is dislocated when its articular surfaces are no longer congruent but wholly displaced one from the other. Anything less than this but without congruency is a subluxation. In the process of a dislocation those structures which normally hold the joint together must in some way be torn apart. The structures are the ligaments, capsule, cartilaginous elements like the labrum glenoidale in the shoulder, and possibly muscle attachments. Nerve and vessel damage must be excluded.

Initial treatment is reduction at the earliest possible moment. Frequently a closed manipulation will achieve this but if the bone button-holes through the capsule an open reduction may be required. Fractures sometimes occur with a dislocation but these are treated on their individual merits once the dislocation has been reduced. Sometimes a major ligament repair may be necessary, e.g. in the knee joint, but otherwise a period of rest to allow pain to settle and the soft tissues to heal followed by vigorous rehabilitation is required.

COMPLICATIONS

These may be considered as local and general:

Local	General
Infection	Venous thrombosis
Delayed union	ARDS (adult respiratory distress syndrome)
Non-union	
Mal-union	
Avascular necrosis	(Joint problems)

Infection

Despite rigorous application of the methods outlined in the treatment of *open* fractures infection of bone is still a problem. The problem has also been alluded to in internal fixation of closed fractures. The real danger is of chronic osteomyelitis which may be impossible to eradicate. The delay in bone healing caused by infection may result in a non-union. A variety of bacteria are responsible but *Staphylococcus aureus, Streptococci, E. coli, Pseudomonas*, and anaerobic species of the bacteroides group are common. Unfortunately in the chronic infections a mixed population of organisms can be present adding to the difficulty of eradication.

Treatment: Drainage, removal of dead bone (sequestrectomy) and the use of antibiotics in various ways are standard techniques. Antibiotics can be given systemically, or locally in suction irrigation systems, or as a slow release from methylmethacrylate beads. The soft tissues need to be rested and bone stabilised to promote healing, and plaster of Paris in the form of resting splints or complete plasters is widely used. There may be a place for the application of external fixation.

Delayed union

There is no absolute time for a particular fracture to heal. However, if a large number of fractures of the tibia are considered union will be found between 12–16 weeks. If a fracture goes beyond this average expected healing time it is called a delayed union. If signs of union are present it may be necessary only to be patient and await union and consolidation. If however there is little sign of union, bone grafting may be considered.

Non-union

Two types of non-union are recognised; atrophic and hypertrophic. The *atrophic* type is a difficult problem (Figs. 23/16 and 23/17).

The *hypertrophic* type, or so-called elephant's foot, will usually respond to simple bone grafting. Compression plating with or without bone grafting is also successful. Basset has claimed that healing can be obtained by the use of wire coils through which electric current is passed so producing a magnetic field. The fracture is placed in the field and induced currents in the fracture environment are said to stimulate healing. Other workers have stimulated a non-union by direct implantation of electrodes into the fracture. Again, success in

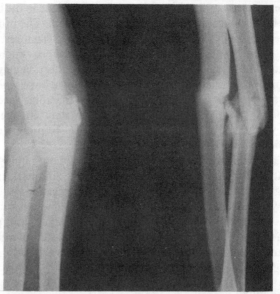

Fig. 23/16 A non-union of the radius and ulna. *Note* there is very little callus around the fractures, especially the radial fracture. These are atrophic non-unions

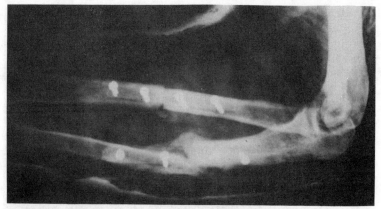

Fig. 23/17 Both fractures have been bridged by cortical grafts taken from the tibia, screwed to the bone. (Although this was successful this is no longer a method of choice)

fracture healing is claimed. The use of functional braces is also advanced as a method of healing non-unions.

Although these methods are mentioned for completeness it must be said that the use of cortico-cancellous bone grafts, with or without internal fixation, is a method which has stood the test of time and will be most appropriate for the majority of centres at this time.

Mal-union

Untreated bones heal but not always in the best functional position: valgus or varus angulation, rotation and shortening should be avoided.

Avascular necrosis

This is a problem related to the peculiar blood supply of certain bones. In the process of fracture or dislocation, when blood supply is so impaired that bone cells die, the bone can be revascularised and the process of creeping substitution (p. 456) may allow healing. The sites at which avascular necrosis most frequently occur are the head of the femur either following fracture of the femoral neck or after dislocation; the proximal half of the carpal scaphoid; or the body of the talus after a fracture through the neck of that bone (Figs. 23/18 and 23/19). The whole lunate may undergo necrosis after a dislocation.

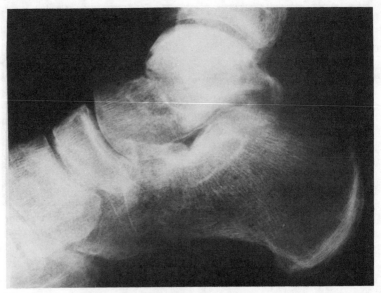

Fig. 23/18 Avascular necrosis of the body of the talus following fracture through the neck. *Note* how dense the body appears compared to the head of talus and the calcaneus below

Attempts to revascularise the dead segment of bone by vascularised bone grafts have been attempted in the femoral head. However, treatment may have to be of a salvage nature if pain or deformity occur.

Adult respiratory distress syndrome (ARDS)

Twelve to 36 hours after an injury of one of the larger bones, or multiple fractures, or pelvic fractures the patient may become incoherent and drowsy. Small petechiae may be found on the chest, on extensor surfaces of the body or in the retina of the eye. The respiration rate may rise and some difficulty with breathing be noticed. A chest radiograph at this time may reveal multiple small opacities. Measurement of the blood gases will show a reduced carbon dioxide content as a result of overbreathing, and a reduced oxygen content as a result of a diffusion problem in the lungs.

It has been suggested that this problem arises because of micro-emboli of fat released from the fracture. These travel to the lung and are sieved out in the alveolar capillaries setting up an

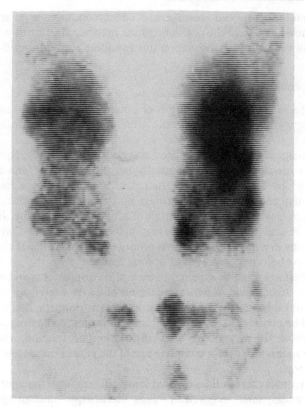

Fig. 23/19   A bone scan of the same talus (right) showing the body to be 'hot' compared to the normal side (left). The perfusion phase of the scan shows that revascularisation is occurring

inflammatory response, while those emboli which are not filtered pass on to form micro-infarcts in skin, brain, kidney and retina. However, a similar picture can be seen in other situations where fat embolism does not occur, and this syndrome is rarely seen after total hip replacement where fat embolisation must occur from medullary reaming and pressure injection of cement. It may, in fact, be a manifestation of the patient having had a sustained hypovolaemia for a period.

Whatever the aetiology treatment with oxygen is required. Sometimes the patient may require tracheostomy and positive pressure ventilation. Even with treatment, the stiffness of the lungs may gradually increase, the partial pressure of oxygen in the blood continue to drop and death ensue. This condition is often not recognised early and the physiotherapist may be called to 'give some chest physio'. In such a situation this condition *must* be considered.

Joint problems

Stiffness may be partly the result of injury, partly the end result of treatment, but hopefully never the result of neglecting the principles of care.

Cartilage is dependent on synovial fluid for its nutrition. Synovial fluid is distributed around joints by movement and is forced into cartilage by load-bearing. If, then, treatment deprives a joint of movement and load-bearing, cartilage nutrition will be affected. If, in addition, treatment deprives muscle of activity it will atrophy. Injury results in scar tissue which tends to gum tissues together and produce adhesions in joints. Inflammation produces oedema which if allowed to persist becomes organised as fibrous tissue.

Our efforts must be directed to each of these problems and where possible treat them. Where supervision of active exercise is taking place and joint stiffness becomes worse, post-traumatic ossification should be considered. The joint where this is most commonly seen is the elbow. It may occur after dislocation or fracture, and its appearance is a signal for complete rest of the joint. Fortunately it is a rare event.

Sometimes there will be marked joint stiffness in all the joints of a hand accompanied by swelling, pain on attempted movement and discolouration of the skin which is glossy. A radiograph shows an inordinate degree of osteoporosis. These appearances are diagnostic of *Sudeck's atrophy*. This can affect hand or foot and is seen after a Colles' fracture and ankle fractures. The sheet anchor of treatment is physical therapy, but successful treatment by sympathectomy (cervical ganglion block), guanethidine block and calcitonin have been claimed.

Osteoarthritis

The loss of joint cartilage is not confined to joints which have been traumatised nor does it necessarily follow an intra-articular fracture. However, damage to adult cartilage leaves an imperfect area in a joint which may lead to progressive loss of its cartilage. This will be manifested clinically by pain and stiffness of the joint. Radiologically the joint space narrows, there may be sclerosis of bone on each side of the joint especially where increased load-bearing is produced, new bone forms at the joint margins (osteophytes) and cysts may form in the bone itself close to the joint surfaces. The severity of these changes is difficult to predict at the time of injury.

The rationale of piecing together intra-articular fractures and holding the reduction with screws and plates is to try to restore the surfaces of the joint accurately in the hope that less osteoarthritic change will occur. It may be, however, that the outcome is dependent on the severity of the initial injury to the cartilage.

Whether treated operatively or non-operatively, intra-articular fractures must be treated by early active movement. Fibrocartilage will form to repair the defects in the cartilage. Surprisingly good results can be obtained by early active movement alone in fractures around the upper end of the tibia and in the elbow in the elderly.

Venous thrombosis

Virchow enunciated three factors which are important in the aetiology of deep vein thrombosis (DVT):
1. Damage to vessel walls.
2. Stasis.
3. Changes in the blood-clotting factors.

These three factors remain true today, and although much more detail of each process is understood the problem remains only partly solved. In the injured patient all three factors are altered. Where surgery is performed they may be altered more, and aggravated if this is followed by a period in bed or a plaster enclosing the lower limb.

The later problems of thrombosis are swelling of the limb on use, pain and skin ulceration. The immediate problem is a pulmonary embolus which may be fatal. For the purposes of this discussion only thrombosis in leg veins will be mentioned. The calf veins form a plexus deep in the soleus muscle and it is here that thrombus forms first. Thrombus may then propagate into the femoral, iliac and deep pelvic veins from this site. It is believed that a clot which breaks off and passes up to the heart and into the pulmonary arteries (i.e. forms an embolus), arises from the femoral or major pelvic veins.

The onset of thrombus formation in an injured patient can be at almost any time, but where surgery is performed it is thought the process begins at, or close to, the time of surgery. The classical expression of thrombus formation clinically is said to occur around 10 days post-surgery. The clinical picture of a DVT is of pain in the calf with oedema. Tenderness in the calf and pain when the foot is passively dorsiflexed (Homan's sign) are classical signs. A small rise in temperature may occur. Unfortunately thrombosis can occur in the

absence of these signs and their presence does not always indicate thrombosis.
The serious consequences of thrombosis have led to a search for prophylaxis, i.e. means to prevent its onset. These are:

1. *Therapeutic*: Methods directed at the alteration in clotting; they include small doses of heparin, aspirin, large molecular weight dextrans and warfarin.

2. *Mechanical*: Methods directed at the prevention of stasis; they include stimulation of calf muscles during surgery by electric currents; boots which enclose the legs and feet and produce intermittent pressure on the limb thus encouraging venous return; early active mobilisation of patients and the use of bandages or stockings which drive the blood into the deep veins and thus promote increased flow in them. Clearly where injured patients may have large wounds and surgery, therapeutic methods of prevention may be inappropriate and more reliance is placed on mechanical methods.

Where a DVT is suspected it should be confirmed by venography. While other methods for confirming a thrombosis exist, venography is more readily available and reliable. When deep vein thrombosis is confirmed heparin intravenously and warfarin orally are given provided there are no other contra-indications.

REFERENCES

McKibbon, B. (1978). The biology of fracture healing in long bones. *Journal of Bone and Joint Surgery*, **60B**, 149–62.

Sarmiento, A. and Latta, L.L. (1981). *Closed Functional Treatment of Fractures*. Springer-Verlag Co Inc, New York.

BIBLIOGRAPHY

Adams, J.C. (1983). *Outline of Fractures, Including Joint Injuries*, 8th edition. Churchill Livingstone, Edinburgh.

Apley, A.G. and Soloman, L. (1982). *Apley's System of Orthopaedics and Fractures*, 6th edition. Butterworths, London.

Meggitt, B.F., Juett, D.A. and Smith, J.D. (1981) Cast bracing for fractures of the femoral shaft. *Journal of Bone and Joint Surgery*, **63B**, 12.

Wilson, J.N. (ed) (1982). *Watson-Jones' Fractures and Joint Injuries*, 6th edition, 2 volumes. Churchill Livingstone, Edinburgh.

ACKNOWLEDGEMENTS

To the Medical Illustration Department of the Robert Jones and Agnes Hunt Orthopaedic Hospital, Oswestry, and the Medical Institute, Hartshill, Stoke-on-Trent for the majority of the illustrations. To Professor B.T. O'Connor who kindly read the manuscript, and to Dr. J. Brennan for pathology specimens. To Mrs J. Jones and Mrs E. Billingham for secretarial work.

Chapter 24

Fractures – 2. Physiotherapy and Charts of Fracture Management

by C.E. APPERLEY, MCSP *and* E.R.S. ROSS, FRCS, FRACS

A fracture is a break in the continuity of a bone accompanied by soft tissue damage. Most bones do not break haphazardly, and the varieties of common fractures are limited. The clinical aspects are discussed in Chapter 23.

Treatment of a fracture begins immediately with first aid, relief of shock and clinical assessment. *Rehabilitation* begins when the fracture comes under definitive treatment. Adams (1983) states that rehabilitation is the most important of the three great principles of fracture treatment:

Reduction is often unnecessary
Immobilisation is often unnecessary
Rehabilitation is always essential.

He also says that treatment of fractures without regard to rehabilitation could be worse than no treatment at all.

Fracture treatment aims at sound union of the bone ends in a good position, i.e. mechanically correct; the absence of stiff joints and atrophied muscles; and full restoration of function with the patient having confidence in using the part.

It is often a violent force that is required to break a normal bone. Therefore there is also damage to other tissues; muscle fibres, fascia and other connective tissues may be torn, blood vessels are ruptured with resultant extravasation of blood, and nerves and skin may be damaged. Thus trauma may lead initially to bruising and oedema with muscle atrophy, stiff joints, disturbed circulation and gross impairment of function following immobilisation.

The principles of physiotherapy aim to prevent this occurring by:
1. The maintenance of normal movement and function of the uninjured structures.
2. The restoration of normal movement and function of the fractured area as soon as possible.

New treatment methods, e.g. functional bracing, have increased patient mobility allowing rehabilitation to be carried out as union proceeds.

THE ROLE OF THE PHYSIOTHERAPIST

To work as part of the multidisciplinary team.
To assess the patient's condition and identify his needs.
To explain any proposed physical treatment, and its aims, to the patient.
To maintain respiratory function especially for those patients with respiratory disease, thoracic cage injury or spinal injury.
To rehabilitate the patient back to independence.
To be aware of likely complications (see p. 467) and to report any untoward signs and symptoms to the nurse in charge of the ward (if relevant) and the doctor.

Assessment

Before commencing treatment the physiotherapist should make an assessment which should be repeated at intervals. This includes reading the medical notes and looking at the radiographs. The following should be noted:
1. Diagnosis and date of injury.
2. Cause of injury.
3. Other injuries, illnesses or complications.
4. Occupation.
5. Home circumstances.
6. *Symptoms*: ask about pain, stiffness and function.
7. *Signs at the fracture site*: (a) local heat; (b) redness; (c) oedema); (d) tenderness.
   Signs in the nearby joints: (a) effusion; (b) range of movement.
   Signs in the whole limb: (a) muscle power/wasting; (b) sensation.
   General examination: (a) functional activity; (b) respiratory function.

FRACTURES IN SPLINTAGE INCLUDING FUNCTIONAL BRACING

The patient must continue to use the injured part as normally as he can. The degree of function related to the fracture area depends on the nature of the fracture, the risk of displacement and the extent of splintage.

Physiotherapy is usually possible from an early stage and will include:

1. Elevation.
2. Active exercises to mobilise all muscles and joints not included in the splintage. For example, a patient with a Colles' fracture must use the fingers, elbow and shoulder as normally as possible.
3. Isometric exercises for the muscles enclosed in the splintage to preserve muscle function and prevent atrophy. These exercises help to pump away oedema thereby avoiding the development of indurated and fibrosed tissues.
4. Encouragement of normal patterns of movement; this will include gait if the lower limb is involved. If the patient is to be allowed non-weight-bearing or partial weight-bearing the use of crutches must be taught; this includes their use in rising from sitting, and from standing to sitting, a reciprocal gait (shadow walking if non-weight-bearing), steps and stairs.

On removal of the splintage a small amount of swelling in the fracture area is normal (being due to callus formation and a small amount of oedema); the physiotherapist must be aware of any signs of non-union or infection, i.e. swelling, heat, tenderness or reddening which indicate an inflammatory state.

Following the removal of splintage the aims of treatment are to mobilise those joints which were immobilised, improve the power of muscles and the condition of soft tissues. Even for patients with simple fractures which do not require physiotherapy instruction on reducing pain and swelling with, for example, contrast bathing, mobilising and strengthening exercises can be beneficial.

In the case of more serious fractures or when a splint is temporarily, or totally, removed before consolidation, supervised physiotherapy is usually necessary. When there is sound union at the fracture site treatment can be increased with exercises being carried out against graduated resistance until normal power is regained.

Throughout treatment exercises should be given for the whole body together with functional activities. This stimulates co-ordination of one part with another and retrains independence. If the lower limb is affected, gait should be re-educated using the heel-toe pattern throughout, and the person rehabilitated until he has reached his normal level of fitness.

FRACTURES TREATED BY EARLY ACTIVE MOTION

Physiotherapy now plays a greater role in the treatment of some fractures which, if immobilised, lead to joint stiffness and loss of function. For example, fractured metacarpals often have minimal displacement but correct alignment is usually sacrificed for the return of good function – a beautiful radiograph but a stiff hand is useless!

Fractures which include cancellous bone, e.g. a crush fracture of the calcaneus, are often treated most effectively by physiotherapy. Ice therapy and elevation reduces pain and swelling, and movement of the ankle and subtalar joints must be early and repetitive. The activity moulds the fragments so that a useful range of movement is usually regained. Tibial condyle fractures also have improved reduction with movement, *but* it must be combined with continuous traction or cast bracing of the leg to prevent angulation at the knee.

Within this category is the elderly patient with an impacted fracture of the neck of humerus. In this instance physiotherapy should include techniques to aid relief of pain, active exercises, and graduated functional activities.

FRACTURES TREATED IN TRACTION

Prolonged traction as a treatment for some fractures is now being replaced, or supplemented, by other methods especially functional bracing. For example, a patient with a fracture of the mid-shaft of the femur may be walking, partial weight-bearing in a cast brace, with a good range of hip, knee and ankle movement and muscle activity possibly within 4–6 weeks of the injury. This is compared to the 12–16 weeks on traction alone, with subsequent stiff joints, especially the knee, and atrophied and fibrosed tissues.

Some fractures still require prolonged traction or internal fixation. These are fractures that are difficult to brace at the 'sticky stage', e.g. a fracture of the junction between the upper and middle thirds of the femur. Fixation of the proximal small segment is difficult particularly when it is influenced by the strong flexor and abductor muscles of the hip.

Physiotherapy

Physiotherapy during traction includes:

1. Maintenance of respiratory function.
2. Circulatory exercises with ankle dorsiflexion and plantar flexion and deep breathing exercises.
3. Maintenance of the general tone of the body's muscles by:
   (a) Strengthening exercises of the arms in preparation for crutch walking.
   (b) Exercises for the unaffected leg. Care must be taken with resisted exercises in the first few weeks, because overflow of muscle activity to the affected leg may alter the position of the fracture and actually delay rehabilitation.
4. Isometric contractions of muscles in the affected limb, especially the quadriceps group.
5. Passive mobilisation of the patella of the fractured leg to prevent patello-femoral adhesions.
6. At union of the fracture, knee flexion exercises may be permitted.

When traction is removed treatment will be continued with graduated exercise until acceptable function for the particular patient's needs is regained.

FRACTURES TREATED BY INTERNAL FIXATION

Internal fixation of a fracture is used when closed methods are *unsuitable*, e.g. holding a transverse fracture of the olecranon; or *inadequate*, e.g. a fractured neck of the femur. It is also indicated when precise reduction is required and is not possible by manipulation, e.g. intra-articular fractures, fractures of the medial malleolus, or the radius and ulna in the adult.

Internal fixation is not always adequate to hold a part, especially with stresses of weight-bearing, as the plate may break; it may be supplemented by external fixation, e.g. a plaster of Paris cast or cylinder. Plating the fracture allows active rehabilitation; the disadvantage of additional external fixation is that joint stiffness may be considerable, especially with the extra trauma of surgery. To avoid this stiffness, delayed splintage is often used. Postoperatively the fracture area may be protected by a plaster of Paris back-slab. Treatment then consists of elevation of the limb and active movements to maintain the mobility of joints and muscles, as well as helping to pump away the inflammatory exudates. The patient is not allowed to weight-bear. After a few days, or when the stitches are removed, the patient should have a good range of movement in all joints. The plaster cast can than be completed, or splintage applied, and treatment continued as already described. There is little or no stiffness when the splintage is removed because the initial inflammation has been resolved, together with reabsorption of exudates.

DISLOCATIONS

Traumatic dislocation can occur at any joint, but those most commonly affected are the shoulder, elbow, interphalangeal and ankle joints. Dislocation may be associated with a fracture of adjacent bones, i.e. a fracture-dislocation. Dislocation cannot occur without damage to the joint capsule and ligaments – these are torn which allows the articular surfaces to separate; or a ligament may be avulsed from its attachment.

Treatment is usually early closed reduction by manipulation, but sometimes surgical intervention is required, e.g. for an open reduction or ligamentous repair. When ligaments and the joint capsule are torn, the joint must be splinted in a position which will aid healing. The time of splintage depends on the part of the body which is affected, for example six weeks for a dislocated knee, one week for a finger; three weeks for the lateral ligament of the ankle.

The aims of physiotherapy are as for fractures, but the affected joint will be stiff when the splintage is removed and may require intensive physiotherapy. During immobilisation circulation of the limb should be stimulated, together with exercises to prevent muscle atrophy. When the plaster cast or bandage is removed, exercises are directed to gaining range, strength and co-ordination of movement.

PHYSIOTHERAPY WITH ASSOCIATED INJURIES OR COMPLICATIONS

If there are other injuries or complications the physiotherapy for the fracture must be adapted or in some cases completely withdrawn. Only complications directly affecting the physiotherapist are considered.

Joint complications

Joint injuries may include dislocation; subluxation; ligamentous rupture or strain; haemarthrosis; disruption by intra-articular fractures; or a penetrating wound into a joint with possible infection.

Joint stiffness is the most common complication of fractures and is predisposed by:

(a) Peri-articular adhesions: Injury to individual tissues, oedema and immobilisation cause adhesions between muscle, ligaments, capsule and bone. Some joints are more vulnerable than others, e.g. knee, elbow and fingers stiffen easily with permanent impairment, while the hip and wrist usually regain movement more easily.

(b) Intra-articular adhesions: These occur when a fracture involves the articular surface, or is near to it. A haemarthrosis will result which may be absorbed, or may organise forming adhesions.

Physiotherapy is usually preventive but if adhesions have occurred then intensive treatment is necessary. Active and stretching exercises; ultrasound; local heat and functional activities may be useful. If the physiotherapist is trying to mobilise a stiff joint before consolidation of the fracture, she must exercise caution, and be quite certain that the movement is at the joint and *not* at the fracture site. If a fracture is close to a joint, e.g. a supracondylar fracture of the femur, knee mobilisation may be delayed until consolidation has been achieved.

If stiffness persists after consolidation and intensive physiotherapy, then manipulation under anaesthesia may be considered.

(c) Infection: This often causes stiffness of long duration.

(d) Mal-union: see page 469.

(e) Myositis ossificans: This is post-traumatic ossification of a haematoma around a joint. The cause is unknown. Passive movement may increase its production, and should be avoided with bone or joint injuries. The most usual site of myositis ossificans is at the elbow joint when, a few weeks after injury, the range of movement is noticed to be decreasing. Treatment is rest.

(f) Sudeck's atrophy: A painful osteoporosis occurring usually in the hand or the foot (see p. 472). Treatment is intensive physiotherapy, and occupational therapy, with active exercise, local heat, and elevation of the part. Interferential therapy has been found to be of value.

(g) Osteoarthritis: This is liable to follow mal-union if the joint surfaces remain incongruous, or following avascular necrosis.

(h) Unreduced dislocation: If treatment is not progressing satisfactorily, then the therapist should check with the surgeon that it
was reduced initially and has not re-dislocated.

Muscle complications

(a) *Torn muscle fibres* are common with fractures and may adhere to
    other structures during the healing process. If the affected
    muscles are treated while the fracture is healing adhesions are
    reduced, and consequently the period of rehabilitation is
    shortened.
(b) *Disuse atrophy* can largely be prevented by repeated active
    exercises from the time of injury.

Tendon complications

(a) *Torn tendons*: These are rare, the most common example being a
    transverse fracture of the patella which is usually associated with a
    tear of the extensor mechanism of the knee; repair is essential.
    This slows down rehabilitation, but unresisted active quadriceps
    exercises are usually permitted from the time of surgery. A
    protective back-slab is worn for walking until active knee
    extension, without a lag, is regained.
(b) *Avulsion fractures*: When the tendon pulls off a fragment of bone,
    e.g. the supraspinatus tendon at the shoulder; if the fragment is
    not severely displaced then gentle, graduated shoulder exercises
    can be started at once. Pendular exercises are especially useful in
    the first few weeks, and elbow and hand exercises. If reduction
    was necessary, rehabilitation will be delayed and movement
    regained more slowly.

Nerve injury

This is not uncommon with fractures. It is usually in the form of a
neurapraxia which recovers quickly. *Axonotmesis* occurs when the
injury imposes a traction force on the nerve, and *neurotmesis* occurs
with open fractures from penetrating injuries.

Nerve injury should be diagnosed at the initial examination.
Sensation and muscle power should be re-tested at subsequent
assessments, because nerve damage may result from treatment or
positioning, e.g. pressure of a below-knee plaster cast on the common
peroneal nerve at the neck of the fibula. Physiotherapy will need to be
adapted and treatment directed to maintain the mobility of those

joints which are usually moved by the affected muscles. An example is an axillary nerve lesion associated with a fractured surgical neck of the humerus. Treatment should be commenced immediately in the form of gentle small-range pendular exercises of the shoulder with the arm supported in a collar and cuff sling. At three weeks post-injury union will have occurred; a greater range of movement can be achieved by careful active-assisted movements. As previously mentioned the physiotherapist must be sure that movement is at the shoulder joint and not at the fracture site. At six weeks the patient should be taught auto-assisted exercises, and the importance of maintaining mobility to prevent a 'frozen shoulder' explained to him. Throughout treatment, mobility and muscle power of the hand and elbow should be maintained. As the nerve lesion begins to recover, physiotherapy should include facilitatory and strengthening exercises.

If recovery of a nerve does not occur as expected, electromyography and exploration of the nerve may be indicated.

Other complications

Pressure sores: If these should occur the physiotherapist may be asked to treat them by ice-cube massage, infra red irradiation, ultraviolet irradiation or ozone therapy.

Infected wounds: These are most likely to happen when the fracture site has been contaminated. Treatment may include extensive wound toilet and skin grafting. Physiotherapy is aimed at maintaining muscle power and, where possible, joint mobility.

Venous thrombosis: If this occurs physiotherapy will be in accordance with the wishes of the particular surgeon. Leg exercises and deep breathing exercises will have their place.

Adult respiratory distress syndrome (ARDS): See page 470 for a clinical description of this condition. The physiotherapist may well be the person who notices the first signs of this, particularly if it presents with typical chest symptoms which call for 'chest physio'. The treatment is oxygen therapy and *not* conventional chest physio-therapy.

Not all fractures require physiotherapy and many patients only require to be taught simple exercises and to be advised to use their fractured limb in as normal a manner as possible. Every surgeon will have variations of treatment and the physiotherapist must always check what is required.

The following pages of charts give indications for the management and treatment of fractures in all parts of the body.

ABBREVIATIONS USED IN THE FOLLOWING CHARTS
IF Internal fixation
MUA Manipulation under anaesthesia
OA Osteoarthritis
POP Plaster of Paris (cast, cylinder or black-slab)
RTA Road traffic accident
THR Total hip replacement

CHARTS OF COMMON FRACTURES

When referring to this section, it is important to recall the previous detail which has been discussed. For example, soft tissue damage will have occurred at the time of the fracture and may well influence the physiotherapy which is given, both in the early and late stages of rehabilitation.

Points to bear in mind when reading the charts

COLUMN 1
A broad anatomical classification is given. For greater detail see relevant texts.

COLUMN 2 USUAL AGE-GROUP
This is, as it says, an indication of the age-group which most frequently sustains this type of fracture. It must be remembered that almost any fracture can be sustained by a person of any age. Epiphyseal injuries are confined to the immature skeleton.

COLUMN 3 HOW INJURY OCCURS
This suggests the most usual but by no means the only way to sustain the fracture.

COLUMN 4 MOST USUAL METHOD OF TREATMENT
The surgeon will consider many factors before selecting his method of treatment. One or two more common methods have been listed here for the guidance of the physiotherapist.

COLUMN 5 MOVEMENT BEGUN

This is, of necessity, only a guide to timing. The surgeon will indicate his requirement, which will be based on local factors such as the general health of the patient, the degree of stability of the fracture, etc. The terms *weight-bearing* and *non-weight-bearing in plaster* indicate the time at which some weight can be expected to be taken on the limb.

Broad outlines only of treatment are given, and the reasons for them. It must be remembered that all injuries are different, as are the people who sustain them. The treatment must be given to meet the needs of the particular patient, *not* as they appear in any book.

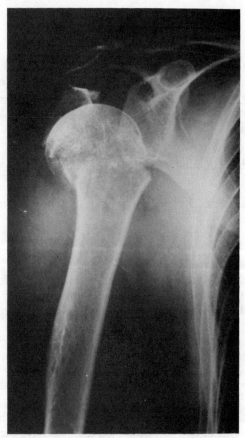

Fig. 24/1   Impacted fracture of the neck of humerus

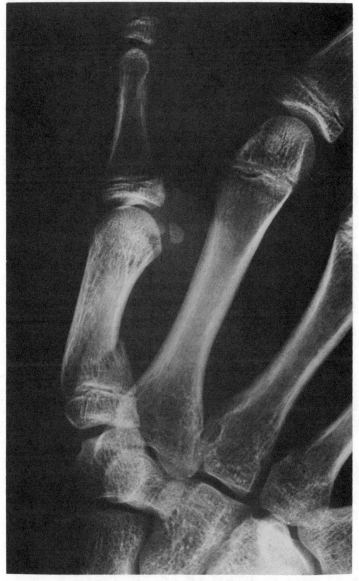

Fig. 24/2   Bennett's fracture of the first metacarpal

FRACTURES OF THE SHOULDER REGION

Site	Age-group	How injury occurs	Most usual method of treatment	Movement begun	Complications	Results and comments
CLAVICLE	All	Birth trauma Fall on outstretched hand Direct injury	Sling	As soon as pain permits	Neurovascular but uncommon	Excellent
SCAPULA – Glenoid – Neck – Acromion – Body	Adult	Direct blow	Sling	As soon as pain permits	—	Excellent
HUMERUS – Upper end – Neck (Impacted) (Fig. 24/1)	All	Fall on outstretched hand	Sling	As soon as pain permits	Axillary nerve lesion	Good especially in children
– 2/3/4★ part-fractures of upper end ± dislocation	Adult	Fall on outstretched hand	Sling Internal fixation Prosthetic replacement	Early	Stiffness Loss of function	Poor but functional demand may be low
– Shaft	Adult	Direct, e.g. gunshot Fall on outstretched hand	U-slab or hanging cast Functional brace	2–3 weeks	Non-union	Good Considerable compensation possible if mal-union

* 2 part=neck (of humerus); 3 part=neck+greater tuberosity; 4 part=neck+both tuberosities

Notes

The soft tissue damage around a shoulder subjected to a fracture is considerable. The importance of early movement cannot be overstressed but where early movement produces much pain it will be counter-productive. Better to allow the soft tissues to settle (2–3 weeks and if pendular active movements can be begun so much the better) then start a vigorous programme.

COMPLICATIONS

Nerve lesions are associated more often than not with specific injuries, e.g. the axillary nerve in dislocation of the shoulder. Where such well-known associations exist the nerve damage will be looked for automatically by examining: (a) the sensory component, i.e. loss of sensation to the skin; (b) the motor component, i.e. loss of muscle action. Pain may exclude adequate examination of both.

FRACTURED CLAVICLE

This can be treated with a 'figure of 8' bandage; this does not support the fracture. It can cause great discomfort in the axillae. It is used less often now. This fracture, if combined with a 'flail' chest lesion, is serious.

FRACTURE-DISLOCATION OF SHOULDER

This is a common injury in the elderly. Range must be maintained. This can be done if great care is taken to support the weight of the limb when the patient is performing movements. Axillary nerve lesion is fairly common. It is not always easy to see whether deltoid muscle is working for several weeks, but the skin sensation of the C5 nerve will be altered. If the nerve is involved the need for maintaining the range of movement is still of the greatest importance. In most instances there is spontaneous recovery from the nerve compression.

FRACTURED SHAFT OF HUMERUS

Blood vessel damage usually associated with open wounds, e.g. gunshot wounds. Usually picked up early in casualty. Radial nerve damage should always be sought and loss of wrist and/or finger extension is easily demonstrated.

FRACTURES OF THE ELBOW REGION

Site	Age-group	How injury occurs	Most usual method of treatment	Movement begun	Complications	Results and comments
Supracondylar	Child	Fall	1. Collar and cuff 2. Dunlop traction 3. K-wire stabilisation	3 weeks	Myositis ossificans Mal-union Volkmann's ischaemic contracture	Good
T- and Y-shaped fractures of lower humerus	Adult	Fall	1. Early active movement 2. Internal fixation with screws and plates	As soft tissue recovery permits	Mal-union Arthritis	Poor
Condylar	Child	Avulsion injuries	(a) Lateral usually fixed with K-wires or screws (b) Medial – may be left to form fibrous union	2 weeks	Non-union Mal-union Late ulnar palsy	Good Good
Radial head	Any	Fall – usually an indication of severe medial soft tissue damage to the elbow	1. Collar and cuff 2. Excision (only in adult if badly comminuted) 3. Very rarely amenable to fixation	As pain permits	Stiffness Late O A	Good

Olecranon	Any	Avulsion or direct blow	Tension band wire Screw	Immediately	Stiff elbow	Excellent (usually some loss of extension)

Notes

RANGE

Forearm rotation (pro- and supination). The functional usefulness of the hand after an elbow injury is proportional to the degree of rotation regained. It is re-educated in functional activity only.

Flexion. The hand must reach the mouth; beyond this, flexion is not essential.

Extension. While full range movements are always the aim, an arm with no extension beyond 90 degrees can be functional if the other movements are good. *Never attempt to increase the range by passive movements.*

COMPLICATIONS

Volkmann's ischaemic contracture. This is rare in its full-blown form resulting in muscle ischaemia and tissue necrosis with subsequent contracture. The flexor muscles of the forearm are specifically involved. The pulse is a poor indicator of forearm muscle ischaemia. It is much more important to heed a complaint of pain (a well-supported fracture will be relatively pain-free) in the forearm especially if that pain is intense on passive finger extension. The capillary circulation to the fingers is also very important. The return of blood to the nail beds when blanched is a good indicator of this.

HAND SWELLING

It is important to avoid this since it may contribute to a poor functional result ultimately. Elevation and early finger exercises with careful attention to plaster or dressing tightness will avoid this.

SOFT TISSUE DAMAGE

In elbow injuries this is often extensive, resulting in considerable swelling. In adults it tends to organise and give rise to permanent limitation of joint movements if it is not treated. Fortunately few elbow injuries of adults need to be in plaster so that ultrasound therapy can be given at once, even if movement is not permitted. In children repeated manipulation must be avoided or myositis ossificans may result. Likewise passive exercising of elbow injuries is to be condemned.

FRACTURED OLECRANON

The triceps will displace a fracture of the olecranon when it acts. However, a tension band will convert the muscle force into an axial compression force on the fracture and, hence, early active rehabilitation should be the rule. Monteggia fractures represent a very severe injury to the whole elbow joint and, even if the ulnar fracture is well stabilised, it may not be possible to begin early movement.

491

FRACTURES OF THE RADIUS AND ULNA

Site	Age-group	How injury occurs	Most usual methods of treatment	Movement begun	Complications	Results and comments
ULNA SHAFT Isolated fracture	Any	Direct blow	Functional brace Long-arm cast	Immediately On cast removal	Non-union in adult	Excellent
Upper third with dislocation of radial head (Monteggia) (see Fig. 23/11)	Any	Direct blow or forced pronation	Child – manipulate POP	On removal of POP at 3–6 weeks	Radial nerve palsy rare	Excellent
			Adult – reduce radial head and plate ulna	As soon as radial head thought to be stable		Poor
Ulnar and radial shafts	Any	Direct blow or fall	Child – MUA and long-arm cast	On removal of POP 3–6 weeks	Mal-union Non-union Cross-union	Good (some loss of rotation will always occur but may be un-important functionally)
			Adult – plate	Immediately		
RADIUS Lower third with dislocation of lower radio-ulnar joint (Galleazzi)	Adult	Fall on outstretched hand	Internal fixation	Early	Loss of forearm rotation	Fair only

				On plaster removal		
Lower ¼	Child	Fall	Plaster		Mal-union	Good. Considerable moulding from growth can compensate for dorsal angulation
Lower 1 inch (Colles') (see Figs. 23/5, 23/6)	Adult	Supination due to fall	Plaster	Fingers, elbow and shoulder straight away	Rupture extensor pollicis longus. Sudeck's atrophy. Osteoarthrosis. Mal-union (common)	Good
Smith's	Adult	Fall	Plaster	As above	Stiffness of wrist	Good
Barton's	Adult	Fall	Internal fixation	Immediately		Can be very poor where mal-union occurs

Notes

RANGE
Flexion and extension of the elbow and wrist are not affected unless the limb is put into a long plaster.

Forearm rotation. The alignment of the forearm bones is crucial to rotation. Also the upper and lower radio-ulnar joints must be correctly aligned. This, combined with uncertainty of union and late development of mal-union, has led to wider acceptance of internal fixation in these fractures. In children the virtual certainty of union means non-operative treatment is advised. There are, however, cases which will require open reduction and internal fixation, e.g. as bone growth slows down in late teens or where rotatory malalignment cannot be corrected by closed means.

Functional bracing in upper limb fractures. Sarmiento has advocated bracing in certain fractures, e.g humeral shaft, isolated ulna and Colles' fractures. There is little evidence as yet that such methods are widely applicable but limited use suggests high union rates with good functional results.

POWER

This is quickly regained once firm union is established. The overall time for complete rehabilitation is often shortened if 'strengthening exercises' for the arm are delayed. The power of the hand in a 'gripping' action should be encouraged from the beginning.

COMPLICATIONS

Blood vessels and nerves are sometimes damaged at the same time since these fractures are usually the result of direct blows and often occur in road traffic accidents. However, they are not complications in the normal sense of the word, in that they do not occur as a result of the fracture.

Non-union is the most likely complication, particularly of the ulna, which is slow to unite. Heat, swelling or tenderness over the fracture area or pain or sudden loss of forearm rotation should be regarded as possible indications of non-union or re-fracture.

PHYSIOTHERAPY

This must be directed towards encouraging use rather than attempting to 'hurry' recovery. These injuries are difficult to treat. Delaying movements may seem to be adding to joint stiffness, yet any attempt to force movements always meets with disaster.

Notes

FRACTURES OF THE CARPUS AND HAND

Site	Age-group	How injury occurs	Most usual method of treatment	Movement begun	Complications	Results and comments
Scaphoid	Young adult	Fall on outstretched hand or direct blow to back of wrist	Plaster immobilisation for 6–12 weeks	Immediate finger and elbow exercises	Non-union Avascular necrosis Late osteoarthritis	90% good results
Metacarpals	Young males	Classical 'punch' injury	None if isolated (may require fixation in severe/unstable injuries)	Immediately		Excellent – loss of knuckle contour may occur but functionally excellent
Bennett's (fracture-dislocation) (Fig. 24/2)	Any	Direct blow	Bennett plaster K-wire or screw	On removal of plaster		Excellent, provided the metacarpophalangeal joint is reduced. Even if fracture not reduced may give little trouble

Phalanges	Any	Direct blow Twisting injury	If stable hold alignment by strapping to next healthy finger May require internal fixation with small screws or wires	Immediate use	Stiffness of fingers	Usually excellent but if there are associated tendon or neurovascular injury can result in a very stiff finger

Notes

FUNCTION

Power and pincer-type grips are the primary functions of the hand. In order to perform these actions effectively, normal kinaesthetic sensation, good joint range and controlled muscle power are needed.

RANGE

The joints of the wrist and hand are a complex structure designed to perform very strong and very delicate movements.

The actual range of movement of each joint varies with the individual, and comparison with the uninjured hand is the only guide to their normal range.

Since function is the essential feature of the hand, it is this, rather than particular joint range, which should be the aim.

POWER

This is very important in the hand. All re-education should be designed towards power. Joint range is of no benefit if it is not controlled by strong muscle power.

COSMETIC APPEARANCE

This is often sacrificed in order to keep the functional range, e.g. fractured metacarpals usually result in the 'loss' of a knuckle because of a slight overlapping of the bone ends. To obtain a cosmetically perfect result would require an operative procedure which could result in a loss of metacarpophalangeal joint range.

SCAPHOID FRACTURES

It is now believed that a scaphoid fracture is only part of an injury to the wrist area. The bony injury may not indicate the severe damage which has occurred especially to important volar ligaments. A condition of 'carpal instability' may exist which if diagnosed early requires the scaphoid fracture to be internally fixed to ensure its union and proper subsequent wrist function.

FRACTURES OF THE FEMUR

Site	Age-group	How injury occurs	Most usual method of treatment	Movement begun	Complications	Results and comments
Sub-capital	60+	Fall but some patients fracture, then fall	1. Internal fixation 2. Prosthetic replacement, e.g. Moore, Hastings or THR	As soon as recovered from anaesthesia and all tubes and drains removed	1. Non-union Avascular necrosis 2. Infection–dislocation	Variable but if case selection is good very acceptable results from both forms of treatment
Inter-trochanteric	Usually elderly	Fall	Internal fixation (a) nail-plate (b) Ender-nail (c) compression screws	As soon as possible	Infection Failure of device	Good. Results depend on type of fracture Compression screw devices appear to have some advantage
Sub-trochanteric	Young adult	High velocity Direct violence Pathological*	Traction Internal fixation, e.g. Zickel nail	Will depend on treatment but early	Mal-union Non-union	Good
Shaft	All	Direct injury	1. Traction 3/12 2. Traction 6/52 – cast brace	The ankle and knee should be exercised on	Mal-union Non-union Infection	Excellent results can be obtained by all methods

3. Internal fixation (IF) plates or intramedullary rods	traction from 10 days onwards With IF mobilisation can be begun on day after surgery. Weight-bearing may be delayed for 12 weeks
4. Plaster spica in children	

the main operative treatment offers early mobility and is therefore widely practised.

RANGE

Usually these patients only want to be able to enjoy 'quiet' living, i.e. the ability to sit (90% of hip flexion), stand and walk (some extension of hip if possible), toileting (30% abduction). A much greater range is desirable, but not essential.

POWER

Personal independence is only possible if the muscle power is sufficient to perform the action. Encouragement to keep practising sitting, standing or walking is very important. The quadriceps, hamstring and glutei muscle groups are the most important ones to maintain.

Notes

*PATHOLOGICAL FRACTURES

A bone may be weakened by disease within the bone itself, e.g. Paget's disease; by disease which produces its effect on bone, e.g. osteomalacia; or by a disease process which only affects bone secondarily, e.g. a breast carcinoma which disseminates and produces skeletal deposits (secondaries). All such processes may precipitate a fracture in bone by an injury which otherwise would not result in a fracture. All fractures in almost any bone in an elderly patient must be regarded suspiciously but spinal fractures, upper femoral fractures and rib fractures especially.

UPPER FEMORAL FRACTURES

The hazards of traction for the elderly are bronchopneumonia, pressure sores and DVT. Selected cases can do very well but in

500

FEMORAL SHAFT FRACTURES

RANGE

The quadriceps muscle must clearly be working normally to gain full extension. Likewise it must not be limited in its excursion to allow full knee flexion. In shaft fractures the muscle may be damaged, be trapped in the fracture, be involved in callus, be adherent to the femoral shaft or be grossly atrophied by prolonged disuse. Some loss of flexion almost always occurs but severe loss of flexion fortunately only rarely. When this happens it may be possible to free the quadriceps (quadricepsplasty) and regain flexion. The importance of maintaining quadriceps bulk cannot be too strongly empha-

sised since it contributes to knee stability which is perhaps even more important than range.

POWER

The quadriceps muscle atrophies very quickly. It is important to encourage its use as quickly as possible after injury.

COMPLICATIONS

Overdistraction on traction is to be avoided. Non-union should not result from treatment but may still occur in compound fractures as a result of the initial severe damage.

Notes

FRACTURES AROUND THE KNEE

Site	Age-group	How injury occurs	Most usual method of treatment	Movement begun	Complications	Results and comments
Supracondylar	Any	Direct in young High violence May be due to twisting injury in elderly	1. Traction 2. Internal fixation (especially if intra-articular component)	Quadriceps exercises early for all Knee mobilisation early, i.e. 10 days following internal fixation but weight-bearing deferred for 9 weeks and full weight-bearing for 12 weeks	Neurovascular to popliteal vessels and nerve	Overall fair If simple non-comminuted fracture, fixation or bracing can give excellent results
Patella	Any	Direct blow Avulsion if quadriceps act strongly but knee unable to extend	Internal fixation Plaster cylinder Excision	Straight away On removal of cast 6 weeks	Retro-patellar arthritis	Excellent
Upper tibia	Adults	Valgus or varus stress drives femoral condyle into upper tibia	1. Perkins method 2. Internal fixation }	In the first few days	Lateral popliteal nerve palsy Mal-union Instability Osteoarthritis	Generally excellent or good

| Tibia shaft | Any | Direct or indirect | Long leg plaster
Functional brace
Internal fixation
External fixation } | Removal of POP
3 weeks
Immediately | Non-union
Mal-union
Compartment syndrome, i.e.
Volkmann's of the calf | The result must be viewed in terms of the initial damage, the age of the patient and the available techniques
No generalisation can be made |

Notes

FRACTURES OF THE FEMORAL CONDYLES OR TIBIAL PLATEAUX

Unless the bone architecture is restored after these fractures, the normal joint is deranged. Instability results in pain and loss of normal joint range. The type of trauma which gives rise to these injuries will usually have caused some degree of dislocation of the joint, often damaging the soft tissue very considerably.

RANGE

Full extension is the primary aim; without this the quadriceps muscles cannot act efficiently. A patient can learn 'to live with' a stiff straight knee, but a loss of 10°, or more, of extension creates a weak painful joint and a poor gait. It is seldom possible to regain full range movements after these fractures in the middle or older age-groups, so that full extension is the most important movement.

POWER

Controlled movements of the knee joint are essential in walking, sitting and standing. Whatever movements are restored to the joint, these are only as useful as the degree of muscle power controlling them. Every effort to maintain the power of the quadriceps muscle must be made, even if the knee joint cannot be moved because of fixation.

FRACTURE OF THE PATELLA

The patella is a sesamoid bone in the tendon of the quadriceps. When fracture occurs it may do so leaving the overlying periosteum and ligaments intact, e.g. stellate fracture in the elderly. These simply require removal of the haemarthrosis, a few days' rest then active exercise. Where, however, the fracture is pulled apart and loss of extension of the knee occurs the fracture must be held together till union occurs or, if too comminuted, removed and the quadriceps mechanism repaired. The patella lends itself to a technique similar to the olecranon, i.e. tension-band wiring. A figure of eight wire passed through the upper and lower poles of the patella over its anterior aspect is all that is required, unless several fragments are present. As soon as wound healing has occurred quadriceps exercises and knee flexion are started. If the patella has been excised, 6 weeks in a plaster of Paris cylinder is necessary to allow the quadriceps mechanism to heal.

It is important to keep the quadriceps muscle as strong as possible. A 'lag' occurs if the patella is removed because of the change in the angle of pull of the muscle. This lag, or loss of full extension, is a feature of most fractures of the patella in the early stages of rehabilitation and must be overcome if the knee is to regain full stability.

FRACTURES OF THE SHAFT OF THE TIBIA

Simple transverse fractures of the tibia occur but road traffic accidents result in high velocity injuries many of which are compound, many comminuted. The problem can be divided into: (a) care of the soft tissues and (b) care of the bone.

Treatment will depend on the degree of damage to each. In severe injuries which might have resulted in an amputation in the past external fixation has allowed stabilisation of the skeleton thus permitting soft tissue repair.

Notes

ANKLE FRACTURES

Site	Age-group	How injury occurs	Most usual method of treatment	Movement begun	Complications	Results and comment
Malleoli	Any	By talus rotating in the ankle mortice	Plaster – long leg Internal fixation	On removal of POP Day 2	Stiffness of the joint Infection Osteoarthritis may occur in either treatment	Results can be excellent but again are dependent on the type of fracture
Talus neck	Young adult	Severe dorsiflexion injury	Internal fixation	Early if well stabilised	Avascular necrosis	Bad. The blood supply is cut off to the body which then dies Revascularisation can occur but damage to the ankle and subtalar joints leads to OA
Calcaneus	Adult	Falls from a height landing on heels	1. Early movement non-weight-bearing } Straight away 2. Internal fixation		Poor function in the subtalar joint	Bad. The involvement of the subtalar joint leads to loss of function,

					i.e. inversion and eversion. If in addition such movement as persists is painful arthrodesis may be necessary	Excellent
Metatarsals (5th)	Adult	Avulsion injury as foot inverts	Below-knee walking plaster for 3/52	As soon as plaster removed	Non-union very occasionally	Excellent

Notes

FRACTURES OF THE ANKLE AND HINDFOOT

The function of the foot on the lower leg is to perform the actions required for propulsion of the body over uneven surfaces at varying speeds. The injuries that can be sustained vary from a simple strain to complex fracture-dislocations involving one or more joints. Unless the bone and joint architecture can be restored to normal, the function of the foot is restricted and usually painful.

restore. Without them walking on uneven surfaces is painful or even impossible.

Loss of dorsiflexion is a serious problem and leads to back kneeing (see Chapter 2).

COMPLICATIONS

Avascular necrosis of the talus is evident within a week or two on bone scanning. Fortunately this is a rare injury.

RANGE

Inversion and eversion are the most important movements to

FRACTURES OF THE PELVIS AND ACETABULUM

Site	Age-group	How injury occurs	Most usual method of treatment	Movement begun	Complications	Results and comments
Stable, e.g. iliac wing; pubic ramus	Adult	Direct blow or fall	Bed rest	As soon as initial pain settles encourage free movement in bed and walk as soon as possible, i.e. 3–4 days	Haematoma	Excellent Sometimes mistaken for a fractured upper femur in the elderly
Unstable, e.g. both rami on one side with dislocation of the ipsilateral SI joint	Adult	Crush injury	Pelvic sling 6–10 weeks Internal or external fixation	On removal of traction Can sometimes sit out after 3–4 days	Haemorrhage Ruptured urethra Ruptured bowel Ruptured spleen Ruptured diaphragm	Variable Long-term back pain, short leg; pelvic disproportion may become a very real problem
±Dislocation of the hip	Adult	Dash-board injury, i.e. blown on flexed knee and hip Direct blow to greater trochanter	Traction 4–6 wks Increasingly internal fixation	Gentle assisted movement while on traction as soon as pain permits Internal fixation can be followed by immediate movement but not weight-bearing	Sciatic nerve palsy Avascular necrosis Myositis ossificans Osteoarthritis	50% good and excellent results claimed for non-operative management 75–80% good results claimed for operative management

Notes

PELVIC GIRDLE

A single fracture of the pelvic girdle (i.e. one ramus or the wing of the ilium) does not significantly alter the stability of the pelvis. Early walking should be encouraged.

Multiple fractures which break the ring in two places, e.g. two rami on the same side plus a disrupted sacro-iliac joint render the pelvic girdle unstable. If non-operative management is used weight transmission through the pelvis must await union of bone. Some exercises may be permitted for the remainder of the limb and the rest of the body. External fixator systems may be strong enough to allow the patient to get up weight-bearing as early as one week.

COMPLICATIONS

The force which fractures the pelvis may either directly injure abdominal organs, e.g. liver, spleen, bowel or bone, may damage bladder and urethra, or the increased abdominal pressure may rupture the diaphragm. Such severe injuries may require, e.g. temporary diversion of the urine or faeces by suprapubic cystostomy and colostomy. These other injuries will determine whether operative intervention for the fractures is possible and will alter possible physiotherapy measures.

FRACTURES OF THE SPINE

Site	Age-group	How injury occurs	Most usual method of treatment	Movement begun	Complications	Results and comments
Flexion injuries	Any	Fall or something falling on patient	Bed rest Cervical collar Traction Fusion	Depends on severity and level of lesion	Neurological	Excellent
Extension injury	Adults	Car accident especially rear-end collisions	Collar	6 weeks +	—	Bad. Usually so-called 'whip lash' injury which has no fracture at all Good if only a fracture of a spinous process
Crush injury	Adults	Force exerted from above or below, e.g. fall from a height	Bed rest Spinal support	Move as pain decreases	Neurological	Good if not associated with severe deformity
Flexion-rotation Fracture-dislocation	All	Direct forces, e.g. RTA	Bed rest 6–8 weeks Fixation with distraction rods	Early passive movements of all joints	Neurological (see Cash's Textbook of Neurology for Physiotherapists, chapters 5–9)	Usually neurological involvement which produces greater or lesser permanent disability

REFERENCE

Adams, J.C. (1983). *Outline of Fractures, Including Joint Injuries*, 8th edition. Churchill Livingstone, Edinburgh.

ACKNOWLEDGEMENTS

The charts on management of fractures have been adapted and enlarged from those first used by Miss M.K. Patrick OBE, MCSP in *Cash's Textbook of Some Surgical Conditions for Physiotherapists*, 6th edition. The authors of the chapter are grateful to her for their use. Similarly Figures 23/6, 24/1 and 24/2 are reproduced by permission of Miss Patrick.

Chapter 25

Soft Tissue Injuries and Sports Injuries

by J.A. FOWLER, BA, MCSP, DipTP, MBIM

Injuries to soft tissue, such as muscles, tendons and ligaments occur from a variety of causes and the effects of injury are legion because people are different. The effects on a sedentary worker will differ from those on one who is active; housewives will be affected differently from their husbands; there are also age differences to be taken into account. The matter is further complicated if those affected participate in sport and more so if it plays an important part in their lives.

EXAMINATION AND ASSESSMENT

The reader is referred to Problem Orientated Medical Systems (POMR) (Weed, 1968, 1971; Graves, 1971; Cross, 1974; Heath, 1978) as a means of keeping medical records and providing a logical format for patients' notes.

This method of note-keeping organises information relating to the patient by providing a continued narrative under the headings of data base, problem list, initial plans and progress notes. The latter is written as 'narrative' notes with sub-headings of:

Subjective — what the patient says
Objective — the physiotherapist's observations and evaluations
Assessment — the physiotherapist's professional opinion as to the short- and long-term goals of treatment
Plan — the development of a treatment programme designed to reach those goals.

Examination and assessment of any region should follow the format outlined by Adams, 1981; Cyriax, 1978; Lee, 1978; with emphasis on inspection, palpation, range of movement and power. The nature of any pain and its distribution should be noted, as should temperature change, local swelling and joint stability. Sensory testing should not be overlooked. Examination of the upper limb should be conducted with the patient stripped to the waist; for the lower limb, shorts or other appropriate attire should be worn. For examination the patient ideally should be in standing, but may be lying or sitting depending on his age, height and degree of deformity, and the height of the physiotherapist. It is very difficult for a short physiotherapist to conduct a full examination on a tall patient who is standing. It is tiring and uncomfortable for the elderly or infirm to remain standing for long periods.

The physiotherapist should have at hand a tape measure, scissors, a safety pin, protractor (or goniometer) to aid the examination and should be familiar with the use of a patella hammer.

Once the examination and assessment are completed the physiotherapist is in a position to make a plan of treatment and can then modify and progress the treatment as often as necessary in conducting an 'audit'.

PRINCIPLES OF PHYSIOTHERAPY

SHORT TERM
The objectives should include:
1. Prevention of further damage
2. Limitation of any bleeding
3. Reduction of pain
4. Reduction of swelling
5. Prevention of immobility/stiffness in joints and soft tissues
6. Maintenance of muscle power

LONG TERM
The objectives should include:
1. Restoration of kinaesthetic/proprioceptive mechanisms
2. Re-education of movement
3. Increase mobility of joint and soft tissue
4. Increase power of muscle
5. Restoration of function and return to daily living
6. Restoration of confidence in affected part
7. Prevention of the return of oedema/swelling
8. Prevention of recurrence of the injury

The modalities of treatment that are used will include ice, compression with or without elevation, exercises, ultrasound, interferential, pulsed and unpulsed short wave diathermy.

Robert Jones bandage (Fig. 25/1)

This type of bandage provides an even pressure and is a well-tried method of applying compression. It has two main objectives:
1. To prevent bleeding.
2. To reduce swelling.

APPLICATION
(a) The pressure is applied firmly and evenly over a wide area above and below the joint even though the pressure is needed locally. (Local pressure is more likely to damage underlying soft tissues and blood vessels and thus prejudice the blood supply.)
(b) The area should be well padded using cotton wool or gamgee in

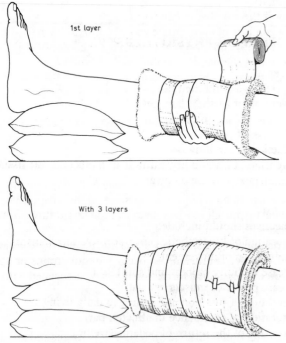

Fig. 25/1   A Robert Jones bandage

three layers. The padding should be retained using a flannelette or crêpe bandage.

1st layer: A thick layer of padding is held on by the bandage which is not taken right to the limit of the padding as this prevents the bandage cutting in. Opportunity is taken at this layer to fill in any hollows, e.g. the coulisses at the ankle.

2nd and 3rd layers: As the first with each layer being covered by the bandage.

(c) The limb should be elevated while the bandaging is applied as this reduces the trapping of blood on the distal part of the limb.

(d) The bandages are applied from distally, working proximally. If possible the limb should be in the neutral or shortened position for the ligaments.

GENERAL RULES FOR APPLYING THE BANDAGE

1. An even pressure should be maintained.
2. Obtain two-thirds to three-quarters overlap of each turn.
3. Keep the edges parallel.
4. Bandage from within out and from below upwards (distal to proximal).
5. Support the part being bandaged.
6. Use a bandage of appropriate width, e.g. 7.5–10cm (3–4in) for the ankle region; and 10–15cm (4–6in) for the knee or thigh region.
7. Ensure that the bandage stabilises the chosen area.
8. A back splint can be incorporated.

CLINICAL TYPES OF SOFT TISSUE INJURIES

To simplify the understanding of soft tissue injuries they can be classified as: strains; sprains; ruptures; and contusions.

Although it is accepted that a strain may be a milder form of a sprain and be applied to both joints and muscles, in this chapter it is defined as damage to muscle of less than complete rupture. Sprains are concerned with ligaments and joints. For example, a biceps femoris strain is distinct from a sprained lateral ligament of the knee joint. It is doubtful whether contusion can occur without strains or sprains of some degree; haematoma formation is always associated with strains.

Strain

Muscle and tendon injuries are referred to as strains and are the result of overstretch. They may be sub-divided as follows:

1. *Chronic strain*: The injury develops over a long period of time which leads to fatigue, muscle spasm, myositis and ischaemia and varying degrees of damage.
2. *Acute strain*: The result of a single violent force to a muscle, usually one that is acting over two joints, which occurs when the contracting muscle is forcibly stretched; for example, the body-weight of a goalkeeper or jumper when landing acts in opposition to the contracting quadriceps.

Ryan (1969) considered strains in four categories; Williams (1979, 1980) describes three, namely, complete, partial intramuscular and partial interstitial. This is not purely an academic exercise, as accurate classification of the extent of the damage (and so by inference the amount of bleeding, muscle spasm and loss of function) will determine the correct line of treatment.

GRADE I: FIRST DEGREE (MILD CONTUSION OR STRAIN)

The initiating trauma is usually crushing and can be the result of a blow from an outside agency, for example the corner of a desk knocking against the thigh on getting up from the chair behind it. There will be tearing of a small number of muscle fibres, the fascia remains intact and bleeding will be minimal. The resulting muscle spasm, pain and tenderness will be localised; pain and spasm in the muscle resists stretching. It is usual with these injuries to have limited local muscle endurance but no interference with function.

If the injury is to an active games player treatment should start immediately after injury by the application of ice for 15–20 minutes followed by a compression bandage applied with moderate pressure. After 20–60 minutes the patient is encouraged to stretch the muscle actively but gently; for example, the quadriceps of a sportsman may be stretched by half squats, partial weight-bearing or he may lie prone and carry out non-weight-bearing knee bending. The maxim is 'little activity taken often'. Ultrasound of low power and dosage may be applied immediately. Ideally the patient should be seen four times a day, or at least morning and late afternoon, then reduced progressively after two to three days. Massage may be given around the site of injury but not directly to it.

If the pain is minimal then light work can be resumed on the next day; pain guides the progression but the site of injury should be protected for two to three days to avoid accidental knocks by the application of a sorbo pad and bandaging. A more conservative approach will restrict activity for longer, usually until the pain and any swelling have been resolved for a week.

GRADE II: SECOND DEGREE (MODERATE STRAIN)

The trauma is more severe – a greater blow is required. There will be a larger number of muscle cells crushed and torn over a wider area. The fascia is still intact and so the haematoma is confined within the muscle even though the bleeding is considerable. The undamaged muscle and subcutaneous fat will be displaced with the formation of a definite palpable mass which is partially liquid and partially clotted blood. The area of the injury will be very tender with considerable pain. The resulting spasm is more severe than it is with Grade I injuries so there is very little muscle extensibility or contractility. There is a longer time scale for recovery with this level of injury.

Initial treatment starts immediately, or at least within 24 hours, by the application of ice, compression with elevation using a Robert Jones bandage or Tubigrip. No active movement or stretching of affected muscle is allowed for at least 24 hours, although active exercises may be encouraged for unaffected parts in an attempt to maintain basic fitness. If the patient can tolerate the discomfort or pain then rhythmical static contractions (auto-resisted if possible) are allowable but no movement of the joints above and below the injury.

The patient with lower limb muscle damage is allowed to be non-weight-bearing on crutches with a pressure bandage. Dispersal agents containing hyaluronidase can be applied to the injury if there is no wound. Gentle effleurage and kneading proximally is particularly helpful. The patient should be seen at least twice, preferably four times, a day.

After 24 hours: After removal of the pressure bandage, active muscle contraction is encouraged. Extensibility is gained by moving antagonist muscles. Proprioceptive neuromuscular facilitation techniques (PNF) such as slow reversals, hold-relax and timing for emphasis are of particular benefit. Stretching may be started within the tolerance of the patient. Non-weight-bearing, massage and rhythmical static contractions may need to be continued; ultrasound, if of low power output and duration, may be used.

48–72 hours: All previous treatment is continued with more emphasis on active unresisted contractions and extensibility, although a hold-relax contract-relax proprioceptive neuromuscular facilitation technique can be adopted. If a good range of movement and full static contraction are obtained then the patient can be progressed to partial weight-bearing if applicable. Transverse frictions to the affected area can be added to the massage manoeuvres.

72 hours: Continue the above treatment regime while allowing increasing progression. The pressure bandage can be removed and need not be replaced unless the swelling increases rapidly. Progressive resisted exercises can be instituted with the weight and load commensurate with pain and discomfort. Fowler (1977) outlined a technique for finding the 10–12 Repetition Maximum (RM) which can be useful later. By trial and error, the amount of weight that can just be lifted (the one repetition maximum – 1RM) once by the patient has first to be found; then the 10–12RM is calculated by taking either two-thirds or three-quarters of the 1RM which is the amount of weight that will allow maximal power to be developed.

If the lower limb muscle is involved then progress to full weight-bearing should start; when full range of movement is attained progress from fast walking to jogging to running is allowed.

Assessment and fitness testing is essential before full training is allowed although the return to work may be very much earlier.

If a hard mass is still present in the muscle after four weeks from injury time, myositis ossificans should be suspected; treatment must be stopped and the patient referred back to the doctor.

GRADE III: THIRD DEGREE (SEVERE STRAIN)
This level of injury involves a larger area of muscle. The fascia is torn at least partially, more than one muscle may be involved and more than one area in the muscle affected. The bleeding, though considerable, is more diffuse due to the fascial tear and an intermuscular haematoma forms.

Treatment: This follows that outlined for Grade II but the patient should be admitted for a period of in-patient care. Progression is much slower; although the patient can mobilise non-weight-bearing in 24–48 hours, partial weight-bearing should not be started too early. Stretching can start five to seven days after injury and active exercises on the second day. Analgesics may be necessary for any pain.

GRADE IV: COMPLETE RUPTURE
The force causing this injury is more than that required to produce Grade III. There is an immediate contraction of muscle ends, with an obvious gap between them. In some instances the sound of rupture may be heard.

Muscle spasm is very severe and widespread with very acute pain. Bleeding is considerable though always proportional to the vascularity of the muscle, and inversely proportional to the spasm of the muscle. There is considerable swelling. Active contraction will be absent;

theoretically, there is no limit to extensibility but the acute spasm will prevent it.

Unless joints are involved in the trauma there is no loss of movement produced by the antagonists except the inhibition by the muscle spasm and pain. There is obvious loss of movement produced by agonists in the active range.

Treatment: It is not considered useful to suture the muscle ends together. It is more important to try and secure the fascial sheath, evacuate blood and secure haemostasis. Then a compression bandage is applied and the muscle immobilised for 10–21 days in a shortened position. Physiotherapy may include movement of all free joints; exercises to all unaffected muscles of other groups; and rhythmic static contractions in the area of the injury if possible. If a lower limb muscle is involved the patient may be allowed up non-weight-bearing after 48 hours. Treatment is as outlined for a Grade III injury with slower progression. The use of low frequency current (e.g. faradism) to produce passive contraction, assist mobility of muscle fibres and affect recovery of muscle fibres probably by influencing fast and slow twitch fibres and the distribution of motor units and fusimotor systems, is still under investigation (Pette, 1980). It should be considered as a treatment modality. Physiotherapists will use short wave diathermy, interferential and diapulse as appropriate.

The regime described refers to the muscle belly but there are other sites where the muscle can be damaged:

1. *Musculo-periosteal junction*: This occurs usually by indirect trauma with pain, little or no swelling and some loss of function. (The degree of swelling will depend upon the extent or degree of damage.)
2. *Musculo-tendinous junction*: Shows similar signs and symptoms but a greater loss of function.
3. *In the tendon*: The tendon is painful and swollen especially if there is a sheath. There is marked loss of function and no high level activity is possible.
4. *At the tendon-periosteal junction*: There is usually very little tenderness or swelling but considerable loss of function.

General signs and symptoms of soft tissue injury

The level of pain, swelling, tenderness and loss of function are determined by the degree of damage.

There will be increased pain on passive stretch and on active contraction. To differentiate between the pain caused by moving an inert structure or by contraction of a muscle it is necessary to cause contraction of the muscle against resistance but allow no movement to take place. If this isometric effort produces pain the possibility of there being a damaged ligament is eliminated (Cyriax, 1978). There is varying loss of function and muscle spasm. Tenderness which is local at first will spread later. Swelling may be of very rapid onset and there will be bruising due to tracking under the influence of gravity.

Treatment: The general aims of treatment will be to relieve pain and muscle spasm, restore function and stop – and limit the effects of – the bleeding. Further damage and injury should be prevented by using techniques which are effective and appropriate for the stage of the injury.

Contusions or bruises

These are usually caused by direct blunt violence, crush or direct contact with another person or a hard landing surface. More often than not the skin is unbroken with extravasation of blood into the subcutaneous tissue due to capillary damage. The normal blood flow is affected because of occlusion of capillaries and pressure of any swelling. Normal tissue nutrition is impaired. There is stiffness of the part because of pain, swelling and muscle spasm.

The aim of first aid is to limit any bleeding and a hyaluronidase/heparinoid type of dispersant such as Lasonil, Hirudoid or Movelat cream or gel, is very useful if used within 48 hours and if there is no wound present. Cold compresses and pressure bandages will also be effective in limiting the bleeding and reducing the pain. Depending on the extent of the bruising there may or may not be loss of function. If there is loss of function then it is reasonable to assume that there is at least Grade II/III muscle damage and appropriate action has to be taken.

Haematoma

In addition to the superficial haematoma of a contusion there are two other types described which are decided by the state of the muscle sheath. Both are caused by damage to blood vessels within the muscle resulting in extravasation.

INTRAMUSCULAR HAEMATOMA (Fig. 25/2)

In this category the blood is contained within the immediate area of the muscle by an intact muscle sheath. After an injury producing bleeding, tension within the muscle increases; the bleeding soon stops and haematoma formation is completed within two hours. It remains friable for two to three days during which time there is danger of further bleeding if more trauma occurs.

INTERMUSCULAR HAEMATOMA (Fig. 25/3)

If the muscle sheath is torn then the extravasated blood seeps into the

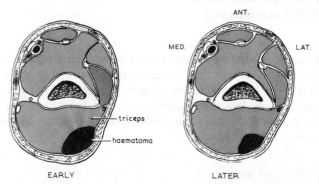

Fig. 25/2 An intramuscular haematoma affecting the triceps brachii

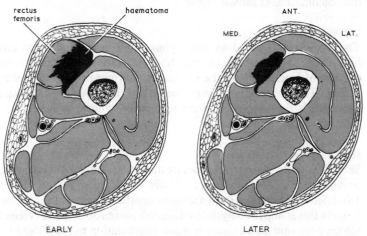

Fig. 25/3 An intermuscular haematoma affecting the rectus femoris

space between muscle in the fascial planes. The resulting haematoma is more diffuse and bleeding continues longer as tension does not build up. The extravasated blood tracks under influence of gravity distally and shows a discolouration beneath the skin.

It is difficult to separate inter- and intramuscular haematoma as they show very similar signs in the first 48 hours or so. After this time they can be differentiated. The characteristics of an *intermuscular* haematoma are:

1. Disappearance, or drastic reduction, of swelling at 48–72 hours; followed by
2. Reappearance of stronger muscular contraction.
3. Evidence of tracking of blood as the bruising shows some distance from the primary lesion.
4. Pain is moderate only.

RESOLUTION OF HAEMATOMA
Organisation of the haematoma occurs because removal of the blood and exudate is impaired by damage to the blood and lymph vessels, especially the arterioles and the venules. Compression of the veins by congestion, and lack of muscular action in the muscle fascial pump due to pain and spasm, impairs reabsorption and allows organisation to occur.

Recovery and repair

Repair involves two processes, the formation of connective tissue and the regeneration of muscle tissue.

CONNECTIVE TISSUE
The tissue is infiltrated by macrophages which are converted into fibroblasts; together with existing fibroblasts these undergo mitosis because of inactivation of the inhibitory enzymes present in healthy tissues. The fibroblasts secrete procollagen, a precursor of collagen which with the fibrocytes forms scar tissue which, as it matures, strengthens and shortens.

MUSCLE TISSUE (Allbrook, 1980)
Skeletal muscle is able to regenerate and in so doing will close a gap providing it is not too large. Muscle fibres grow at the rate of 1.0–1.5mm per day and need a smooth interface along which to grow. Usually this is impaired by the proliferation of fibroblasts and collagen forming too much scar tissue to allow regeneration to occur, and the defect is usually too large. It has been shown that after minor damage

due to pressure there is rapid recovery and within 24 hours after injury damaged fibres cannot be distinguished from the undamaged.

The cycle of events following severe damage to fibres with associated haematoma is muscle fibre necrosis, phagocytosis and regeneration.

Much of the research work has been performed on animals, and in 1966 Allbrook et al noted that . . . 'it would appear that in clinical cases activity is an important factor in speedy and effective muscle recovery. Active joint and muscle movements provide a suitable environment for muscle and soft tissue regeneration'.

Further work is needed to determine if the repair process can be enhanced and a suitable environment for repair produced by using low frequency electrical stimulation, e.g. faradic type currents. There is evidence to show that trophic changes occur when muscles are stimulated electrically (Hudlicka et al, 1980).

Tendon injury

REPAIR

The major problem following laceration and repair of a flexor tendon is that functional recovery is hindered by the formation of adhesions which restrict tendon excursion. Potenza (1962) showed that adhesions to repaired tendons occur at each point where the physical integrity of the tendon is disrupted. Excision of the synovial sheath following tendon repair appears to have no adverse effect on the healing process nor on the functional result but if the bony floor of the digital tunnel is damaged through removal of the flexor tendon and disturbing the vincula brevia then extensive adhesions form. Matthews and Richards (1976) demonstrated that adhesions tend to form in the presence of a combination of suturing the tendon, removing the digital theca and immobilisation. (See also Matthews (1979) and Potenza (1980).)

When flexor tendons are divided within the flexor digital sheath there is proliferation of fibroblasts and vascular elements of the surrounding tissues which are damaged at the time of injury. At the same time resting tenocytes are transformed into tenoblasts within the cut ends of the tendon. Repair is then effected by the proliferation of these cells and the synthesis of new collagen fibres (Matthews and Richards, 1974). The initial collagen is laid down at right angles to the long axis of the repaired tendon. In 18–21 days the collagen is re-aligned and in response to tension lies parallel to the long axis. During this time the synovial sheath regenerates. Within 21–25 days there is enough collagen deposited to allow gradual active movement and unrestricted use can be allowed after five weeks; at 128 days the wound is completely matured and it would be difficult to identify the scar histologically (Potenza, 1980).

The optimum time to commence active mobilisation of a repaired digital tendon is 23–25 days when the scar tissue is sufficiently strong to withstand stress.

JOINT INJURIES

Bass (1969) describes an injury to a joint as having three potential effects; (a) on ligaments only, (b) to the joint producing a synovitis and effusion, and (c) a combination of (a) and (b).

Ligaments

Injuries to ligaments are conventionally described as sprains and are classified in three degrees of severity. These injuries are caused by overstretching at the extreme of the range and are either acute or chronic; most acute lesions will occur in the lower limb or the spine. The medial ligaments of the ankle are damaged during eversion and the lateral ligament by inversion. Damage to the collateral ligaments at the knee occurs during rotary stress on a flexed knee or by a person falling over an outstretched leg, the medial ligament being the one most commonly affected.

GRADE I: FIRST DEGREE (MINOR SPRAIN)

With a Grade I sprain there will be minimal damage with some pain and tenderness at the site of injury. Swelling will be slight and there will be some loss of function. The differential test is to put the ligament at stretch and thus a knowledge of functional anatomy is essential to the physiotherapist.

Treatment: Ice, followed by the application of a Tubigrip bandage, crêpe bandage or other type of support, and limitation of use for the first 24 hours. If the injury is to a lower limb ligament then the patient may be allowed to walk but to do little else with the injury during this time. Early commencement of static muscle contractions is desirable for two reasons: first, the blood flow is maintained and the swelling reduced; second, developing strong muscles will develop strong ligaments (Inglemark, 1957).

GRADE II: SECOND DEGREE (SEVERE SPRAIN)
A greater force is required to produce this level of injury: many more fibres are involved or a ligament may be partially detached from its attachment. The patient should be assessed medically or (in certain clinics/departments) by an experienced physiotherapist. Swelling is considerable but takes time to develop. Pain and tenderness are more acute. Movement is limited and, if in the lower limb, the patient is unable to bear body-weight even if the knee or ankle is kept stiff and straight. Function is very limited.

Immediate treatment: This involves the use of ice, compression and elevation if appropriate. To reduce pain the doctor may inject a local anaesthetic but activity must be restricted until later when the effects have worn off.

GRADE III: THIRD DEGREE (COMPLETE RUPTURE)
With a Grade III sprain there is rapid onset of effusion, very considerable pain and tenderness, the joint is unstable and there is complete loss of function. This must be assessed medically as the ligament rupture may result in displacement.

Treatment: First aid treatment involves the use of ice and compression with splinting and rest. If the ligament *is* displaced it is repaired surgically and the limb put in plaster of Paris for six to eight weeks. If it is *not* displaced plaster of Paris is applied to the limb and retained for six to eight weeks.

Static exercise must be started at once and all non-affected areas must be exercised. After about a week isometric movement can be attempted inside the plaster cast. For a lower limb injury weight-bearing is restricted and the patient is instructed in the use of sticks. When the splint is removed tissue mobility is encouraged and ultrasound, transverse frictions, and hydrotherapy are used. Effusion is controlled by the use of pressure bandaging correctly applied. At the appropriate time the patient joins classwork in the gymnasium.

Synovitis (Fig. 25/4)

Cyriax (1978) stated that this term should be abandoned as it is a symptom common to many disorders; it is not a diagnosis. Wiles (1959) said very much the same, especially in the chronic sense. Synovitis is an inflammation of the synovial membrane due for example to trauma, chondromalacia, loose bodies, arthritis, tuberculosis, syphilis or haemophilia. Depending on the site it will mean that there is also damage to ligaments around the joint. The extent of trauma will decide the degree of synovitis; within the knee the menisci, cruciate or collateral ligaments may be involved. If all three are involved the description 'unhappy triad' has been applied (O'Donahue, 1970).

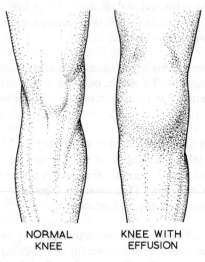

NORMAL
KNEE

KNEE WITH
EFFUSION

Fig. 25/4   Traumatic synovitis of the knee joint

Dislocation will damage the synovial membrane, so will 'nipping' of the membrane between the bony ends, even though it is thought that this is not possible. Direct blows will certainly damage. In some patients arthritis may lead to acute synovial rupture. Typically, synovitis is seen in the vigorous person who attempts to carry on despite the effusion.

SIGNS AND SYMPTOMS
There is characteristic swelling which has taken some time to develop. The joint area will be hot and red and the swelling will fluctuate on palpation. Pain may be present over the injured structure but more often there will be a feeling of tension or pressure due to the swelling. The joint will be held in a relaxed position away from the extremes. Muscle atrophy will occur rapidly especially when the knee joint is involved.

In a synovial rupture of the knee the patient typically describes getting up from a chair, going upstairs or circuit training, such as step-ups or stride jumps, and feels a sudden pain at the back of the knee which rapidly swells, spreading into the calf causing an increase in girth of 5–7.5cm (2–3in) after several hours. The synovial fluid is irritating and leads to an inflamed oedematous leg. Homan's sign is positive and the condition is often mis-diagnosed as deep vein thrombosis. The signs of synovitis are similar to those of a haemarthrosis (blood within the joint).

DIFFERENCE BETWEEN HAEMARTHROSIS AND SYNOVITIS

With haemarthrosis the swelling is generalised and occurs rapidly indicating that there is significant intra-articular injury. Less serious injury produces an effusion which is manifest by swelling occurring over a period of hours; the effusion is serous. The classic type of injury to a joint has been described as capsular sprain which can be identified with the Bass classification (Williams, 1964). Thus capsular sprain can involve the whole joint, a specific capsular structure or ligament either as partial or complete sprain.

Signs: Pain on certain movements and extremes associated with local spasm. Clinical instability will only be demonstrable in a complete tear and even then it may be difficult due to muscle spasm. Swelling is usually slight although in some cases gross superficial swelling may be present, e.g. in damage involving the fibular collateral ligament.

TREATMENT

Ligament damage alone: The affected area is rested with a Robert Jones type compression bandage. Ice is useful to help reduce any swelling. Transverse frictions may be given to the site after insonation with low power ultrasound for 3–5 minutes as the latter will have anaesthetised the part. Graduated activity is begun at once and isometric action of muscles around the joint is essential.

Synovitis: Ice and compression with elevation as appropriate. Relative rest with specific instructions as to what can and cannot be done. If swelling persists for 48 hours, and if it interferes with mobility, then the joint may be aspirated. After aspiration the joint may be infiltrated with 25–50mg hydrocortisone which may be repeated if necessary. Other anti-inflammatory drugs such as phenylbutazone (Butazolidin) or ibuprofen (Brufen) may be prescribed. After aspiration isometric exercises should be encouraged progressing to a graduated exercise regime when the effusion has cleared. Where necessary weight-bearing must be reduced to a minimum.

HEALING OF LIGAMENTS

When there is a complete tear or a rupture of a ligament the ends retract and the gap fills with blood, not because of bleeding from the ligament but from the damaged subcutaneous tissues. Eventually the clot organises by invasion from fibroblasts, collagen is laid down joining the ends within two weeks. There is insufficient strength to be fully functional until six to eight weeks have passed with restoration of collagenous continuity.

It has been reported that the unstressed length of ligaments is the same if allowed to heal without suturing as it is if the ligament is sutured (Potenza, 1980). If, for example, the medial ligament at the right knee is stressed by pushing the thigh medially with the left hand and the leg is pulled laterally with the right hand the sutured ligament will not give or lengthen but the unsutured ligament will do so, the stretch depending on the amount of fibrous tissue between the ends. The suggestion is that for maximum stability of joints, especially in the young and in athletes, the damaged ligament should be sutured.

Combined synovitis and ligamentous damage

The synovitis is given priority of treatment and the injured ligament is protected from further damage.

Bursitis

Bursae are membranous sacs lined with synovial membrane and sited so that they prevent friction or wear and tear of muscle and tendons as they pass over bone. They are of two sorts:

1. *Normally occurring (true) bursae* are found subacromially, and at the elbow, knee and heel.
2. *Adventitious bursae* occur in response to new friction on tendons over bone and can occur anywhere, e.g. hip, ischial tuberosity or at the medial side of the great toe.

   The response to injury or disease of both types is the same, inflammation, which may be the result of mechanical irritation or bacterial infection.

IRRITATIVE

The inflammation arises because of excessive pressure, friction or gouty deposit. The wall of the bursa becomes mildly inflamed as a result of unaccustomed activity, exercise or ill-fitting shoes. The sacs become filled with clear serous fluid and are not usually painful unless pressured, e.g. a bunion or calcaneal bursitis.

Treatment: Rest, perhaps in a sling for the upper limb and restricted weight-bearing for the lower limb. Short wave diathermy, ice or infra red irradiation as appropriate. Muscle strengthening if necessary (PNF is useful, using slow reversals); mobilising if there is any limitation in joint freedom. The doctor may inject hydrocortisone into the bursa; this requires reduced activity for two to three days afterwards. In intractable cases of chronic pain the bursa may be removed surgically.

INFECTIVE

This may be an acute infection with a pyogenic organism, or a chronic infection with a low grade organism such as tuberculosis.

Treatment: Rest; appropriate antibiotics with surgical drainage or excision. If there is an operation then pre- and postoperative physiotherapy is indicated. Short wave diathermy and massage may be given to the scar but not to the bursa.

Tenosynovitis

This is inflammation of the synovial lining of a tendon sheath but not the fibrous sheath. This condition also presents as an irritative and infective tenosynovitis.

IRRITATIVE

This form is due to excessive overuse and friction. There are no adhesions, no limiting movement but there is pain and crepitus on palpation. The sheath is mildly inflamed and there is a watery effusion into it. It is likely to occur at the wrist and ankle. Racquet players are particularly prone.

Treatment: Movements must be restricted and the part rested by the use of splints, bandaging or plaster of Paris. If the paratendon of the tendo calcaneus is affected then the heel of the shoe is raised about 2.5cm (1in) for males, and females are encouraged to wear shoes with a moderate heel. Ultrasound, short wave diathermy, and/or ice may be effective. Cyriax (1978) states that as the cause is longitudinal friction then transverse frictions will cure. Stubborn cases may respond to hydrocortisone injections and for other patients surgical intervention by slitting the sheath may be performed. In this event there will be pre- and postoperative physiotherapy.

BACTERIAL (INFECTIVE)

The acute lesion is caused by a pyogenic organism and produces a purulent exudate. The chronic lesion is caused by a low grade organism or tuberculosis.

Treatment: The appropriate antibiotic is prescribed once the causative organism is known. The part is immobilised for up to two to three months after which physiotherapy may be advocated.

Tenovaginitis

The tendon sheath rather than the synovial sheath is affected. Adams (1981) states that although the cause is unknown it is not due to infection. Cyriax (1978) suggests it may follow repeated strains. Crepitus never occurs but use of the part causes pain.

Treatment is similar to that for tenosynovitis. If the condition affects the extensor pollicis longus or abductor pollicis longus it is referred to as De Quervain's disease.

UPPER LIMB CONDITIONS

Rotator cuff injuries (Figs. 25/5, 25/6)

Whether called rotator cuff injuries or, less commonly, tendinous cuff injuries the muscles involved are supraspinatus, infraspinatus and subscapularis. All of them blend with the capsule distally.

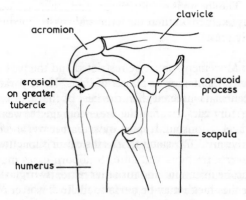

Fig. 25/5 Rotator cuff lesion

PAINFUL ARC SYNDROME

Adams (1981) gives five causes of the pain caused by abduction at the glenohumeral joint during the middle range of movement. The supraspinatus tendon is usually nipped between the tuberosity of the humerus and the acromion process (Fig. 25/6).

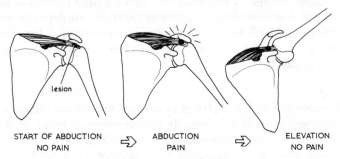

START OF ABDUCTION
NO PAIN ⟹ ABDUCTION
PAIN ⟹ ELEVATION
NO PAIN

Fig. 25/6   Painful arc syndrome

1. Injury to the greater tubercle (tuberosity) of the humerus, either an undisplaced fracture or contusion to this site.
2. Partial tear of the supraspinatus tendon at the teno-periosteal junction. Cyriax (1978) states that the lesion must lie superficially at this junction for the painful arc to be elicited. If a painful arc occurs during passive elevation then the lesion traverses the distal end of the tendon.
3. Supraspinatus tendinitis.
4. Calcified deposit in the tendon.
5. Subacromial bursitis.

(Cyriax would add infraspinatus and subscapularis tendinitis because involvement of these structures is indistinguishable from that of supraspinatus.)

TREATMENT

Detailed treatment is found in Cyriax (1978) and Adams (1981). Suffice to say that where there is an undisplaced fracture or contusion, it is treated by early mobilising and strengthening exercises. The supraspinatus lesions are treated by rest, transverse frictions, short wave diathermy, ultrasound, exercises, or injection of hydrocortisone.

A subacromial bursitis is not usually treated by frictions as this form of treatment is ineffectual or tends to make it worse. Muscle spasm may be reduced by effleurage and kneading. Rest in a sling, hydrocortisone injection, ice, short wave diathermy or infra red irradiation may be palliative.

Supraspinatus tendon

A complete tear of this tendon entirely disrupts abduction at the glenohumeral joint. The partial tear elicits a painful arc, i.e. pain around 90 degrees of abduction. The extent of the pain depends on the degree of tearing. If full passive movement is relatively painless, and if there is no painful arc, then the musculo-tendinous junction is probably affected.

CAUSES
The injury may be due to a fall on an outstretched hand or a slippage of a heavy load while lifting. Often the patient is over 60, unless an older sportsman; he experiences pain at the tip of the shoulder which later becomes intolerable; it is usually worse at night. Local tenderness is elicited just below the acromion. The limited abduction possible is produced by scapula rotation and maintained by deltoid.

TREATMENT
In the elderly patient it is usual to avoid an operation because of arthritic changes developing in the shoulder and the poor state of the tendon, but there are no such restrictions on younger patients.

After repair the arm is rested in a plaster of Paris splint with 90 degrees of abduction, 60 degrees of flexion and 45 degrees of lateral rotation for three weeks. Following immobilisation intensive active exercise will be necessary. Massage, heat or ultrasound can be used as adjuncts to mobilisation and restoration of function. The prognosis is fair if repair is carried out immediately, and poor if delayed.

Infraspinatus

Although this muscle which inserts into the middle of the three impressions on the greater tubercle of the humerus may be ruptured completely, suffer strains or tendinitis, such conditions are rare. The only reference to a rupture is in Cyriax (1978) when he describes it as presenting with painless weakness and a painful arc which is very noticeable at first but then ceases over two to three years. When this occurs 30 degrees of lateral rotation is lost.

Tendinitis and strain of the muscle is more common than a rupture although still rare. The lesion will lie either at the insertion into the greater tubercle or in the body of the tendon. A full range of passive movement will be present at the shoulder; resisted lateral rotation will hurt while all other resisted movements will not. In addition, if the lesion is deep and distal, full passive elevation will be painful because the tendon is nipped between the tubercle and the acromion. If the lesion is superficial there will be a painful arc. If neither of these movements produce pain then a lesion exists in the middle part of the tendon.

TREATMENT

This will consist of rest for the *traumatic* lesions with ice, ultrasound and, when appropriate, transverse frictions. The treatment of choice for *tendinitis* is transverse frictions or injection of a steroid suspension at the site of the lesion.

Subscapularis

Damage to the subscapularis muscle, which inserts into the lesser tubercle (tuberosity) of the humerus, will usually be a stress injury caused by over-strain or continued overuse.

There is usually a full range of passive movement but resisted medial rotation is painful and adduction is usually pain-free unless pectoralis major, latissimus or teres major are involved. The site is tender to the touch. There may be a painful arc of movement which suggests that the upper part of the muscle is involved or, if full passive adduction in flexion is painful, the tendon of subscapularis is trapped against the coracoid process (Cyriax, 1978).

TREATMENT

Rest, ice and ultrasound for the recent injury and, when indicated, transverse frictions to the tender site. If tendinitis due to repeated overuse is present then the treatment is transverse frictions or an injection of a steroid suspension by the doctor.

Capsulitis of the shoulder

Other terms for this condition are 'diffuse capsular lesion' (Cyriax, 1978); a manifestation of arthritis or adhesive capsulitis (Neviaser, 1945); and periarthritis or frozen shoulder (Adams, 1981).

The condition is ill-defined and not understood. It is characterised by limitation of passive and active movements. Pain appears as the limit of the range is reached. Resisted movements do not hurt. There is no evidence of infection and injury is not a constant feature. There is loss of capsular resilience with a hardish end-feel like leather being stretched. The patient complains of severe aching pain in the shoulder and upper arm which comes on gradually. In some instances sleep is disturbed as the patient turns during the night. Abduction, extension, flexion, medial and lateral rotation are all limited by as much as half normal range. Radiography reveals no abnormality and there is no evidence of inflammatory or destructive changes.

There is a tendency to spontaneous recovery within 6–12 months with reduction of pain and shoulder joint stiffness.

TREATMENT
This is relative rest in a sling which should be removed for short periods to allow gentle active-assisted exercises. Anti-inflammatory drugs such as aspirin or phenylbutazone may be prescribed.

Provided Cyriax's criteria are matched, and the prescribing consultant agrees, then passive stretching may be commenced, the aim being to stretch the capsule only enough to cause an increase in pain for one to two hours. Steroid injections may be given into the joint and are said to improve movements and reduce pain dramatically. As pain lessens, active exercises are increased and muscles strengthened. In some instances short wave diathermy, ice and ultrasound may be useful.

Long head of biceps brachii

Tendinitis at this site is due to overuse or one severe strain affecting the mid-part of the tendon. Resisted movements at the shoulder are painless and passive movement are full and pain-free. Resisted supination and flexion of the elbow produce pain at the intertubercular sulcus.

Cyriax (1978) suggests treatment by transverse frictions and says that steroid injections are usually unnecessary because massage is frequently effective. Alternatively, ultrasound may be used.

Rupture of the long head of biceps does not occur under normal stress unless the tendon is weak due to age and is aggravated by friction as it runs through the intertubercular sulcus. The patient is usually male and past middle age and complains of moderate pain with the feeling that something is giving way when he pulls or lifts. Later a bulge may be noticed in the front of the arm (Fig. 25/7). There is localised tenderness in the intertubercular sulcus. Resistance to elbow flexion produces bunching of the long head of the muscle. The strength of flexion and supination will not be greatly affected.

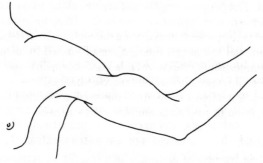

Fig. 25/7   Ruptured long head of the biceps brachii

TREATMENT

The disability is usually so slight that operation is not required. If repair is needed then it is usual to suture the distal stump into the bicipital groove and ignore the proximal end. Immediate treatment is aimed at encouraging active movements, especially at the shoulder, elbow and radio-ulnar joints. Any pain that is felt will be reduced by analgesics, or by using a sling which can be discarded after two to three days. If, after this time, it is still necessary to rest the limb the patient can carry it in his pocket. Short wave diathermy and resisted muscle work to the antagonists will help overcome spasm and reduce pain. It is essential to strengthen the muscle and to have it restored within two to three weeks.

Tennis elbow (lateral epicondylitis)

This is a common well-defined clinical entity and the term is used to cover all non-specific lesions affecting the wrist extensor group or muscles at their common origin at the elbow

The cause is overuse or strain of the extensor origin, often caused by a tennis player with a top spin backhand or using a badminton racquet with too small a handle.

A painful scar usually lies at the teno-periosteal junction due to a partial tear of the aponeurotic fibres at the anterior part of the lateral epicondyle. The elbow is unaffected. Pain and tenderness are felt on the outside of the elbow with radiation down to the wrist. Passive and resisted elbow movements are full and painless; resisted extension and radial deviation at the wrist hurt at the elbow. Flexion of the wrist and ulnar deviation are pain-free. A radiograph will reveal no alteration from the normal.

TREATMENT
In mild cases the limb is rested using a plaster of Paris sling for four to six weeks. Hydrocortisone injection may be given and the part rested for a short time afterwards. Deep transverse frictions may be given. Prior to using a Mills' manipulation (the forced extension of the elbow advocated by Cyriax), short wave diathermy may be of use in mild cases as well as following manipulation. If the injury does not improve, or fails to respond to conservative methods, then operation is performed when the extensor origin is stripped from its attachment and allowed to fall back.

Other sites where this lesion may occur include:
(a) in the body of the tendon 5–10mm below the epicondyle, or (b) on the supracondylar ridge in the origin of extensor carpi radialis longus.

The opposite lesion – golfer's elbow (medial epicondylitis) – can occur at the common flexor tendon origin on the medial epicondyle or at the musculo-tendinous junction about 6.25–12.5mm below the epicondyle.

LOWER LIMB CONDITIONS

Hamstrings (biceps femoris)

The signs and symptoms following injury to this muscle will vary in degree and be related to whether the injury is a Grade I, II or III strain. If the damage is at the fibular insertion then there may be spasm of the muscle and the knee will appear locked, mimicking the effect of a torn lateral meniscus. There may also be damage to the common peroneal nerve.

Resisted flexion of the knee will be painful at the side; there will be spasm in the muscle belly; and the knee will be held in slight flexion to gain the shortened position. Extension of the knee joint will be limited or painful. Weight-bearing will be uncomfortable at Grade I level but will be impossible at Grade III or IV.

TREATMENT
The initial treatment will be ice, rest and compression. For Grade II or III low-powered insonation may be useful with or without faradism. Later, massage using effleurage, kneading and then transverse frictions will be beneficial. Early rhythmical static contractions are advisable in Grade I and II but best delayed for 24–48 hours in Grade

III. Progression to free and resisted activity using progressive resisted exercises and PNF, such as slow reversals, hold-relax timing for emphasis as appropriate, follow the normal course.

Quadriceps

The rectus femoris is the muscle most often damaged, usually at the musculo-tendinous junction, although with, for instance, a more forceful take-off in a sprint start, mis-kick or direct blow, the belly may be affected. Many so-called 'pulled muscles' are the result of haemorrhage from a ruptured vein (Smillie, 1978).

In Grade I (minor strain) injuries there is discomfort on extension of the knee and flexion of the hip. This will be disabling in Grade II (moderate strain). In either case performance and function will be affected. In Grade III (severe strain) injuries a definite gap will be felt; and in Grade IV (complete rupture) injuries the gap is clearly visible at about the middle of the thigh. Weight-bearing and function is unaffected in Grade I injuries but is increasingly a problem in Grades II–IV. There will be an area of tenderness at the site of injury. The general signs and symptoms have already been outlined and by applying anatomical knowledge to them it becomes possible to decide which muscle is affected and the degree of damage sustained.

Gross injury to the vastus medialis can occur following trauma relating to the limb having been trapped. Vastus lateralis is seldom injured because it is protected by the ilio-tibial tract but may be involved through herniation of the muscle following inguinal hernia repair by removal of a strip of the ilio-tibial tract. The vastus intermedius is damaged by a direct blow with subsequent haemorrhage which may lead to myositis ossificans.

Quadriceps apparatus

Except as outlined above disruption of the quadriceps apparatus may occur at one of three points:
1. avulsion of the tendon from the upper pole of the patella
2. through the patella
3. at the attachment to the tibial tubercle.
In all of them the applied force is unexpected flexion resisted by contraction of the quadriceps group.

AVULSION OF TENDON FROM THE PATELLA
This injury usually happens to obese, middle-aged or elderly men. The patient stumbles going down stairs, starts to fall and a strong

reflex contraction of the quadriceps occurs. In the middle-aged or the young either the tendon can be avulsed or the patella fractured, in the elderly avulsion usually occurs.

Treatment: This consists of repair with stout non-absorbable sutures or stainless steel wire. A plaster of Paris cylinder is applied and after five days isometric quadriceps exercises are allowed. The patient is usually allowed up non-weight-bearing after 10 days and progressed through partial to full-weight-bearing over a period of four to six weeks. The plaster is removed after two to three weeks and is replaced by a back-slab until 90 degrees flexion and full extension of the knee joint is obtained. Low frequency current stimulation, for example, interrupted direct current (IDC) or faradism, and ultrasound may be used as and when appropriate.

DISRUPTION THROUGH THE PATELLA

This usually occurs transversely through the mid-patella in middle-aged adults who stumble with a reflex contraction of the quadriceps. The knee is swollen and tender with a tense haemarthrosis. A gap can be felt which fills with blood. The patient is unable to straight leg raise or to move the leg at the knee.

Treatment: This varies widely according to the individual surgeon. It can range from supportive bandaging to surgical interference. The physiotherapist must apprise herself of the surgeon's wishes. In all methods isometric quadriceps muscle drill should be taught.

AVULSION AT THE TIBIAL TUBERCLE

This injury is the least common and occurs in children and young adults. It is very painful and slow to heal. The condition is treated by suture of the patella tendon and a plaster of Paris cylinder applied for six weeks. Gentle quadriceps drill is started five to seven days after operation and gradually increased.

The patient is allowed up non-weight-bearing progressing to partial weight-bearing for a period of four to six weeks finally being allowed full weight-bearing. A back-slab is worn until 90 degrees of flexion is obtained.

PRINCIPLES OF PHYSIOTHERAPY

1. Reduction of pain
2. Reduction of swelling
3. Maintenance of muscle strength
4. To obtain joint stability
5. To obtain joint mobility

6. Avoidance of quadriceps lag
7. Re-education of gait
8. Continuous assessment and testing for fitness

Swelling is usually a problem at the time of injury and following repair. This is controlled by the plaster of Paris or the pressure bandage together with quadriceps drill as appropriate and when allowed. Swelling is likely to occur when the support is removed and when weight-bearing is started; this can be best controlled by quadriceps drill in elevation together with massage such as effleurage, kneading and squeezing-kneading.

The pain will gradually subside but analgesics may be prescribed at first.

Improving muscle strength will also obtain stability of the joint and avoid quadriceps lag. It is achieved by a system of quadriceps drill, progressive resisted exercises, PNF technique of maximal resistance, with slow reversals, timing for emphasis and stabilisations when a weak part of the range is met. To help in the healing process and the correct interplay of muscles it is essential that a normal walking pattern is obtained as soon as possible by emphasis on the equality of weight-bearing, length of stride and the time spent on each. It is also important that the proprioceptors are challenged by using a wobble board, uneven ground, jumping, running and weaving.

Rupture of the tendo calcaneus

This particular injury is very often overlooked as one of the other muscles, such as plantaris, is often suspected of being strained. The rupture is always complete and occurs as a result of forced dorsiflexion when the gastrocnemius is contracting strongly. Many domestic and sporting situations can lead to the damage, e.g. jumping off the bottom step of the stairs, jumping to 'smash' at tennis and landing with full weight on one leg. The injury can occur in all age groups, male or female. It may occur spontaneously in the middle-aged who are taking unaccustomed exercise, probably due to disuse weakness. In the female it may occur while participating in keep fit classes.

CLINICAL SIGNS
A sudden agonising pain rather like a kick is felt and a gap can be palpated some 5cm above the insertion into the calcaneus. There will be some swelling and the patient can walk with a limp or with difficulty. There will be tenderness at the site and some thickening in the area due to the bleeding. The muscle belly will show some spasm. Plantar flexion is possible but is much weaker when performed in long

sitting or lying and is produced by the other posterior tibial muscles and the peronei.

Two tests are of use in the diagnosis:

(1) If the tendon is intact, squeezing the relaxed calf will contract gastrocnemius reflexly causing slight plantar flexion.

(2) The patient is asked to raise the heel from the ground while standing on one leg. If the tendon is ruptured this is impossible.

Treatment: This will depend upon the individual surgeon and once again the physiotherapist will need to apprise herself of his wishes. Apart from the variants in treatment techniques, the choice will be further governed by whether the injury is recent or old. In general the post-treatment management may be summarised as follows:

A below-knee plaster of Paris cylinder is applied with the foot plantar flexed, for three to four weeks; during this time the patient is allowed up non-weight-bearing with crutches. The plaster is then changed and the foot position changed to plantigrade for a further two to three weeks.

At about four to six weeks the plaster is bivalved to allow active non-weight-bearing exercises. Non-weight-bearing walking with crutches continues, and after a further two to six weeks progression to partial weight-bearing is allowed, and then weight-bearing.

OBJECTIVES OF PHYSIOTHERAPY

1. To strengthen the gastrocnemius muscle particularly, and other muscles in general, while the ruptured tendon is healing.
2. To mobilise the ankle joint and foot.
3. To re-educate walking.
4. To develop spring, running and jumping.
5. To limit any swelling.
6. To break down adhesions and overcome their effects.
7. To stimulate the patient's response.
8. To test for fitness – functionally and physiologically if applicable.

Treatment techniques to achieve the objectives of physiotherapy are those of standard orthopaedic practice. Care should be taken not to progress the exercises too soon to avoid breakdown of the repairing tendon. Exercises will progress from non-weight-bearing to partial and then full weight-bearing.

A most important aspect of treatment is that of continuous assessment and fitness testing basing the progression of treatment on the findings. Joint mobility can be aided passively (Maitland, 1977) and actively. Physiological stretching techniques, i.e. reach grasp incline (or lean) support standing; holding with foot in dorsiflexion at the position of discomfort for one to two minutes and then resting for the same period (Fig. 25/8). The manoeuvre is repeated two to three times each session two or three times a day.

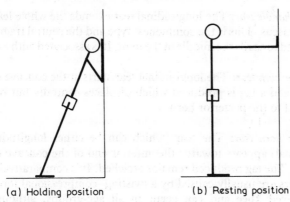

(a) Holding position   (b) Resting position

Fig. 25/8   Physiological stretching of the tendo calcaneus

Massage such as effleurage, wringing, squeezing-kneading to the calf muscle in elevation helps to limit and reduce swelling. Kneading and transverse friction will be necessary to break down any adhesions and to mobilise the tendo calcaneus and other tendons around the ankle.

The tendon should be well and truly healed within 128 days (4 months) and should be fairly strong at five to six weeks; at the appropriate time exercises and activities can be used to develop spring, running and jumping. Circuits may be incorporated into the regime.

Torn meniscus of the knee

The menisci are semilunar cartilaginous structures attaching centrally to the tibial condyle. They are thicker at the periphery than the central margin. The medial meniscus is broad posteriorly and narrow anteriorly. The lateral meniscus is, by comparison, thicker and has a wider more uniform width than the medial meniscus. The medial meniscus is more fixed than the lateral one. The functions of the menisci can be summarised as weight-bearing, shock absorbing, stabilising and facilitation of rotation.

CLASSIFICATION OF TEARS (Fig. 25/9)
Basically there are three types of tear and they all begin as a longitudinal split.

Bucket handle tear: The longitudinal tear extends the whole length of the meniscus. This is the commonest type and the central fragment is displaced towards the middle of the joint. It is associated with locking.

Posterior horn tear: The longitudinal tear starts at the concave central border and a tag is produced which displaces centrally but remains attached to the posterior horn.

Anterior horn tear: The tear (which can be either longitudinal or horizontal) appears towards the anterior end of the concave central border. The tag produced remains attached. It is comparatively rare. The tears are usually caused by a twisting, compressional force on a semi-flexed knee and can occur in all age-groups, although the longitudinal injury is more likely in the younger person.

The most common conditions producing abnormal stress and strain on the knee joint are on the football field and, to a lesser extent, in coal mining; any activity involving twisting on a flexed knee will render the menisci liable to damage.

CLINICAL FEATURES
The average age for all meniscectomies between 1940 and 1974 has risen from 27.6 to 43.7 years for males and from 22 to 50 for females and the most common meniscal tear is of degenerative origin (Smillie, 1978). The medial meniscus is affected more often than the lateral.

The twisting injury causes the patient to fall and complain of pain on the antero-medial aspect of the joint and there is inability to continue the activity. There is difficulty in straightening the knee and in walking bearing weight. Overnight the knee becomes swollen; this resolves over two weeks with rest and bandaging. During this period the patient regains the ability to straighten the leg. At some later date the knee gives way during a twisting movement with consequent pain and swelling. These incidents occur repeatedly and eventually the patient will say that the knee 'locks' that is, a sudden interference with extension during rotation occurs. The locking has been shown to be due to interposition of a section of the meniscus between the femur and the tibia at a point anterior to the coronal plane of the joint. It occurs when the longitudinal tear extends to the anterior section and is

MENISCUS DAMAGE

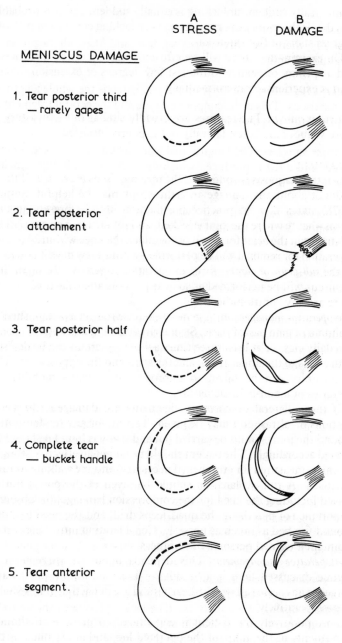

A
STRESS

B
DAMAGE

1. Tear posterior third
   — rarely gapes

2. Tear posterior
   attachment

3. Tear posterior half

4. Complete tear
   — bucket handle

5. Tear anterior
   segment.

Fig. 25/9   Tears of the menisci

dramatically sudden; unlocking is equally sudden, and it is probably this that is the more important sign. True locking occurs about 10–40 degrees short of full extension.

On examination there will be effusion, wasting of the quadriceps and a springy resistance to the last few degrees of extension. Sharp pain is experienced antero-medially.

Lateral meniscus: The features are broadly similar but the history is more vague. Pain is felt laterally but is poorly localised.

TREATMENT
When the diagnosis is confirmed the torn meniscus is excised. If there is doubt about any damage an arthroscopy may be helpful. Smillie (1978) states that 'in practice the menisci injuries present in two forms – acute where the joint is locked, and sub-acute or chronic'. The treatment in the *acute* form will be to unlock the knee within 24 hours. Operation for removal will be performed within a few days if possible. In the *sub-acute or chronic* form an operation to remove the offending meniscus will be performed as soon as possible after diagnosis unless there are any contra-indications.

Pre-operative management: A general exercise routine is established to maintain or gain basic fitness. Strong rhythmical quadriceps exercises in a daily class or at least three times a week. A circuit can be devised with a bias to the upper trunk and the arms and the opposite leg. The opportunity can be taken to improve the patient's mobility by exercises of a non-ballistic nature.

If the collateral or coronary ligaments are damaged transverse frictions or ultrasound may be given. Testing for any tendon injury around the joint should be carried out and if any is found it should be treated accordingly. The patient should be taught an effective straight leg raise, measured for crutches (if necessary) and the walking routine practised. A full explanation should be given of the postoperative period including the need for the compression bandage, the absolute importance of practising the quadriceps drill, and the need to move around the bed as much as possible. Consideration must be given to maintain a trained person's basic fitness.

Postoperative management: This depends upon the surgeon. The regime discussed here is a 'middle of the road' approach. (Many surgeons advocate full weight-bearing and greater activity immediately postoperatively.)

Postoperatively the patient is encouraged to practise rhythmical movements of the ankle of the operated leg, and at all joints of the opposite limb to maintain the circulation. Quadriceps drill is encouraged and straight leg raising without lag is attempted. The patient may be non-weight-bearing until this is achieved. The patient may be confined to bed for 48–72 hours and movement around the bed must be encouraged as much as possible. Later he will be walking, progressing from non-weight-bearing to partial weight-bearing and then to full weight-bearing in about 10 days with a compression bandage and emphasis on proper gait. If there is any quadriceps inhibition low frequency current stimulation, e.g. faradism, is usually effective. The knee is mobilised to full flexion as soon as possible using ice, heat or ultrasound to supplement the exercise regime.

In the final stages of treatment there is a need to progress exercise for basic fitness by the use of circuits and weight training, with a bias to activities of the lower limb; use of a wobble board is essential. Massage, such as kneading, transverse frictions and effleurage may be required for the scar, ligaments and the effusion. Full range of mobility of all joints especially the hip, knee and ankle must be maintained. Fitness should be tested using the Harvard step test or other test (De Vries, 1970). In the early stages mobility is measured by using a goniometer, and later by the ability to squat and sit on the heels. Stability is tested early by hopping, and various figured manoeuvres, e.g. weaving, and later progressing to jumping from varying heights, bounding and hurdling. Skills should be tested by dribbling with a football, kicking, jumping, tackling and dancing.

Testing for ligamentous injury

Care must be taken not to test too vigorously otherwise further damage can follow. The patient is supported on a plinth.

MEDIAL (TIBIAL) COLLATERAL LIGAMENT
The lower limb is held at the knee (in extension), the fingers of the holding hand at the back and the palm at the lateral condyle of the femur; the other hand grasps the tibia just above the ankle and while the lower hand pushes laterally the upper pushes medially.

LATERAL (FIBULAR) COLLATERAL LIGAMENT
The viability of this ligament is tested in the same way as the tibial ligament but with the hand positions reversed. The upper hand is on the medial condyle of the femur and the lower hand on the fibular side of the ankle. The upper hand pulls laterally and the lower hand pushes medially.

CRUCIATE LIGAMENTS (DRAWER SIGN)
The knee must be flexed to 90 degrees and the foot fixed on the couch by sitting lightly on it to prevent it sliding. The quadriceps muscle must be relaxed. The fingers are placed on the upper posterior part of the tibia and the thumbs on the anterior femoral condyles. The upper end of the tibia is pushed and pulled.

If the anterior cruciate ligament is damaged then the anterior glide may be in excess of 0.5cm and if the posterior cruciate ligament is lax then the posterior glide will be increased by a similar amount.

Noyes et al (1980) discuss the amount of laxity present as being dependent upon the integrity of the secondary restraints on joint movement, e.g. if the medial ligament is torn the amount of laxity present will depend on the damage to the cruciate or the lateral ligaments.

Primary restraint	*Secondary restraint*	*Clinical test*
Torn Laxity——→ Intact ————————→		Slight laxity
↘ Stretched ——————→		Large laxity

Tibial collateral ligament (Fig. 25/10)

This ligament is usually damaged as a result of rotary stress on a flexed knee. In football it will occur during a face-to-face tackle when the ball is being taken from a player who is dribbling and a valgus force occurs, or force will be applied to the lateral side of the knee forcing the leg into abduction. As already described, ligaments can sustain minor and major injury including complete rupture. The degree of damage depends on the extent of stress or trauma.

In younger patients the damage is nearly always traumatic and with the older patient chronic strain often complicates an impacted loose body at the knee. There will be effusion which will take time to develop. If the joint swells rapidly a haemarthrosis is present and a total rupture should be suspected. There is tenderness at the site of injury. In the younger patient a slipped epiphyseal plate may occur and in damage to the femoral attachment a condition known as Pellegrini-Stieda's disease may arise due to ossification of the partially avulsed ligament from its upper attachment.

At first the patient can walk, but within the hour may only be able to do so with assistance. Many hours later the pain is worse and the joint very swollen. The amount of disability and pain depends upon the extent of the injury, i.e. whether Grade I or II. Acute traumatic

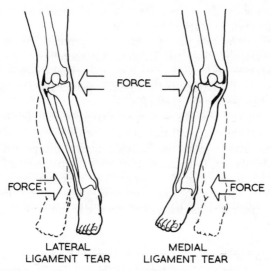

Fig. 25/10 Tears of the collateral ligaments of the knee joint

arthritis is present and may prevent the valgus strain test. If untreated by physiotherapy the pain and swelling gradually subside over 3–8 weeks and recovery will be effected in 8–12 weeks with movement slowly returning.

COMPLETE RUPTURE

In cases of suspected total rupture the decision, whether it is complete or one of overstretch, must be made as a matter of urgency. If the slightest doubt exists then preparations are made for operative repair. The final diagnosis is not assumed until the presence of abduction in extension is demonstrated (Smillie, 1978). Pain in a complete rupture is usually less than if there is a partial tear. There will be haemarthrosis.

Treatment has already been outlined. Where there is only minor damage the mainstay of it will be quadriceps drill. This may be started at once, but if there is haemarthrosis or if immobilisation in a plaster cylinder is necessary it will be delayed. Transverse frictions, ultrasound or short wave diathermy may be helpful.

Fibular collateral ligament (Fig. 25/10)

This ligament is a strong rounded cord attached to the lateral epicondyle of the femur and to the head of the fibula. It is closely associated with the biceps femoris attachment and the common peroneal nerve. It is relaxed in flexion.

Injury is relatively uncommon as it is protected from adduction strain by the opposite limb. Damage may therefore only occur if the leg is forcefully adducted on the thigh as in a rugby tackle. Very often such force will also damage the common peroneal nerve which is less likely to happen if the knee is flexed.

Complete rupture seldom occurs as an isolated injury but involves the capsule, the cruciate ligaments and/or the nerve (Smillie, 1978). There may also be lesions of the attachment to biceps femoris and/or the ilio-tibial tract. If damaged, the severity of pain and inflammation will depend upon the grade of strain. The knee will feel warm to hot, with an effusion, yet an almost full range of movement; valgus strain will hurt and palpation will reveal the site of injury.

TREATMENT

1. Ice applications for 15–20 minutes two to four times a day. Rather than have the patient attend four times a day, it is proper to give precise instructions to him so that he may carry it out for himself. The application of ice can be quickly reduced to twice daily and then daily. Later still to three times a week.
2. Pressure bandage to control effusion.
3. Transverse frictions when the inflammation has subsided.
4. Isometric quadriceps exercises progressing rapidly to resisted exercises.
5. Non-weight-bearing walking with crutches will be allowed at first, progressing quickly through partial weight-bearing to full weight-bearing with emphasis on correct gait.

Cruciate ligaments (Fig. 25/11)

Damage to the cruciate ligaments can cause severe biomechanical disturbance, mainly in an antero-posterior direction. They also control lateral mobility, rotation, hyperextension and hyperflexion.

ANTERIOR CRUCIATE LIGAMENT

This ligament is injured as the result of direct violence when:

1. dislocation of the knee occurs;
2. the femur is driven backwards with the knee at right angles and the tibia fixed;
3. there is a sudden block to rotation; or
4. in abduction it occurs as the medial ligament is damaged.

Ligamentous rupture can occur in four distinct forms: at the inferior and superior attachments within the body of the ligament; and partially antero-medially or postero-laterally. If the injury occurs in isolation the capsule is intact. There is effusion of blood or bloodstained synovial fluid. The haemarthrosis is slight. The risk of injury to the anterior cruciate ligament is increased when there is a torn meniscus present and more violent activity is undertaken.

The clinical picture is usually the slight haemarthrosis in a slightly flexed knee with a possible momentary locking at the time of the injury. Pain and muscle spasm are marked and the joint is tender to touch. The spasm will prevent the drawer sign (see p. 546) being performed though it can be tested after aspiration and anaesthesia.

Established instability will need surgical repair. Much of the instability can be overcome by developing the thigh muscles especially the quadriceps muscles; this can be sufficient in all but the highest levels of sporting activity.

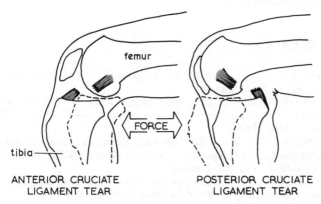

Fig. 25/11 Tears of the cruciate ligaments of the knee joint

POSTERIOR CRUCIATE LIGAMENT

Rupture of the posterior cruciate ligament together with damage to the posterior part of the capsule is 'of common occurrence' but is very often missed or misdiagnosed (Smillie, 1978). The cause of damage is a force which drives the tibial head backwards when the knee is flexed and most commonly occurs in road traffic accidents when the knee strikes the dashboard.

The site of injury is at its inferior or superior insertion. Clinically there are contusions, abrasions and lacerations on the anterior aspect of the knee or tibial head (Trickey, 1968). The amount of swelling varies. It will be greater if the capsule is intact. There is tenderness to deep palpation in the popliteal space.

In rupture of the posterior cruciate ligament, the drawer sign occurs spontaneously as the head of the tibia sags backwards when the knees are at right angles and the feet on the couch. Hyperextension will be present if the capsule is ruptured posteriorly.

Conservative treatment will involve strengthening all the thigh muscles to provide stability to the knee. If surgical repair of the ligament is performed a compression bandage is applied post-operatively with the joint in a few degrees of flexion maintained by a plaster of Paris back-slab. When the stitches are removed a plaster cylinder is applied for up to eight weeks, and weight-bearing is allowed.

Physiotherapy will be directed to strengthening all the muscles of the lower limb, especially those of the thigh, and gaining knee flexion and extension. Any effusion which may occur following removal of the plaster cylinder can be treated by massage, ice and elevation and an elastic stocking.

REFERENCES

Adams, J.C. (1981). *Outline of Orthopaedics*, 9th edition. Churchill Livingstone, Edinburgh.

Allbrook, D.B., Baker, N. de C. and Kirkaldy-Willis, W.H. (1966). Muscle regeneration in experimental animals and man. *Journal of Bone and Joint Surgery*, **48B**, 153–69.

Allbrook, D. (1980). *Muscle Breakdown and Repair*. In *Scientific Foundations of Orthopaedics and Traumatology*, (ed Owen, R. et al). William Heinemann Medical Books Limited, London.

Bass, A.L. (1969). Treatment of muscle, tendon and minor joint injuries in sport. *Proceedings of the Royal Society of Medicine*, **62**, 925–8.

Cross, H.D. (1974). The case for problem oriented medical records. *British Journal of Hospital Medicine*, **1**, 65–79.

Cyriax, J. (1978). *Textbook of Orthopaedic Medicine*, Vol 1: *Diagnosis of Soft Tissue Lesions*, 7th edition. Baillière Tindall, London.

De Vries, H. (1970). *Physiology of Exercise for Physical Education and Athletics*, chapter 12 (Physical Fitness). Staples Press, London.

Fowler, J.A. (1977). Fitness and its components. *Physiotherapy*, **63**, 10, 316–19.

Graves, S. (1971). Better records: First step to better quality. Problem oriented record is key to better medical practice. *Modern Hospital*, **116**, 105–8.

Heath, J.R. (1978). Problem oriented medical systems. *Physiotherapy*, **64**, 9, 269–70.

Hudlicka, O., Tyler, K.K. and Aitman, T. (1980). *The Effect of Long-Term Electrical Stimulation on Fuel Uptake and Performance in Fast Skeletal Muscles*. In *Plasticity of Muscle*, (ed Pette, D.). De Gruyter, New York.

Inglemark, B.E. (1957). Morphophysiological aspects of gymnastic exercises. *Bulletin Federation Internationale d'Education Physique*, **27**, 37.

Lee, J.M. (ed)(1978). *Aids to Physiotherapy*. Churchill Livingstone, Edinburgh.

Maitland, G.D. (1977). *Peripheral Manipulation*, 2nd edition. Butterworths, London.

Matthews. P. (1979). *Biological Factors in the Management of Flexor Tendon Injuries*. In *Recent Advances in Orthopaedics – 3*, (ed McKibbin, B.). Churchill Livingstone, Edinburgh.

Matthews, P. and Richards, H.J. (1974). The repair potential of digital flexor tendons. *Journal of Bone and Joint Surgery*, **56B**, 618.

Matthews, P. and Richards, H.J. (1976). Factors in the adherence of flexor tendon after repair. *Journal of Bone and Joint Surgery*, **58B**, 230.

Neviaser, J.S. (1945). Adhesive capsulitis of the shoulder: A study of pathological findings in periarthritis of the shoulder. *Journal of Bone and Joint Surgery*, **27**, 211.

Noyes, F.R., Grood, E.S., Butler, D.L. and Malek, M. (1980). Clinical laxity tests and functional stability of the knee: Biomechanical concepts. *Clinical Orthopaedics and Related Research*, **45**, 84–9.

O'Donahue, D.H. (1970). *Treatment of Injuries to Athletes*, 2nd edition. W.B. Saunders Co, Philadelphia.

Pette, D. (ed) (1980). *Plasticity in Muscle*. De Gruyter, New York.

Potenza, A.D. (1962). Effect of associated trauma on healing of divided tendons. *Journal of Trauma*, **2**, 175–84.

Potenza, A.D. (1980). *Tendon and Ligament Healing*. In *Scientific Foundations of Orthopaedics and Traumatology*, (ed Owen, R. et al). William Heinemann Medical Books Limited, London.

Ryan, A.J. (1969). Quadriceps strain, rupture and 'Charlie horse'. *Medical Science and Sports*, **1**, 106–11.

Smillie, I.S. (1978). *Injuries of the Knee Joint*, 6th edition. Churchill Livingstone, Edinburgh.

Trickey, E.L. (1968). Rupture of the posterior cruciate ligament of the knee. *Journal of Bone and Joint Surgery*, **50B**, 334.

Weed, L. (1968). Medical records that guide and teach. *New England Journal of Medicine*, **3**, 593–600.

Weed, L. (1971). Quality control and medical records. *Archives of International Medicine* (January number).

Wiles, P.W. (1959). *Essentials of Orthopaedics*, 3rd edition. Churchill Livingstone, Edinburgh.

Williams, J.G.P. (1964). Knee injuries on the field of sport. *Rheumatism*, **20**, 76–87.

Williams, J.G.P. (1979). *Injuries in Sport*. Bayer (UK), Haywards Heath, England.

Williams, J.G.P. (1980). *A Colour Atlas of Injury in Sport*. Wolfe Medical and Scientific Publications, London.

BIBLIOGRAPHY

Colson, J. (1969). *Progressive Exercise Therapy in Rehabilitation and Physical Education*, 2nd edition. Butterworths, London.

Gray's Anatomy, 36th edition. (jt eds Warwick, R. and Williams, P.L.) (1980). Longman, Edinburgh.

Heilig, A. and Pette, D. (1980). *Changes Induced in the Enzyme Activity Pattern by Electrical Stimulation of Fast Twitch Muscle*. In *Plasticity of Muscle*, (ed Pette, D.). De Gruyter, New York.

Kapandji, A. *The Physiology of the Joints*. Churchill Livingtone, Edinburgh.
(1982) Vol 1: *Upper Limb*, 5th edition.
(1970) Vol 2: *Lower Limb*, 2nd edition.

Kessel, L. and Boundy, U. (1980). *A Colour Atlas of Clinical Orthopaedics*. Wolfe Medical and Scientific Publications, London.

Matthews, P. (1976). The fate of isolated segments of flexor tendon within the digital sheath: a study in synovial nutrition. *British Journal of Plastic Surgery*, **29**, 216.

Palmer, I. (1938). Injuries to the ligaments of the knee joint. *Acta Chirurgica Scandinavica*, **81**, Supplement iii.

Sreter, F.A. and Mabuchi, K. (1980). *Effects of Chronic Stimulation on Cation Distribution and Membrane Potential in Fast Twitch Muscles of Rabbits*. In *Plasticity of Muscle*, (ed Pette, D.). De Gruyter, New York.

Tidy's Massage and Remedial Exercises, 11th edition. (ed Wale, J.O.) (1968). John Wright and Sons Limited, Bristol.

Wright, D. (1976). Testing for fitness. *Physiotherapy*, **62**, 8, 260–5.

Wright, D. (1981). *Fitness Testing After Injury*. In *Sports Fitness and Sports Injuries*, (ed Reilly, T.). Faber and Faber, London.

ACKNOWLEDGEMENTS

The author expresses his thanks to Miss Eileen Thornton BA, MCSP, DipTP Assistant Principal, Royal Liverpool Hospital College, School of Physiotherapy and Mr Richard Calver MChorth, FRCS, Consultant Orthopaedic Surgeon, Walton and Fazakerley Hospitals, Liverpool, for their valuable help and advice in the preparation of these chapters. He also thanks Miss Sue Davies for her patience in preparing and typing the manuscript.

Chapter 26

Sports Medicine

by J.A. FOWLER, BA, MCSP, DipTP, MBIM

Sports medicine, as defined by the Council of Europe, is 'The appreciation of the art and science of medicine from a preventive and therapeutic point of view to the practice of sports and physical activity in order to utilise the opportunities afforded by sport for maintaining or improving health and to avoid any possible dangers'.

Health can be defined as the ability of individuals to mobilise their resources physically, mentally and spiritually for the preservation and advantage of self, dependants and the society to which each belongs (Miles, 1977). Self is deliberately mentioned first because those who are unhealthy or unfit cannot be wholly valuable either to their dependants or to society. However, even in disability certain other attributes can be brought to bear as disability need not be a bar to physical activity or sport.

The idea of physical, mental and spiritual well-being is summed up in the motto of the Royal Navy Physical Education Branch, *Mens Sana in Corpore Sano*, (healthy mind in a healthy body). This attitude should prevail in all people engaged in or supporting sport. Part of the physiotherapist's role is to foster this attitude and to encourage the approach of hard but fair play both on and off the field or arena. It is possible to be ruthless in play, giving or taking no quarter within the rules and to be non-aggressive, and to be friendly and sociable after play is finished. Sport and physical activity should attempt to develop in their adherents the graciousness inherent in good sportsmanship.

According to Miles (1977; 1981) there is an interplay of forces determining health and action in the management of ill-health or injury. In the former, chance, environment and personal factors decide health levels, and assessment, treatment and rehabilitation determine management. The idea of cause of injury or illness is expressed in a formula: $I=CE$ prf/tms, i.e.

Injury=

$$\text{Chance}\times\text{Environment}\times\frac{\text{Accident proneness}\times\text{risk acceptance}\times\text{personal training}}{\text{Training}\times\text{maturity}\times\text{safety precautions}}$$

It would not be amiss to consider, briefly, what is meant by fitness. Fit for what?–normal activities, low-level sporting achievement, Olympian levels?

The World Health Organisation defines fitness as the sense of social and physical well-being. Sir Roger Bannister, eminent neurologist and first four-minute miler, suggests that it is 'The state of physical harmony which enables someone to carry on his or her occupation to the best of ability with greatest happiness'. Professor Asmussen, the physiologist, defines it scientifically as having an absolute and relative meaning. In absolute terms the person that can run fastest, jump highest, lift and handle the heaviest loads and attain the highest output during a working day must be the most fit for that particular activity. Fitness takes on another meaning when applied in a health programme. Here, the word is relative. A person of small size may not be able to lift as much weight as a large person and his maximum output may be less, but physiologically he may be the most fit. Fitness is thus an ambiguous expression and limits have to be set to define it accurately.

Physical fitness is a degree of conformity to accepted standards of given criteria which are mobility, muscle strength, anaerobic and aerobic power, endurance and neuromuscular co-ordination. Standards must be given for each case and more detailed study recommended (Fowler, 1977; De Vries, 1966).

FITNESS TESTING

It is essential, before returning an athlete to competition or training, that adequate safeguards are taken to avoid an injury occurring again or the original injury breaking down. A system to see that muscles, tendons, ligaments, joints and bones will stand up to stresses and strains imposed by high-level activity must be devised.

The fitness testing must be part of the assessment at all stages of the treatment and, as in all things physiotherapeutic, progression is dependent upon whether certain goals are achieved. It is unrealistic to test muscle power and active joint range alone; it is essential also to test passive ranges, accessory movements, elasticity and extensibility, and to ensure that movement is symmetrical and co-ordinated, both with the opposite limb and with the whole body. Balance and poise must be restored. It may be that the final fitness test is the level of activity demanded by the event and the competition. The answer to the initial question, What caused the injury? must ultimately be used to provide the answer to the subsequent question, Is the performer fit enough to start training/competing again? Wright (1976; 1981) discusses this fully; as a guiding principle it is better to delay full activity for a few days than to chance further breakdown with the risk of increased disability time, loss of games fitness or, more importantly, loss of confidence in the remedial organisation. Further guidelines could include, that the athlete (1) has no running limp (if a lower limb), or, if the injury is to the upper limb that there is no comparable loss of timing of that limb; (2) can jump from a height of 1 metre with good technique, progressing to jumping and landing on the injured limb. (A little thought and application will give an equivalent test to the upper limb or one can even be devised for the trunk involving the combination of the upper and/or lower limbs.); (3) has full pain-free active movements or slight pain at extremes against resistance for muscle; (4) has full squat on both or one leg, or full press-up; (5) can, before running, extend the knee with 20 lb × 10 in 45 seconds. (Before contact sport the athlete should be able to lift 45 lb × 10 in less than 45 seconds.); and (6) should have no support or strapping except to hold on a dressing. If support is needed then the athlete should not train or play.

CLASSIFICATION OF SPORTS INJURIES

The logical treatment of injuries and their prevention is difficult unless the type of injury as well as its pathology is determined. Williams (1971) offers a classification of two basic categories; 1. consequential, and 2. non-consequential (Table 1).

There are numerous studies of the incidence of sports injuries and the author particularly commends those of Williams (1979) and Hornor and Napravnik (1973).

Table 1 Classification of sports injuries (Williams, 1971)

1. Consequential   (Example)

  A. Primary
    (1) Extrinsic
      (a) Human   – Rugby: black eye of front row forward
      (b) Implemental   – Incidental: blow from hockey ball

                             Overuse: blisters from oars

      (c) Vehicular   – Cyclists: fracture clavicle or friction burns from crash
      (d) Environmental   – High board divers: sprung back
      (e) Occupational★   – Cyclists: chondromalacia

                             Long distance runners: tendo-calcaneous tendinitis

    (2) Intrinsic
      (a) Incidental   – Muscle tears
      (b) Overuse   – i. acute: canoeists tenosynovitis of wrist extensors

                             ii. chronic: stress fracture

★ I would consider this as a consequential primary extrinsic cause of injury which is not in the original Williams' classification. However, it could be argued that this should appear under the intrinsic overuse heading.

  B. Secondary
    Short term   – Weak quadriceps syndrome
    Long term   – Degenerative joint disease

Under this category injuries occur which are due to direct participation in sport.

2. Non-consequential
  Injuries in this class are those which affect athletes and their performance but are the result of some other non-competitive activity, e.g. tripping at home and injuring an ankle or the back.

Another classification of sports injuries is given by Vaughan Thomas
(1977):

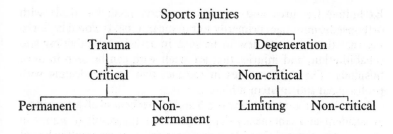

MECHANISM OF INJURY (Fowler, 1979) (Fig. 26/1)

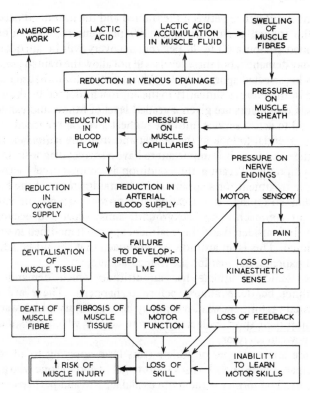

Fig. 26/1 A mechanism of injury

REHABILITATION OF THE SPORTS INJURY

Excluding fractures and psychoses, sports medicine deals with orthopaedic minutiae, primarily soft tissue trauma. It would be fair to say that there is little new to be seen in actual physiotherapy and rehabilitation, and injuries that are dealt with can be seen in most hospitals. The *difference* lies in the fact that we are dealing with professional and amateur athletes.

It has been found that between 5 and 10 per cent of all attendances at accident and emergency departments are the result of injury in sport. It is estimated that 10 per cent of sports injuries result in loss of work time, in addition to loss of training/playing time (Williams, 1979).

Philosophy and motivation

The main difference between the trained and the untrained person is that the trained person demands 100 per cent recovery. For the untrained person a 60 to 80 per cent recovery will be adequate for everyday demands, but these levels will not allow the trained person to follow his selected sport at the level he is aiming for or had achieved. There is, therefore, a similarity to the approach adopted by the armed forces. Combatants are given a graded level of fitness and cannot be returned to active service until the highest levels are reached.

It is essential to look at the *patient* and treat the *individual* rather than the condition. It is important to have a correct diagnosis and not just symptoms. Treating the condition is comparatively easy, for example treatment for a sprain of the lateral ligament of the knee is rest and strapping, but treating the *person* requires an entirely different approach. The background, aims, sport and occupation need to be considered and the treatment approach modified to suit the individual. This is an attitude and approach that should be adopted for all patients, not just for the trained athlete.

The dedicated athlete has an attitude which demands that something be done almost before it happens. There are some dedicated performers who, when they have an injury which warrants they stop their sport, will search for an answer which suits them so that they can carry on.

There are two types of athlete (this term applying to all sports' participants): the one who uses sport to get fit and the one who gets fit for sport. The former is the more casual athlete and perhaps typifies the archetypal 'Britisher' – the amateur-minded approach where taking part is the most important factor. Injuries to this athlete usually result from inco-ordinate actions and failure of technique. The latter person is the more dedicated; he tends to be more selfish or single-minded; he does not like being injured, not because of the pain and discomfort, but because of the inability to follow his chosen sport. It is the dedicated athlete who usually needs, and demands, extensive treatment for overuse injuries.

Sport is a part of all our lives and has a long history of participation, both active and passive, for pleasure, entertainment and reflected glory. It is a pity, therefore, that athletes are so poorly served with essential facilities for the treating of injuries.

The ideal situation in which to look after injured athletes is in a full-time dynamic rehabilitation routine within a controlled environment. Thus professionals do best and prosper, especially American footballers and ballet dancers. The Eastern bloc athletes, though defined as amateurs, bring a professional approach to their sport and have superb sports injury clinic support. There is some doubt about facilities for professional footballers in the UK. Some clubs have splendid facilities and staff for the treatment of injuries, but in the majority physiotherapy cover is left to the unqualified. Perhaps the facilities that exist in some football clubs could be set up in sports centres and staffed accordingly. This would have the merit of allowing for constant observation by staff, and there would be close contact between all members of the rehabilitation team thereby allowing for changes in rehabilitation at any stage of recovery. An alternative solution would be to employ general practitioners, who are interested in sports medicine, as clinical assistants in local hospitals under the guidance of a consultant and assisted by departmental physiotherapists. This could mean an out-of-hours' routine, i.e. clinics very early or late Saturday afternoon or Sunday morning. Yet another solution is to have a physiotherapist actually available in the accident and emergency department at critical times, and then most soft tissue injuries could get more specialised treatment. On this point of specialisation, if and when the medical profession decides to make a specialty of sports medicine then progress will be possible for all concerned, for if physiotherapists fail to involve themselves then the governing bodies of the various sports will set up their own 'masseur' system and another profession will develop.

Staff

Interstaff relationships are very important. Successful treatment and satisfaction depend on team-work, with the doctor, therapist and coach all working for the patient. The doctor plays only a small role in organisation and, as with all team members, personality and an intimate knowledge of sport are as important as qualifications.

Economics

At high performance levels an athlete spends 90 per cent of his allocated sports time in training and 10 per cent in competition. Professional footballers train for 1½–2 hours daily for four days, less on Fridays. However, they may play two to three times a week; then there is no training that day (the match day) and, if there is late-night travelling back from a game, then none the next day. A little more time is devoted to training during late off-season (July). A good amateur 1500 metre runner or cyclist trains and works harder for about 18–30 hours each week. A continental professional cyclist will finish the road season in October, take to six-day track racing for four months, and then start road-race training in February ready for the main season in March. Not all ride six-day racing, some just ride a bicycle for hours each day and start serious training in January.

Tennis players have similar outdoor and indoor seasons. The rewards are high. A lot of top sports people can earn vast sums, while others reap only prize money. Consider what injury will do. A professional footballer worth £1m in a team worth £3–5m has to face enormous problems especially if the team is involved in contesting the league, both domestic cups and European competitions. Injury to such a player will produce enormous pressure on all sides; there is a danger that short cuts will be taken unless firm expert medical advice is given. The motivation of the individual is very high and nothing is gained by injury. In addition, all sports people have short careers and security has to be built up before the age of 30.

For the gifted amateur an injury can ruin a whole season, four years' preparation for the Olympics, or the chance of a place in the team. In addition, consider the amount knocked out of the 10 per cent competition time; basic fitness can be maintained but the skill factor deteriorates and may, in activities such as gymnastics or basketball, take some time to reach a former level.

PSYCHOLOGY OF ATHLETES

It is important to read the specialist books and articles on the subject. Malcolm (1971) and Sanderson (1981) are good starting points and give many other references.

REHABILITATION

The reader is referred to the articles by Williams (1962; 1965), Maddox (1981), Bass (1966), Sperryn (1969) and Corrigan (1968). According to Williams (1962) there are three principles of management:

1. *Recognition*: This means understanding/recognising the causative mechanism. It does not need expertise in all sports, but a basic knowledge of kinesiology and practical anatomy plus the awareness of body movement in injury which will lead to a more accurate assessment.

2. *Prevention*: If the causes of injury are recognised, it is possible to reduce the risk by some form of control. These will include establishing a code of rules and obedience to them; gaining fitness and skill; and by the provision of soft landing areas and protective clothing. Road traffic accidents are said to be caused by an inability to recognise a developing dangerous situation – why not sports injuries?

   For a variety of reasons injury may be caused by protective clothing. The player wearing such apparel may go into a tackle harder; a bulkier body has more momentum and will hit the opponent with greater force thus causing damage. Conversely, bulky clothing/equipment makes for less freedom of movement and inability to move out of danger.

3. *Treatment*: The patient is a person not a condition. The treatment for a torn muscle in a housewife will differ from that for an active younger female athlete. The aim, however, is the same, namely to restore the person to full fitness, competitive or otherwise, as soon as possible. This will include the basic and specific fitness levels and the necessary skills.

Role of the physiotherapist

The role of the physiotherapist is three-fold: professional, educational and managerial, the boundaries of which are not clearly defined and there must be some overlap.

PROFESSIONAL
As a result of their training all physiotherapists are *capable* of treating sports injuries. What is lacking is *experience* in the practical application of their basic knowledge. The best way to further this and

to attain more professional expertise is to become involved in sport and to attend as many post-qualification courses as possible.

The patient is afforded a strong measure of protection because the physiotherapist is bound by the ethical rules laid down by the Council for the Professions Supplementary to Medicine (CPSM) State Registration Board and the Chartered Society of Physiotherapy (CSP). The physiotherapist is given some support by the CSP and by the medical profession.

The syllabus of the CSP together with its approved courses and those of the Association of Chartered Physiotherapists in Sports Medicine ensure the highest professional ability because of their high practical, clinical and theoretical standards. The inherent professional nature of physiotherapists and the care and concern they demonstrate for patients guarantees that the treatment given will be as effective as possible. It also enables them to know their limitations and to decide when to get help.

EDUCATIONAL

Along with the supporting therapeutic team the physiotherapist has a part to play in educating the athlete in the prevention of injury and training for sport, as well as dealing with problems of a domestic and psychological nature.

MANAGERIAL

The athlete, perhaps more so than the untrained person, requires management. Williams (1962) gives guidelines on the fairly strict approach that must be brought to the injured athlete. There are precise instructions to be given at each stage of treatment as to what a person can and cannot do. There are fitness tests and assessments. All of this involves managing the patient rather than just giving treatment.

On a personal note, I think that, in line with the whole-person approach to patients, this is an area to which physiotherapists will have to give more consideration and, consequently, in which they will have to develop greater expertise.

REFERENCES

Bass, A.L. (1966). Rehabilitation after soft tissue injury. *Proceedings of the Royal Society of Medicine*, 653–6.

Corrigan, A.B. (1968). Sports injuries. *Hospital Medicine*, 2, 1328–34.

De Vries, H.A. (1966). *Physiology of Exercise for Physical Education and Athletics*. Staples Press, London.

Fowler, J.A. (1977). Fitness and its components. *Physiotherapy*, 63, 316–19.

Fowler, J.A. (1979). Physiology of exercise and injury. *Physiotherapy in Sport*, III, 1.

Hornor, Z. and Napravnik, C. (1973). Mechanisms, types and treatment of injuries. *British Journal of Sports Medicine*, 1, 45–6.

Maddox, B.T. (1981). *Rehabilitation in Sport*. Chapter in *Sports Fitness and Sports Injuries*, (ed Reilly, T.). Faber and Faber, London.

Malcolm, A.R. (1971). The athlete and his injury. *Physiotherapy*, 8, 352.

Miles, S. (1977). The management of injury. *British Journal of Sports Medicine*, 1, 45–6.

Miles, S. (1981). *A Formula for Health*. Chapter in *Sports Fitness and Sports Injuries*, (ed Reilly, T.). Faber and Faber, London.

Sanderson, F.H. (1981). *Psychology of the Injury Prone Athlete* and *Psychological Implications of Injury*. Chapters in *Sports Fitness and Sports Injuries*, (ed Reilly, T.). Faber and Faber, London.

Sperryn, P.N. (1969). Athletic injuries. *Rheumatology and Physical Medicine*, 11, 246.

Thomas, V. (1977). Fitness within sport. *British Journal of Sports Medicine*, 1, 46–9.

Williams, J.G.P. (1962). Principles of rehabilitation of injured athletes and sportsmen. *Practitioner*, 189, 335–8.

Williams, J.G.P. (1965). *Medical Aspects of Sport and Fitness*. Pergamon Press, Oxford.

Williams, J.G.P. (1971). Classification of sports injuries. *British Journal of Sports Medicine*, 4, 228–9.

Williams, J.G.P. (1979). *Injury in Sport*. Bayer (UK) Ltd, Haywards Heath, England.

Wright, D. (1976). Testing for fitness. *Physiotherapy*, 62, 260–5.

Wright, D. (1981). *Fitness Testing After Injury*. Chapter in *Sports Fitness and Sports Injuries*, (ed Reilly, T.). Faber and Faber, London.

Chapter 27

Advanced Rehabilitation Following Trauma

by S.H. McLAREN, FCSP, Dip Phys Ed

This chapter on rehabilitation concerns therapy of people by people and not by machine. There is obviously a place for treatments from highly sophisticated electro-medical equipment and, possibly, a niche for computerised statistics on patient numbers and types of remedial procedures available, but *not* in this chapter! Here is considered 'person to person' therapy – where the *method of approach* to the injured human being and the *tone of voice* used are of paramount importance in the treatment regime.

In a more leisurely past (the so-called 'good old days') the individual with a problem could find a sympathetic listener and confidant in his home doctor or parish priest but now, sadly, pressure of work (frequently of the 'paper' variety) tends to close the door on this source of 'face to face' communication. The therapist should be able to fill this role in part – *time* should be allowed during the rehabilitation programme for conversation. Often a vital glimpse of the patient's innermost soul may be gained and a reason elicited for his apparent excessive pain or a reluctance to return to his work situation or even to his family.

The previous chapters have dealt with the patients' regime both pre- and postoperatively and the charts on pages 488 to 510 provide an excellent guide to the type of fracture the therapist may be expected to encounter. Also included are the various methods of treatment employed (both surgical and non-surgical) and the length of time required before each case is likely to be ambulant. With all this information to hand and the surgeon's permission to act it's 'all stations go' for the Advanced Rehabilitation stage!

THE END OF THE BEGINNING

Rehabilitation of the patient commences at the moment of accident. For example: A middle-aged man takes his dog for a customary walk along the usual route. Uppermost in his mind is a personal problem with which he is wholly preoccupied so that he crosses a familiar road without due care and attention into the path of an oncoming vehicle.

The first person on the scene should speak the truth to the injured man – 'You have broken your right leg but we will soon have you in St Blogg's Hospital and on the road to recovery. We will contact your wife/mother with the news of your mishap as soon as possible and, don't worry, your little dog is quite safe and is in good hands.' The dazed, frightened victim now knows:

1. *What* has happened to his limb and *why* he is experiencing pain.
2. *Where* he is going and
3. That his dependants are aware of his plight and, by no means least,
4. That his much loved dog is perfectly safe.

With all these immediate problems 'solved' his mind is then more receptive to the re-planning of his temporarily altered life-pattern and, out of recent chaos, organised rehabilitation for his future has begun!

Causes of accidents

Many people have accidents because they are:
(a) physically exhausted
(b) mentally depressed
(c) suffering intense feelings of anger, or
(d) in a temporary state of euphoria.

All these conditions render the human body more prone to traumatic incident. The careless pedestrian, the bored machine operator, the frustrated car driver and the love-sick adolescent are all high on the list of homo sapiens most likely to 'meet with an accident going somewhere to happen'.

Advanced rehabilitation is not just a restoration of the patient to his or her pre-accident state – but to a much healthier, more *vital* life altogether (Fig. 27/1).

'Category' of patient

It is the therapist's job to 'rehabilitate' but the methods and approach may vary with each type of patient.

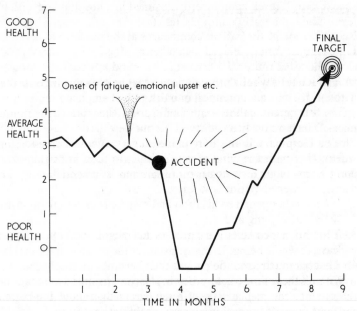

Fig. 27/1 Diagrammatic representation of restoration to a better degree of health following an accident

EXAMPLES

1. The amputee needs extra *time* to make the required psychological adjustment to an altered physical state.
2. The patient who has undergone surgery to arthrodese an ankle or knee joint must master a new technique of propulsion.
3. The patient who has had a joint replacement must also master a new technique of walking.

    Usually these patients have suffered a painful circulatory or arthritic condition for some considerable period of time before the surgical intervention and the type of rehabilitation required would be a continuation of the pre-operative treatment programme with progression as feasible.
4. Pre- and postnatal rehabilitation require a somewhat different technique from the therapist – assuming that the condition in which the patient finds herself is an anticipated event imposed upon her voluntarily!

These example patients have all experienced a doctor's surgery or a hospital department and are acclimatised. Not so the normally healthy victim of a road traffic accident (RTA) who, in a state of surprised shock, finds himself compulsorily detained in a hospital bed with his leg residing in a warm damp plaster cast!

TREATMENT REGIME

'A man is not fully rehabilitated until he is again paying income tax'. There is therefore a great deal of work to be completed by both the victim of trauma *and* the therapist before the former is able to resume a normal, fully active life.

'The dictionary is the only place where success comes before work'. It is therefore vital that the patient understands that *active participation* in his own treatment programme is essential.

Patient involvement

Rehabilitation is one continual process and must involve the complete person as a whole being. In many instances too much emphasis is laid on the injured part and the patient then becomes morosely absorbed by the presence of the fractured limb. It is the therapist's job to restore the patient's confidence in the affected part and *not* allow it to become the focal point of morbid fascination to that patient.

The success or failure of advanced rehabilitation depends almost entirely on the *atmosphere* in which it is conducted:

ENTHUSIASM IS CAUGHT AND NOT TAUGHT!

The ingredients for the making of a good rehabilitationist might well be:
(a) An extrovert personality
(b) A sense of humour
(c) A delight in taking classes of patients for group exercise and
(d) A commanding voice which will carry conviction!

SENSE OF HUMOUR – OR LACK OF IT
Frequently the patient's sense of humour has wilted or even disappeared by the time his plaster cast has dried out and restoration of the ability to laugh at tribulation – *and* at himself – is *vital*. A good therapist will be able to thread humour back into the treatment pattern.

> LAUGHTER IS A GOOD ABDOMINAL EXERCISE
> and
> HE WHO LAUGHS – LASTS!

To advance is to 'encourage the progress of . . .' and, from the outset, the patient should be involved in a forward-thinking regime. This pattern of activity should be designed not only to prime him for his 'bread and butter' work but also to consider his free time expenditure of energy.

SOCIAL NEEDS

The patient may push a pen in an office from 09.00h to 17.00h Monday to Friday but lead an energetic golf-playing, sailing, cycling, footballing, dancing or gardening life in the evenings or at the weekend. Any one of these activities requires a very high standard of stamina, co-ordination and general physical fitness. Into the majority of these extra-mural exertions creeps an element of competition. This is important and can be utilised with success when injected into the patient's treatment programme:

(a) Patient versus therapist.
(b) Patient versus patient in a one-to-one capacity.
(c) Patient versus several other patients in a group situation.

REHABILITATION CENTRES

'A REHABILITATION CENTRE IS FOR A MAN WHO IS RUN DOWN TO GO TO BE WOUND UP'.

Throughout the United Kingdom there are specialised units where traumatic cases are admitted for concentrated treatment. Some centres are for patients requiring 24-hours-a-day, seven days a week attention, e.g. the Spinal Injuries Centre at Stoke Mandeville, Bucks.

A number accommodate both residential and day patients from Monday to Friday, e.g. Hartford Hall, Northumberland and The Hermitage, County Durham.

Many are day centres only, e.g. the Medical Rehabilitation Centre, Camden Road, London NW1 9HL.

In these centres the patient learns to be a 'little fish in a big pond' instead of being the 'only pebble on the beach'. In his own home he may be surrounded by a doting family, waited on hand and foot, until such time as the ambulance transports him two or three times per week to a hospital outpatient department. The conscientious, non-compensationitis fellow will practise his basic home exercises between hospital visits but the awareness of his injured limb is heightened when there is no other traumatised person present. He has no one with whom to share the experience of trauma, nobody similarly afflicted with whom to discuss the subsequent pain or discomfort and the obvious limitation of movement in normal activity. He may well become introspective.

'THE MAN WHO GETS WRAPPED UP IN HIMSELF MAKES A VERY SMALL PARCEL'.

A rehabilitation centre/unit provides a varied daily programme which covers most activities over the period of a full working week.

TREATMENT VARIATIONS

Group exercise classes (a) Competitive
                       (b) Non-competitive.

Individual treatment sessions (as required).

Hydrotherapy A. Passive – aeration baths
              1. One limb
              2. Whole body immersed
            B. Active
              1. Organised group exercise (in treatment pool excluding swimming)
              2. Swimming and diving in standard size swimming pool.

Circuit training   (a) Non-weight-bearing
(Variations)   (b) Weight-bearing
                    (c) For general activity
            or   (d) To work specific area only competing against other members of the group
            or   (e) Working to improve an individual score.

Weight lifting   (a) For correction of lifting techniques *only*
            or   (b) To develop strength and endurance – brick-layers, etc.

Weight and pulley   (a) To encourage joint mobility and/or
work: (b) Increase muscle power.

Functional tests   1. In a specially devised area, e.g. scaffold climbing, rough ground walking and crawling – pushing and pulling (a) 'free' (wheelbarrow loaded or empty), (b) vehicle on rails containing variable weights.
                    2. In a workshop situation (a) woodwork (b) car maintenance.

'Outdoor' work	1. Walks – various
	2. Gardening
	3. Logging
	4. Leaf sweeping, snow clearing, etc.

Games   1. Indoor   ⎫ both in teams, or with a partner
                 2. Outdoor ⎭ and individually against an opponent (see Chapter 28).

The rules for 99 per cent of all games can be adjusted to suit a specific need. The patient with normal intelligence is usually able to adapt his thought processes rapidly and easily to the altered situation and gain added enjoyment from the 'new' approach to an 'old' game.

The rehabilitation centre provides many advantages whether residential or not. The patient may see the medical staff in situ instead of making a tedious journey to a hospital to wait in a frustratingly long queue. He may contact the administration staff concerning sick notes or benefits without travelling to some distant ministerial building there to wait in another long queue, at the end of which is an unfamiliar face.

The unit administrator is available to discuss alternative employment using the patient's existing skills or to arrange re-training for more suitable work developing some latent or new dexterity. All these points assist the patient to regain his equilibrium mentally as well as physically, especially if his injury is likely to render him permanently disabled to some degree. There are at least two sides to everything and conflict between one therapist and another as to the correct approach to rehabilitation is inevitable. Provided the ultimate aim of 'restoring the patient' is achieved, then 'let variety be the spice of life!'

DEBATABLE POINTS

The following 'debatable points' are designed deliberately to provoke controversy. As well as a standard comment, the author's own point of view is expressed and openly invites criticism!

STANDARD COMMENT	AUTHOR'S VIEWPOINT
A1 The same exercises should be repeated at each session so that the patient achieves a high stan-	*A2* Different exercises should be given at each session so that boredom is avoided (for both the

dard of performance in one particular movement before progressing to another.

patient *and* the therapist) and, with a wider range of general activities, a greater variety of joint movement is obtainable.

B1 The patient should have individual gait training to prevent a limp-pattern forming and no attempt should be made to progress to a trot until a limp-free walk is established. This prevents the formation of bad postural habits.

B2 The patient should be encouraged to trot, run and jump, swerve and possibly fall over; laugh, get up off the floor and try again regardless of a limp or any other irregular pattern of movement. By this means he will prove to himself that he is ambulant once more and only *then* should formal correction of gait be introduced into his treatment programme.

C1 The patient's clothing should be reduced to the minimum to allow for freedom of movement and so enable the therapist to observe the precise working of muscles and joints.

C2 The patient should be allowed considerable freedom in the choice of clothing worn during treatment sessions. This prevents embarrassment or other mental discomfort which could inhibit natural movement. Muscle groups contract and relax whether or not they are visible to the therapist!

D1 All exercises and activities in group therapy should be non-competitive thus preventing over-strain of the injured limb. This ensures that the less competent patient never feels inferior to his fellow patients.

D2 A high proportion of exercises and activities in group therapy should be competitive so that the patient exerts himself to the fullest extent as soon as possible. This aim of competition prepares him for a return to the 'outside world' and the inevitable rat race. Learning to laugh at himself when he fails dismally in some minor game or contest will stand him in good stead once he leaves the sheltered hospital environment behind.

E1 When patients are required to work in pairs during a treatment session always ensure that (a) the injuries of each are at the same stage of recovery; (b) the two patients are of the same sex and within the same age group; and (c) that both are of similar build to one another.

E2 Make sure that everyone partners everyone else regardless of injury, sex, age or size. Life in the world outside the hospital walls is not designed to accommodate people in neat pigeon holes! 'The wind blows as hard on the weak as it does on the strong.'

F1 The patient should be treated two or three times each week in a hospital outpatient department. This enables him to continue a normal life at home with his family and friends thus aiding his recovery in a familiar environment. Good training in basic home exercises is sufficient to guarantee development of mobility and muscle power both in the affected limb and in the body generally.

F2 The patient gains most benefit when he is outside his home environment and may learn to become independent more rapidly when he is living and working with others similarly disabled. Very few patients work their muscles and joints to full capacity when performing formal exercises solo at home!

G1 A man's hobby is his own concern and no time should be allotted to this during a treatment session. His ability to perform leisure-time activities will return naturally with time. All effort should be concentrated on the work situation.

G2 The average man works one-third of a 24-hour span in order to play for the second eight-hour period and sleep, to recover from both types of exertion, commandeers the remaining one-third! To promote full rehabilitation, time should be allowed for the patient to discover whether or not his leisure activities – be they boisterous football, peaceful fishing or relatively strenuous gardening – are again possible.

DOS AND DON'TS

The following 'dos' and 'don'ts' are not laws so much as comments. They are designed to stimulate discussion and provoke argument out of which may arise a new approach or a treatment scheme ideal for the particular unit or department.

DOS

1. DO believe in what you are doing!
2. DO keep the final aim in view, i.e. to rehabilitate the patient back to a 24-hours-a-day life.
3. DO remember rehabilitation is a team effort with the patient as the focal point.
4. DO work to restore confidence, stamina and co-ordination; a sense of community living and, above all, a sense of humour.
5. DO use 'contact exercises' wherever possible. So many jobs these days are computerised, mechanised and conveyor-belted and person to person contact is often absent. Advanced rehabilitation can help to restore this deficiency.
6. DO remember that 'the injured man is stronger than the average woman' and female therapists should not underestimate the ability of patients – severely injured or not. So much time is wasted by giving 'feeble' exercises.
7. DO remember full and correct use of the voice is vital if success is to be maximal. **'Enthusiasm and laughter are like the measles – infectious!'**

   Let the patient laugh at *you* so that you are then entitled to laugh at him too. Develop the power of repartee which can be used to great advantage in class work.
8. DO use the patient's name! This is a personal touch and reduces his feeling of being merely a number on a filing card. Introduce yourself to your class whenever a new patient is injected into it.
9. DO offer the patient a challenge and the latent *caveman instinct* will rise to the occasion!

   (a) Let them cheat a little – but catch them at it!

   (b) Let them make a noise whenever it is feasible to do so – a cathedral atmosphere is not conducive to merriment – but make sure there is silence when you wish to give a command or correction.

   (c) Always remember to announce the winners of a race or competition – a little praise goes a long way!

   (d) Devise a 'penalty or prize plan' – a press-up is an excellent exercise in itself and may be utilised as a 'penalty' for anything from being late for class to 'cheating' in a game. Most male patients *delight* in the opportunity to display their prowess in this direction! The therapist also must be prepared to pay the same penalty for a misdemeanour. It is not 'one rule for them and another one for us'. The 'prize' need not be an enormous one. Sometimes a mere reduction in the number of penalty press-ups which may have accrued is sufficient reward! (Some rehabilitation units provide a *Personalised Prize* in the shape of a keyring, a coaster or a bookmark with suitable words inscribed, and the effort expended by the majority of patients in the attempt to win these 'favours' is well worth any initial financial outlay involved. A simple inexpensive item stamped *Super Star of the Year Award* becomes tantamount to the World Cup in value. Try it!)

10. DO 'trick' him into using his injured limb during group therapy. During individual treatments it is more advantageous to allow the patient to demonstrate a movement with his unaffected limb which will then 'teach' the injured limb what is required of it.

11. DO remember to have enough apparatus for everyone in the class to work simultaneously:

(a) This equipment should be basic, inexpensive and easily obtainable for use in the home so that activity can be continued outside the hospital or centre. Many children would delight in the opportunity to 'play' with Daddy or Grandpa when he returns from hospital and teaches the family the exercises and activities he has been doing.

(b) Use a piece of apparatus if it either makes the exercise more interesting (Fig. 27/2) or distracts the patient's attention from the injured area (Fig. 27/3).

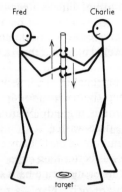

Fig. 27/2 Challenge for patients with painful hands, arms or shoulders. Charlie attempts to pull the pole downwards towards the target while Fred prevents him. The challenge offered to both men is sufficient to overcome a 'normal' pain; at any point either man can concede victory to his opponent by merely 'giving in' to the superior opposition and so prevent overstrain of a joint or muscle group

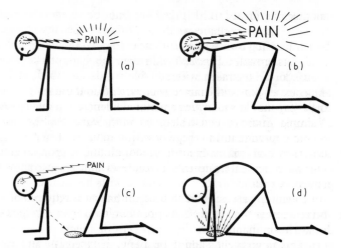

Fig. 27/3 (a) Patient in prone kneeling in preparation for a hip and spine flexion exercise (to mobilise joints following removal of plaster jacket or the equivalent). (b) Increase in awareness of pain on movement of one hip. (c) Add a piece of apparatus, e.g. a rubber quoit or bean bag (*not* a ball). The 'awareness' is now divided between pain and the piece of apparatus. (d) Flexion of same hip pushing the bean bag with knee toward the thumb. *Target*: to propel the bean bag beyond the thumb and double the range of movement is achieved. 'Pain' is now in the bean bag as the thought processes concentrate on knee and thumb regions

12. DO try to keep the number of patients down to a maximum of 12 for class work.

    This allows for: (a) greater use of available space and reduces the risk of collision, etc and (b) with a small number there is a better chance that the individual patient can be seen and praised – or corrected – and the personal level is maintained.

13. DO remember to keep the patient on the move, especially if an outpatient where time is limited. 'Waiting for one's turn' in a game or activity is a time-waster.

14. DO teach lifting techniques as part of any class activity regardless of injury. 'Prevention is better than cure.' Hopefully, the correct lifting of stools, forms or medicine balls will become automatic eventually.

DON'TS

1. DON'T give 'lethal' exercises:

    (a) where one patient is 'fixed' to another and, therefore, unable to free himself when he so wishes.

Examples: (i) arms linked (Fig. 27/4) and
(ii) 'wheelbarrows' (Fig. 27/5)
(b) (i) leapfrog over a partner's back (Fig. 27/6)
(ii) somersaults (Fig. 27/7) and even
(iii) double leg raising (Fig. 27/8)
These are all potential 'hazard exercises'. **Avoid them!**

2. DON'T stop the class following a minor incident, e.g. a grazed knee, a 'jumped' finger or a nose bleed. Send the patient to the nearest first aid department, in company with a volunteer from the same class, and carry on as before. School children, sportsmen and housewives are prone to minor accidents and are used to 'just getting on with it'.

3. DON'T demonstrate an exercise badly or half-heartedly. If you can *do* the exercise – do it well. If not – don't do it at all. Instead, declare your inability to do a press-up or touch your toes, or whatever, to your class and the patients will gleefully attempt to succeed where you have failed.

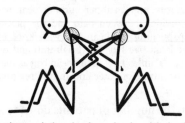

Fig. 27/4 Two patients sitting back to back with both arms linked and pulling in opposite directions. ○ = area likely to be overstrained with *no* chance of escape from an opponent's grip

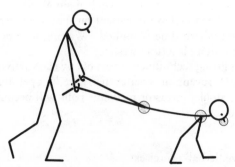

Fig. 27/5 Two patients acting as wheelbarrows. ○ = areas likely to suffer injury if the wheelbarrow 'pusher' is over-enthusiastic

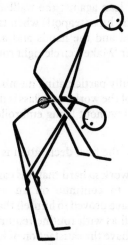

Fig. 27/6 Leap frog. ○ = area which could succumb to forced flexion especially in the patient who is not expecting his partner to 'land' on his back

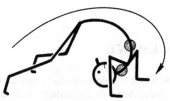

Fig. 27/7 Somersaults. ○ = areas most vulnerable to damage when the weight of the body, travelling at speed, hits the ground

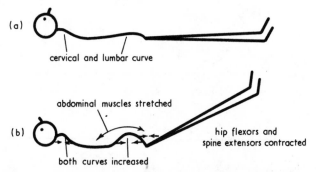

Fig. 27/8 Double leg raising. (a) Body in normal back-lying position; (b) Double leg raising. The patient usually holds his breath, thereby increasing his abdominal pressure to abnormal heights

4. DON'T sit down or lean against the wallbars with arms folded or hands resting on the hips (teapot!) when taking a class. The *voice* gives the command and the hands and arms should be used to emphasise the order 'Make a circle right round the room' or 'Jump up'.

5. DON'T join in as a fully participating member of the group activity. You will see more of the work your class is doing if you are an active spectator, involved without being embroiled.

After all these DON'TS, the final declaration is a DO:

Make your patient work *so* hard that it is easier for him to return to his work than it is to continue on an advanced rehabilitation programme! He will have proved to himself that he is able to cope with the unexpected as well as with routine requirements in his daily life and the therapist will have the satisfaction of knowing that it has been human endeavour and not a machine-wrought treatment that has brought the patient to 'the end of the beginning'.

ACKNOWLEDGEMENT

The author acknowledges the co-operation, inspiration and toil of all the patients, staff and students at The Hermitage; without it this chapter would not have been written.

Chapter 28

'Maxercises'

by S.H. McLAREN, FCSP, Dip Phys Ed
Illustrated by M. RUTTER, BA, Dip Visual Communication

A **Maxercise**=maximum physical and mental exercise combined with an element of fun in a competitive atmosphere within the group. A Maxercise is not a formal exercise, nor is it purely a game. Patients are placed in a one-to-one situation working either against an opponent or together with a partner versus other competing pairs within the group.

These particular Maxercises each utilise one or two pieces of basic apparatus:

a pole
a pole and a quoit
a strong blanket
a plastic football or
a large medicine ball

After many years of experimentation at The Hermitage Rehabilitation Centre the idea of using the same equipment for a 30–40-minute group treatment session has been found to be more advantageous than exchanging one piece of apparatus for another at the end of each exercise. A different piece of equipment may be used the following day (see A2, p. 570). The introductory cartoon figures (Fig. 28/1) – burly, affable Alf and thin, aesthetic, humourless Ernest – typify two patients one at each end of the 'brawn v. brain' range. Variety in the choice of Maxercises should ensure that both Alf and Ernest each win one or more events so that the honours are equally divided. Success and achievement count for a great deal in total rehabilitation.

The key to the amount of difficulty each Maxercise offers is shown in the facial expression (Fig. 28/2). A *smile* indicates the easier situation, e.g. where Alf is sitting passively on the blanket waiting to be pulled across the floor by the lighter weight Ernest who is

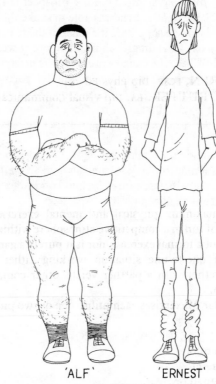

'ALF'　　　'ERNEST'

Fig. 28/1

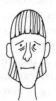

Fig. 28/2

(understandably) *frowning* at the daunting prospect (Fig. 28/19, p. 599). In Figure 28/17 (p. 595) Ernest is able to shake the quoits over Alf's wrists more easily because he is the taller of the two men and has the advantage that extra height gives him, therefore *he* wears the *smile* and Alf the *frown*. Where the facial expressions are *neutral* the effort is shared equally between Alf and Ernest who are partners and not opponents in this instance (Fig. 28/29, p. 617). The amount of co-ordination and physical stamina required to bounce and catch a ball from the surface of a second ball is no greater for one than for the other.

You have now made the acquaintance of Alf and Ernest: let them introduce you to some simple Maxercises which are suitable for the rehabilitation of many different injuries and conditions in male and female patients from teenage upwards.

GROUP 1 MAXERCISES USING POLES

APPARATUS REQUIRED

Industrial weight broom-shanks 30–36-inch long. These are reasonable in price and will last for many years if linseed oil is applied liberally some days before the initial use. A full length new shank makes two adequate pieces of equipment for this type of activity.

SPACE REQUIRED

Sufficient to prevent accidents when moving poles are involved, particularly at head level (Fig. 28/17, p. 595). Preferably an area large enough to move at least 3 metres from one side of the room to the other.

FLOOR SURFACE

For exercises shown in Figures 28/12–16 inclusive there should be no carp.ts or rugs and the floor should be scratchproof. A good polyurethane-type coating is sufficient to prevent permanent marking when the poles are used in direct contact with the floor surface.

Maxercise No. 1 (Figs. 28/3, 28/4, 28/5, 28/6)

Type:	Competitive – against one opponent.
Use:	General strengthening with emphasis on upper limbs.
Apparatus required:	1 pole per person.
Space required:	Minimal.

AIMS

Alf

To maintain the poles in the starting position.

Ernest

To pull one or both poles downwards until the ends touch the floor.

TEACHING POINTS

1. Check that Alf and Ernest are holding the poles correctly – Alf near the top and Ernest at the bottom.
2. Give a clear command to Ernest 'Ready-Pull!' – slowly and steadily without jerking towards the floor. Alf stands still. If Ernest reaches floor level with the pole ends he is the winner.
3. Give a clear, decisive 'stop' after 15–20 seconds – resting briefly before Ernest holds the poles at the top and Alf pulls downwards.
4. Congratulate the winner by *name* – for all to hear. (See Chapter 27, p. 573, 9c.)
5. Remember to change partners frequently (see E2, p. 572). Figure 28/7 shows quick methods of partner changing.

This Maxercise may be performed in a variety of starting positions. Some examples are shown in Figures 28/4, 28/5 and 28/6.

If both partners are non- or partial weight-bearing or wheelchair bound this Maxercise may be performed in long sitting on the floor or sitting on a chair. Remember to apply the brakes firmly if the patient is in a wheelchair. The advantage is nearly always with the partner who is keeping the poles stationary. The flexor muscles are much more powerful than the extensors in the region of the shoulder girdle. The exception will be Alf who will probably unfurl Ernest without undue strain!

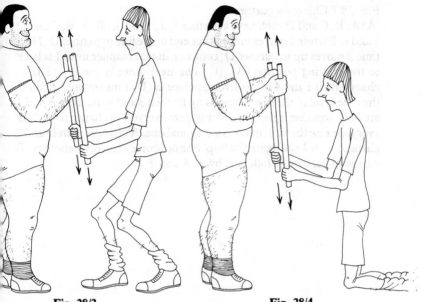

Fig. 28/3   Fig. 28/4

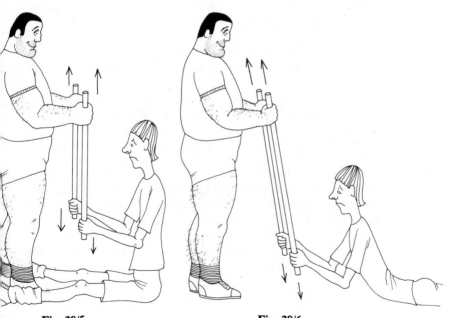

Fig. 28/5   Fig. 28/6

Fig. 28/7 Changing partners

(A) A, B, C and D each have a partner 1, 2, 3 and 4. (B) A, B, C and D stand still while 1 moves to the other end of the line to partner D. Next time 2 moves up to partner D; continue in that manner until 1 is back to the starting position (A). (C) The next move is for B and D to change with 2 and 4 respectively, before in (D) 1 moves once again to the other end of the line followed by B; then 3 and so on until A and 1 are back together again. In order to give everyone a chance to partner everyone else the final move is a diagonal one. A changes with D and 2 changes with 1 and again the 'top' line of people remains stationary. B moves to partner 4, followed by 3, A and 2

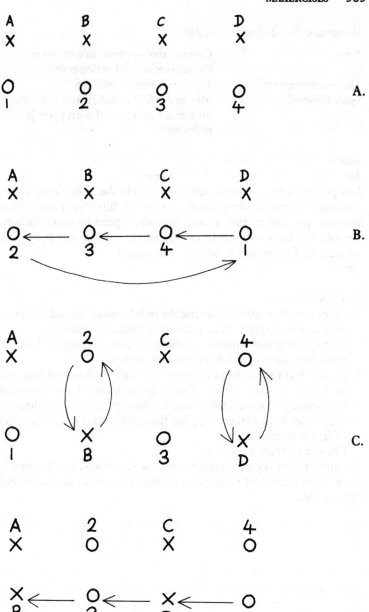

Fig. 28/7

Maxercise No. 2 (Figs. 28/8, 28/9)

Type:	Competitive – against one opponent.
Use:	Co-ordination and reflex training.
Apparatus required:	1 pole per pair of patients.
Space required:	Minimal. (If Alf and Ernest both stand on a mat the sound of a dropped pole is reduced.)

AIMS

Alf

To open his arms unobtrusively allowing the pole to drop from between his finger tips down towards the floor without prior warning to Ernest of his intention.

Ernest

To catch the pole from above before it hits the floor which requires speed of action in conjunction with a good eye for movement.

TEACHING POINTS

1. Make sure that Alf is balancing the pole between his index fingers only and is staring Ernest in the eyes before he drops it.
2. Check that Ernest's hands are above the pole and that he does not turn them palm upwards in order to catch it.
3. Ensure that Ernest drops the pole next time regardless of winning or losing on Alf's drop. This way each will have an equal opportunity to score. Allow time for both partners to try three or four times each before stopping the activity and enquiring who caught how many.
4. Change partners as before.

Variation: Other apparatus (rubber quoits, bean bags) may be used in place of the heavy and noisy poles especially by teams of chairbound participants.

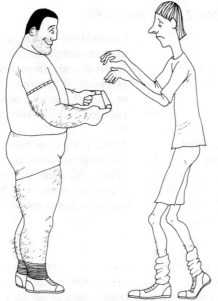

Fig. 28/8

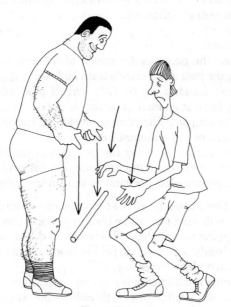

Fig. 28/9

Maxercise No. 3 (Figs. 28/10, 28/11)

Type:	Competitive – working with a partner against other pairs in the group.
Use:	General body movement at speed: (a) elevation of shoulder girdle; (b) knee and spine flexion; and (c) training in running and fast turning (if space permits).
Apparatus required:	1 pole per pair of patients.
Space required:	Minimal if standing still. (If space allows, Alf runs across the room to the stationary Ernest and back to the starting point between each pole action.)

AIMS

Alf

To grip the pole tightly at each end and pass it over Ernest's head, down behind his knees and under his feet three times as quickly as possible without leaving go of the pole at either end.

Ernest

To step over the pole at the appropriate moment without endangering Alf's front teeth with an over-enthusiastic knee and hip flexion movement.

TEACHING POINTS

1. Emphasise the necessity for *control* of movement to Alf's team wielding the pole and Ernest's team high-stepping to avoid it.
2. Watch out for cheating by Alf's line of pole-holders who will probably learn at an early stage that taking one hand off the pole makes life simpler! The press-up makes an excellent penalty – if not a deterrent – to dishonest folk!
3. Alter the race by reversing the direction of the movement, i.e. starting at Ernest's feet and finishing over his head.
4. Note and congratulate the winners and change partners as before.

Variations: This Maxercise allows for umpteen variations on the same theme. The following may all be used to perform this activity:

    (i) a skipping rope folded in half or, indeed, several times.

    (ii) team bands; a metre of carpet binding stitched to form a circle.

    (iii) a twisted blanket (see Fig. 28/24a, p. 607)

With these pliable materials it is possible to alter the starting positions so that Alf is kneeling while threading the skipping rope (or equivalent) over the head (or feet) of a *sitting* or *back lying* Ernest.

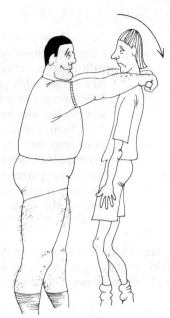

Fig. 28/10

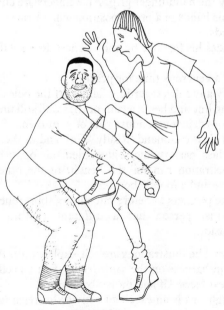

Fig. 28/11

Maxercise No. 4 (Figs. 28/12, 28/13, 28/14)

Type:	'Ski-ing' with variations – working with a partner – (non-competitively to begin with and then, when skilled enough, as a race against other pairs).
Use:	Development of balance, co-ordination and rhythm with essential physical support from partner. Very strong arm work required by Ernest while Alf develops his ankle muscles.
Apparatus required:	2 poles per partnership.
Space required:	Large clear area to move across from one side to the other while balancing on 'skis'.

AIMS

To re-establish a sense of 'team-work' – through physical contact. It requires considerable confidence in one's own muscle power (if you are Ernest's weight!) to maintain Alf's bulk upright on a pair of cylindrical poles!

TEACHING POINTS

1. Clarify the hand/finger grip. Alf's fingers are curled over Ernest's with his hands in a prone position while Ernest's palms are facing upwards.
2. Alf slides his feet one by one – Ernest does *not* tow him across the floor.
3. Allow a generous time for practice.
4. Specify any rules regarding falling off the poles, e.g. (a) return to starting line and begin again, or (b) stand still until re-mounted on poles or (c) invent a house rule of your own.
5. Give a clear command 'Ready – Go!' and, if the winners achieve a first class performance, give them an opportunity to make a demonstration run for the benefit of the others. This is extra exercise and a morale booster!
6. Change partners as before but allow a short rehearsal time as each individual person has a different rhythm and method of propulsion.

Variations: The illustrations are self-explanatory. Alf and Ernest are working in harness on the same 'skis' – first travelling forwards and then Ernest faces Alf and moves backwards.

Although this is an excellent activity for regaining control of foot and ankle movements for rough ground work and scaffold climbing, it is often too painful for a bare foot to tolerate. Do *not* insist on the removal of shoes.

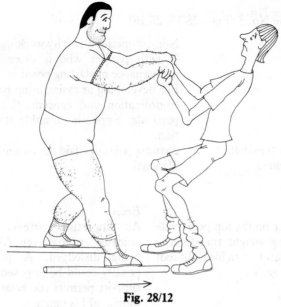

Fig. 28/12

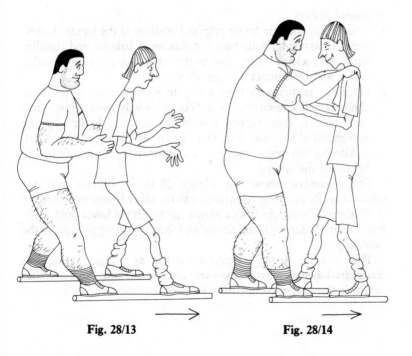

Fig. 28/13   **Fig. 28/14**

Maxercise No. 5 (Figs. 28/15, 28/16)

Type:	Non-competitive activity working closely with partner who is essential for maintenance of starting position.
Use:	For developing or maintaining balance, co-ordination and concentration with particular emphasis on ankle stabilisation.
Apparatus required:	2 strong poles one laid across the other.
Space required:	Minimal.

AIMS

Alf

To balance on the top pole while performing weight transference from his left foot to his right foot and back again.

Ernest

As supporting partner, works twice as hard to prevent Alf from being dislodged. A press-up penalty could be imposed if the support permits the balancer to topple off his perch.

TEACHING POINTS

1. Once again note the finger grip and position of the hands. Ernest needs to assume a wide base for maximum balance and stability while Alf rocks from one foot to the other tilting the pole until it makes audible contact with the floor.
2. Once the participants have learnt to rock adequately let them choose a well-known tune – e.g. 'For he's a jolly good fellow' – and each note is then tapped out in the correct rhythm by the movement of alternate feet. Once again the champion 'musician' and his partner might enjoy giving a command performance for the benefit of the others!

The Maxercise shown in Figure 28/16 is difficult but not impossible. By lungeing from one leg to the other Ernest assists Alf to 'roll' himself from side to side across the revolving lower pole. Alf's feet remain stationary while Ernest and the supporting pole act as the moving parts.

This is *not* a suitable exercise for use as a race. It requires concentration and control to be a safe activity and both these qualities vanish in the face of competition at speed!

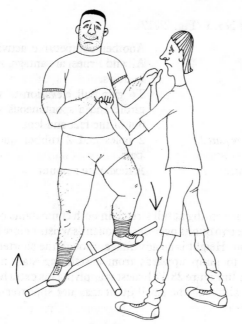

Fig. 28/15

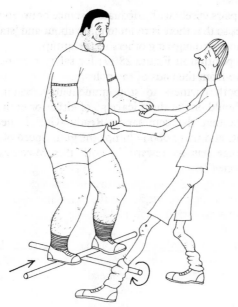

Fig. 28/16

Maxercise No. 6 (Fig. 28/17)

Type:	Another competitive activity in which Alf and Ernest are antagonists instead of buddies.
Use:	To gain full elevation of the shoulder girdle and a spontaneous spring action out of the feet and legs.
Apparatus required:	2 poles and 2 rubber quoits for each pair.
Space required:	A moderate amount.

AIMS

To encourage spring at full stretch in both combatants by attempting to hook the two quoits over the opponent's wrists before he can do the same to you. Height is an advantage, though the shorter person with an ability to jump upwards from a standing start may often be successful. In Figure 28/17 Ernest is applying his extra height to good advantage although the small quoit may not slip over Alf's chunky fists too easily!

TEACHING POINTS

1. Space the pairs wisely with adequate distance between neighbouring couples so that there is room to jump about and 'stab' with the poles without endangering others in the group.
2. Note grip position in Figure 28/17: for safety reasons the hands never move from the ends of the poles.
3. Remind both partners to stop immediately, again for safety reasons, should one of them leave go of either or both poles.
4. Make sure that the command – 'Ready – Go!' is heard by all participants and that nobody jumps the gun. Speed of reaction to the challenge has its reward in both this Maxercise and the following one (7).

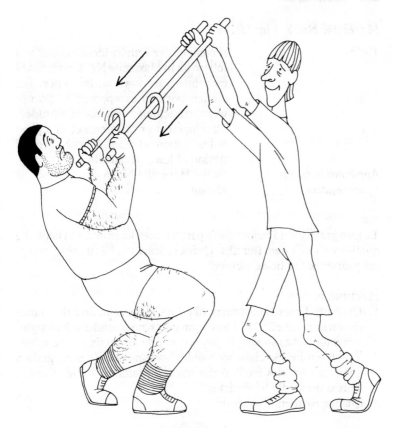

Fig. 28/17

Maxercise No. 7 (Fig. 28/18)

Type: A competitive activity ideally suited as a follow-on to Maxercise No. 6 as the body movements are downwards in a flexed or crouch position as opposed to an upward, stretching-in-extension attitude.

Use: Development or maintenance of a good reflex action combined with general flexion of knees and ankles.

Apparatus required: As for Maxercise No. 6.

Space required: Minimal.

AIM

To gain gravity's aid before one's partner does so, in order to hook the quoits over one's own thumbs. Quick reflexes (and a cunning streak) are guaranteed to bring victory!

TEACHING POINTS

1. Dissuade Ernest and others like him from assuming the stance shown in Figure 28/18. The command 'Knees bend-Back straight' was intended as an *upright* position to prevent strain on the spine!
2. Watch out for the cheat who slides his hand along a pole, grabs a quoit and scuttles back to the starting position with his trophy. This is decidedly 'not cricket'!
3. Change partners frequently.

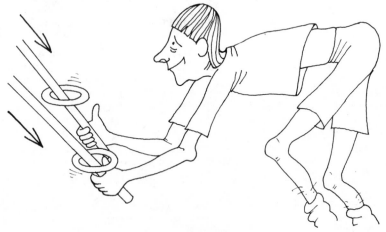

Fig. 28/18

GROUP 2 MAXERCISES USING BLANKETS

APPARATUS REQUIRED
Blankets. Army-type grey blankets – single-bed size – are designed to withstand stress and strain and are virtually indestructible. Even the voracious moth appears to avoid them. Any energy expended in obtaining such blankets is amply rewarded by the amount of useful life they provide.

SPACE REQUIRED
A large hazard-free area such as a gymnasium or an assembly hall. Plenty of ventilation is advisable as fluff and dust can accumulate and cause distress to people with chest problems.

For safety reasons the number of participants in this Maxercise should *not* exceed 12 regardless of floor space available.

FLOOR SURFACE
As for the pole Maxercises, i.e. a smooth, ideally wooden, floor with a good quality polyurethane coating. No carpets or rugs.

Maxercise No. 8 (Fig. 28/19)

Type: Competitive – working in conjunction with a partner not against him.

Use: To provide strong back extension work and powerful finger-grip action for people returning to heavy labouring jobs.

Apparatus required: 1 strong blanket per partnership.

Space required: A large area.

AIM

Alf

To remain balanced at the end of the blanket without holding on with hands or feet.

Ernest

To tow Alf's passive weight smoothly across the room until he can touch the wall – at which point the roles are reversed and Alf pulls Ernest back to the starting point.

TEACHING POINTS

1. *It is essential that a trial run in slow motion precedes this competition at speed.* Ernest must be reminded throughout the activity to lean forwards. Should he tilt backwards and suddenly lose his grip or should Alf roll off the end of the blanket then Ernest is liable to fall heavily.

2. On the return journey when Alf is towing Ernest's negligible weight emphasise that *control* is the keyword. If Ernest rolls off because Alf is careless and jerks the blanket thoughtlessly then the press-up penalty comes into its own.

Variation: Instead of remaining passive, the passenger can sit holding on with hands and feet and a greater yet safe towing speed can be achieved.

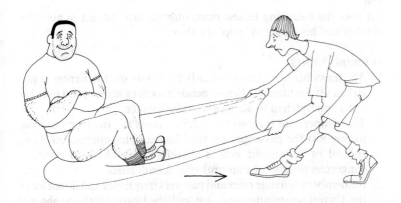

Fig. 28/19

Maxercise No. 9 (Fig. 28/20)

Type:	Co-operating partners in a competitive situation.
Use:	For strengthening of shoulder girdle muscles, hip abductors and evertors of feet.
Apparatus required:	1 blanket.
Space required:	As for Maxercise No. 8.

AIM

Alf tows the balancing Ernest using only his crossed feet to hold the blanket and his hands to 'grip' the floor.

TEACHING POINTS

1. Alf draws his feet slowly towards his hands so that Ernest is not jerked off the blanket. Ernest bends his knees slightly and uses his arms outstretched to act as a counter-balance.
2. The winners are the two who arrive across the floor first *without* having lost the passenger off the blanket. This encourages more control of movement and is therefore less likely to create a dangerous situation by an unthinking enthusiast.
3. Remember to change roles and partners frequently and do *not* leave the Maxercise asymmetrical, e.g. pull the blanket with the *opposite* foot on top during the second run.

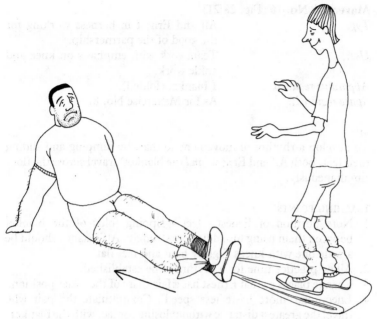

Fig. 28/20

Maxercise No. 10 (Fig. 28/21)

Type:	Alf and Ernest in harness working for the good of the partnership.
Use:	Teamwork with emphasis on knee and ankle work.
Apparatus required:	1 blanket (folded).
Space required:	As for Maxercise No. 8.

AIM

To develop a rhythm of movement so that, by jumping and sliding their feet, both Alf and Ernest (*and* the blanket) travel across the floor simultaneously.

TEACHING POINTS

1. Note position of Ernest's feet – gripping folds of the blanket between them using his adductors strongly. Alf's stance should be a wide one with knees slightly bent and feet flat.
2. Allow practice time for a rhythm to be established.
3. Change places so that Ernest has a fair share of the easier position.
4. Encourage 'more haste less speed'. Congratulate the pair who travel the greatest distance without losing contact with the blanket.

Variation: This is an energetic 'fun' activity if attempted in lines of four each holding on to the body in front. The leader grips the blanket with his feet and the back marker calls 'mush, mush'. The team moves forward as one unit on each 'mush'. Practice time is essential! It is very difficult to stay on the front end of the blanket when three stalwarts are pushing with enthusiasm from behind! The winning team is the one which arrives intact.

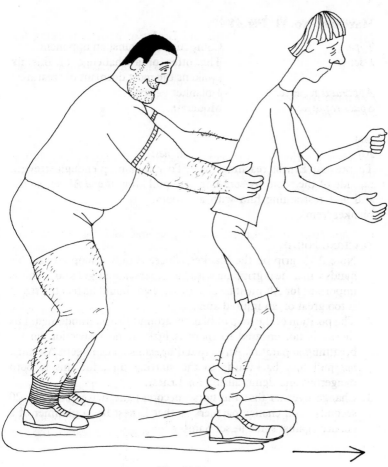

Fig. 28/21

Maxercise No. 11 (Fig. 28/22)

Type:	Competitive – against an opponent.
Use:	The offer of a challenge of this ilk awakens the most dormant of creatures!
Apparatus required:	1 blanket per pair.
Space required:	Moderate.

AIM

Alf	*Ernest*
To prevent Ernest reaching the far side of the room by standing still and restraining him with a blanket 'rein'.	To summon up enough strength to pull himself *and* Alf across the room.

TEACHING POINTS

1. Note Alf's grip on the blanket. There is only a loop around his hands which he is gripping with his fingers, *not* a rigid knot. This is important for Alf must be able to leave go should he feel the strain is too great on an injured area.
2. The position of the loop of blanket around Ernest's abdomen. His thorax is not encased so there is little or no restriction on his breathing apparatus. Any ground he gains he can keep: Alf must *not* pull him backwards to the starting line, for this is both dangerous and demoralising for Ernest.
3. Change over so that the horse becomes the driver after 15–20 seconds – and change partners so that Ernest has a glimmer of a chance against some lesser Samson.

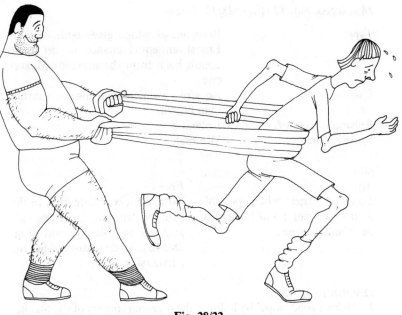

Fig. 28/22

Maxercise No. 12 (Figs. 28/23, 28/24)

Type:	Brain teaser which gives both Alf and Ernest an equal chance to get their breath back from the previous Maxercise.
Use:	An activity which develops brain rather than brawn.
Apparatus required:	1 blanket.
Space required:	Minimal.

AIM

Alf

To assist Ernest where possible without leaving go of his end of the blanket 'rope'.

Ernest

To make a complete knot in the blanket without loosening his grip on the blanket end (Fig. 28/24B). To do so disqualifies the partnership.

TEACHING POINTS

1. Make a good 'rope' by holding the diagonal corners of the blanket and swirling it round (Fig. 28/24A).
2. Insist that the fingers are entwined in a 'wasps' nest' position (Fig. 28/24A).
3. Allow 'thinking' time.

This Maxercise does not make a good race as it encourages cheating from the not-so-bright participants who find it impossible to reason along scientific lines! Ernest should shine brightly in this activity.

Variations: (i) Alf makes the first knot while the blanket 'rope' is at its longest. Ernest being the thinner of the partners ties the second knot on top of the first. It is not impossible to tie three knots in some blankets.

(ii) Untie knots with feet only – either standing up or sitting down. The winners are the two who have all their knots untied without being tempted to use their hands or teeth.

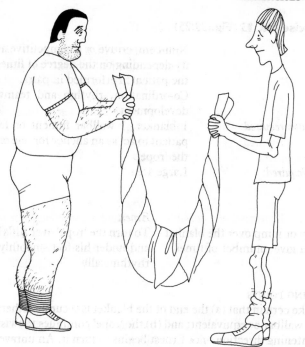

Fig. 28/23

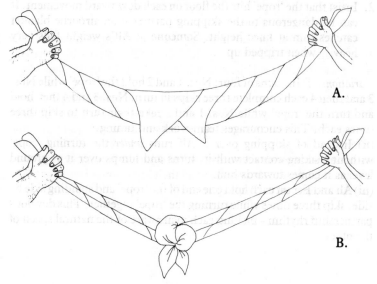

Fig. 28/24

Maxercise No. 13 (Fig. 28/25)

Type:	Non-competitive *or* a competitive activity depending on the degree of fitness of the patient. Performed in pairs.
Use:	Co-ordination, rhythm and teamwork development.
Apparatus required:	1 blanket, 1 wallbar fitment or fellow patient to act as an anchor for one end of the 'rope'.
Space required:	Large area.

AIM

Alf	*Ernest*
To step or jump over the blanket 'rope' a given number of times.	To turn the 'rope' over Alf's head and under his feet smoothly and rhythmically.

TEACHING POINTS

1. Make certain that (a) the end of the blanket is securely tethered to the wallbar or equivalent; and (b) the 'rope' continues to twist in a tightening direction once Ernest begins to turn it. An unravelling blanket can become a hazard.
2. Insist that the 'rope' hits the floor on each downward movement. It can be dangerous to the skipping partner if an airborne blanket catches him at knee height. Someone of Alf's weight falls very heavily when tripped up.

Variations: (i) In teams of four: Nos. 1 and 2 hold the 'rope' while Nos. 3 and then 4 each complete three skips in turn. Nos. 3 and 4 then hold and turn the 'rope' while Nos. 1 and 2 take their turn to skip three times each. This encourages team-work and timing.

(ii) Instead of skipping over it Alf runs *under* the turning 'rope' without making contact with it, turns and jumps over it at ground level as it comes towards him.

(iii) Alf and Ernest each hold one end of the 'rope' and standing side by side, skip three times while turning the 'rope' together. This develops partnership rhythm – making each man aware of the natural speed of the other.

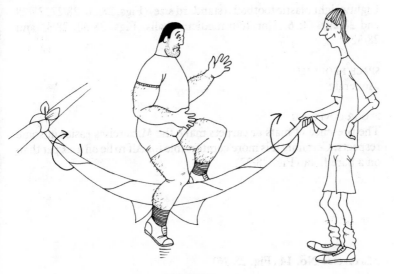

Fig. 28/25

GROUP 3 MAXERCISES USING BALLS

APPARATUS REQUIRED
Lightweight plastic footballs (standard size) (Figs. 28/26, 28/27, 28/28 and 28/29). Or 6, 7 or 10lb medicine balls (Figs. 28/30, 28/31 and 28/32).

SPACE REQUIRED
Moderate.

FLOOR COVERING
The presence of mats or carpets make the Maxercises easier in some respects. Certainly it is more comfortable for Alf to lie on a carpet than on a bare floor (Fig. 28/27).

Maxercise No. 14 (Fig. 28/26)

Type:	Competitive against partner.
Use:	To test the ability of the patient to withstand jarring actions.
Apparatus required:	1 plastic football each.
Space required:	Moderate in size, and without hanging light fitments and uncovered windows!

AIM

Alf	*Ernest*
To knock Ernest's ball down-wards in order to make Ernest drop his ball without letting go of his own ball.	To grip the ball tightly so that Alf cannot dislodge it with his ball.

TEACHING POINTS
1. Note position of Alf's hands which are slightly curved over the top surface of his ball while Ernest cradles the ball from underneath.
2. The feet remain more or less stationary while Alf taps Ernest's ball lightly several times before increasing the amount of power behind the blows. Should Alf lose his grip while hitting Ernest's ball, Ernest becomes the winner through default.

3. Noses, front teeth and spectacles may all be in danger if this Maxercise is not taught correctly. Do *not* allow hitting from below the ball unless each participant is fully aware of the danger of behaving in an uncontrolled manner.

4. Change the ball over as well as the partners. A football with less air in it is easier to hold between the palms and so becomes an unfair advantage if not circulated round the group!

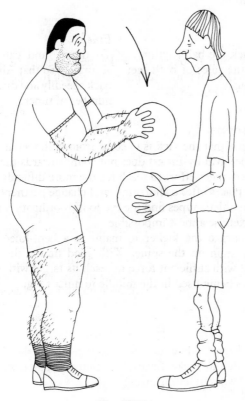

Fig. 28/26

Maxercise No. 15 (Fig. 28/27)

Type:	Competitive – working in conjunction with a partner.
Use:	Development of co-ordination in eye, hand and foot.
Apparatus required:	1 plastic football per pair.
Space required:	Moderate.

AIM

Alf

To kick back the ball rhythmically using the soles of both feet simultaneously.

Ernest

To throw (and catch) the ball accurately so that Alf can kick it back speedily and directly a given number of times.

TEACHING POINTS

1. Emphasise that the kick is to come from both feet at once.
2. A dropped ball by Ernest does not count towards the final score. This encourages effort to reach for the more difficult catch.
3. Change places after a short time and change partners frequently. Some unathletic types find the eye/foot co-ordination required for this Maxercise almost impossible.
4. Do encourage the kicker to maintain a bent-knee position to prevent strain on the spine. With good timing the ball can be returned with sufficient force to reach its target without the knee extensors being used in the middle to inner range.

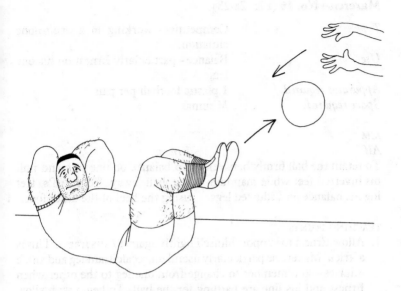

Fig. 28/27

Maxercise No. 16 (Fig. 28/28)

Type:	Competitive – working in a one-to-one situation.
Use:	Balance – particularly Ernest on his one leg.
Apparatus required:	1 plastic football per pair.
Space required:	Minimal.

AIM

Alf	*Ernest*
To retain the ball firmly between his inverted feet while maintaining his balance on adducted legs.	To balance on one foot and pull the ball away from Alf's feet using the heel of the other foot.

TEACHING POINTS

1. Allow Ernest to support himself lightly against Alf's frame. This is a 'trick' Maxercise particularly useful for recalcitrant leg and ankle injuries – so remember to change from one leg to the other when Ernest and his line are battling for the ball. To begin with allow Ernest to choose which leg he wishes to use to pull the ball away from Alf's feet. The second one works doubly hard to support his weight while he is concentrating his effort on the 'active' limb! Use the other leg on the second attempt to win the ball.
2. Coach Alf by suggesting he should bend his knees and turn his toes inwards after Ernest's leg has passed through the space above the ball.
3. Instruct Ernest to 'pull' rather than 'kick' the ball out – this is less traumatic for the stationary Alf!
4. Change over after 15–20 seconds so that Ernest has a chance to grip and keep the ball.
5. Change partners to give those with less weight behind them a chance to succeed!

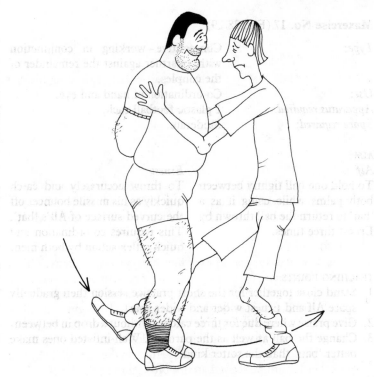

Fig. 28/28

Maxercise No. 17 (Fig. 28/29)

Type:	Competitive – working in conjunction with a partner against the remainder of the couples.
Use:	Co-ordination of hand and eye.
Apparatus required:	1 plastic football each.
Space required:	Moderate.

AIM

Alf

To hold one ball tightly between both palms while using it as a 'bat' to return the ball thrown by Ernest three times.

Ernest

To throw accurately and catch quickly as his missile bounces off the curved surface of Alf's 'bat'. This requires co-ordination and quick reflex action by both men.

TEACHING POINTS

1. Stand close together for the short practice session then gradually space Alf and Ernest wider and wider apart.
2. Give praise where due for three catches without a drop in between.
3. Change the ball as well as the partners. Well-inflated ones make better 'bats' than the softer kind.

Variations: Only possible on hard surface without carpets.
(i) Ernest *bounces* the ball diagonally down to the floor towards Alf who sends back a catch from his 'bat'.
(ii) Ernest *throws* the ball and Alf *bounces* it back.
(iii) Ernest *bounces* the ball to Alf who *bounces* it back off the 'bat'.
(iv) Alf throws the ball high into the air and 2 seconds later Ernest attempts to knock it out of the sky by throwing his ball as if it were a missile. This is *not* suitable for highly excitable people in a room with unprotected windows on all sides or hung with chandeliers. Be sensible in the use of it as a Maxercise.

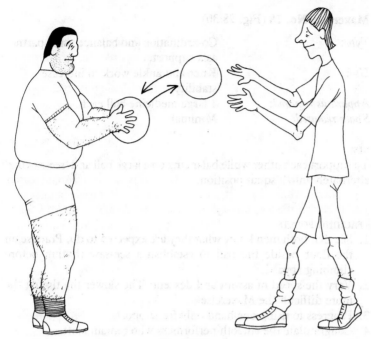

Fig. 28/29

Maxercise No. 18 (Fig. 28/30)

Type:	Co-ordination and balance using partner as a support.
Use:	Knee and ankle work to increase stability.
Apparatus required:	1 large medicine ball each.
Space required:	Minimal.

AIM

To support each other while balancing on a large ball and 'see-sawing' alternately into a squat position.

TEACHING POINTS

1. See that both men know what they are expected to do. Practise on the floor beside the ball to establish a see-saw rhythm before climbing aboard.
2. Vary the speed of ascent and descent. The slower the timing the more difficult the Maxercise.
3. Progress to using one hand only for support.
4. Congratulate the smooth performers who remain aloft.

Variations: (Figs. 28/31, 28/32)
(i) Ernest remains on the ball and, helped by Alf, rolls it under his feet alternately so that he (and it) move forwards slowly and steadily.
(ii) Both Alf and Ernest are mounted on medicine balls and, working as a team, propel themselves across the room without falling off. The speed of progress depends on the skill of the one travelling backwards – he has the most difficult task. Reverse direction after a short period so that each partner experiences the sensation.

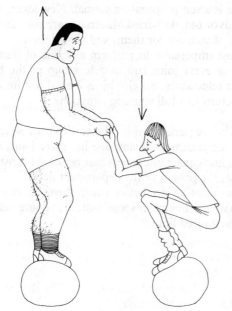

Fig. 28/30

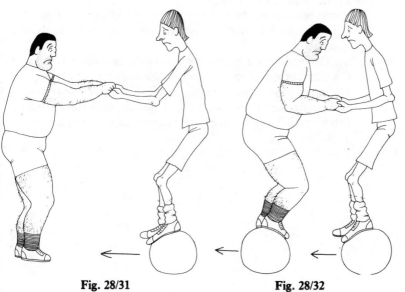

Fig. 28/31   **Fig. 28/32**

A Maxercise is a self-propagating animal. New ideas, developments and variations on old, well-tried Maxercises are born during advanced group work. Watch out for them, and record them.

It is almost impossible to perform any one of these Maxercises without using every joint and muscle group in the body at some stage – albeit reluctantly. Surely this is a good test for a patient who intends to return to a full working situation?

Therapists who are purists dislike Maxercises because (a) they are not specific for the treatment of any one injury or joint; and (b) when taught in an inadequate or careless manner could constitute a risk to the therapist, the patient or the department décor.
Patients who want to get better enjoy them because they offer a challenge to which they can respond and, in so doing, tend to forget or disregard the injured limb.

Select Bibliography

The following selection of books and papers is a random choice from a vast literature. The interested reader is advised to use the *Index Medicus* to locate relevant papers and to consult the various library classifications to identify books.

BOOKS

Brooks, H.L. (ed) (1982). *Scoliosis and Allied Deformities of the Spine*. John Wright and Sons Limited, Bristol.

Browne, P.S.H. (1981). *Basic Facts in Orthopaedics*. Blackwell Scientific Publications Limited, Oxford.

Browne, P.S.H. (1982). *Basic Facts of Fractures*. Blackwell Scientific Publications Limited, Oxford.

Currey, H.L.F. (ed) (1980). *Mason and Currey's Clinical Rheumatology*, 3rd edition. Pitman Books Limited, London.

Currey, H.L.F. (1983). *Essentials of Rheumatology*. Pitman Books Limited, London.

Downie, P.A. and Kennedy, P. (1980). *Lifting, Handling and Helping Patients*. Faber and Faber, London.

Duckworth, T. (1980). *Lecture Notes on Orthopaedics and Fractures*. Blackwell Scientific Publications Limited, Oxford.

Duthie, R.B. and Bentley, G. (eds) (1983). *Mercer's Orthopaedic Surgery*, 8th edition. Edward Arnold (Publishers) Limited, London.

Dyson, G.H.G. (1977). *The Mechanics of Athletics*, 7th edition. Hodder and Stoughton, London.

Edmonds, J.P. and Hughes, G.R.V. (1982). *Lecture Notes on Rheumatology*. Blackwell Scientific Publications, London.

Golding, D.N. (1979). *Concise Management of the Common Rheumatic Disorders*. John Wright and Sons Limited, Bristol.

Golding, D.N. (1981). *Tutorials in Clinical Rheumatology*. Pitman Books Limited, London.

Golding, D.N. (1982). *A Synopsis of Rheumatic Diseases*, 4th edition. John Wright and Sons Limited, Bristol.

Handling the Handicapped, 2nd edition (1980). Woodhead-Faulkner Limited, Cambridge, in association with the Chartered Society of Physiotherapy.

Harris, N.H. (ed) (1982). *Textbook of Clinical Orthopaedics*. John Wright and Sons Limited, Bristol.

Huckstep, R.L. (1981). *A Simple Guide to Trauma*, 3rd edition. Churchill Livingstone, Edinburgh.

Hughes, G.R.V. (1976). *Modern Topics in Rheumatology*. William Heinemann Medical Books Limited, London.

Hughes, G.R.V. (1979). *Connective Tissue Diseases*, 2nd edition. Blackwell Scientific Publications Limited, Oxford.

Huskisson, E.C. and Hart, F.D. (1978). *Joint Disease: All the Arthropathies*, 3rd edition. John Wright and Sons Limited, Bristol.

Klenerman, L. (ed) (1982). *The Foot and its Disorders*, 2nd edition. Blackwell Scientific Publications Limited, Oxford.

McCarty, D.J. (ed) (1979). *Arthritis and Allied Conditions. A Textbook of Rheumatology*, 9th edition. Lea and Febiger, Philadelphia.

McRae, R.K. (1981). *Practical Fracture Treatment*. Churchill Livingstone, Edinburgh.

Martindale: The Extra Pharmacopoeia, 28th edition. (1982). The Pharmaceutical Press, London.

Moll, J.M.H. (ed) (1980). *Ankylosing Spondylitis*. Churchill Livingstone, Edinburgh.

Morgan, R.E. and Adamson, G.T. (1961). *Circuit Training*, 2nd edition. G. Bell and Sons, London.

Roaf, R. (1980). *Spinal Deformities*, 2nd edition. Pitman Books Limited, London.

Roaf, R. and Hodkinson, L.J. (1980). *Textbook of Orthopaedic Nursing*, 3rd edition. Blackwell Scientific Publications Limited, Oxford.

Rowe, J.W. and Dyer, L. (1977). *Care of the Orthopaedic Patient*. Blackwell Scientific Publications Limited, Oxford.

Scott, J.T. (ed) (1978). *Copeman's Textbook of the Rheumatic Diseases*, 5th edition. Churchill Livingstone, Edinburgh.

Thompson, M. (1982). *The Rheumatic Diseases*. Chapter in *Long-Term Prescribing: Drug Management of Chronic Disease and Other Problems* (ed Wilkes, E.). Faber and Faber, London.

Williams, J.G.P. and Sperryn, P.N. (1982). *Sports Medicine*, 2nd edition. Edward Arnold (Publishers) Limited, London.

PAPERS

Anderson, M.I. (1972). Physiotherapeutic management of patients on continuous traction. *Physiotherapy*, 58, 2, 51–4.

Burgess, D., Wood, B., Graham, K. and Dickson, A. (1978). Orthopaedics: 2. Congenital dislocation of the hip. *Nursing Mirror Supplement*, 14 December.

Fractures (1978). *Nursing Mirror Supplement*, 7 December.

Owen, R. (1972). Indications and contra-indications for limb traction. *Physiotherapy*, 58, 2, 44–5.

Powell, M. (1972). Application of limb traction and nursing management. *Physiotherapy*, 58, 2, 46–51.

BIOGRAPHY

Aitken, D.M. (1935). *Hugh Owen Thomas: His Principles and Practice.* Oxford University Press, Oxford.

Hunt, A. (1938). *This is my Life.* Blackie, London.

Robert Jones Centenary Volume (1957). *The Journal of Bone and Joint Surgery*, **39B**, 2, 179–217.

Watson, F. (1934). *The Life of Sir Robert Jones.* Hodder and Stoughton, London.

Watson, F. (1934). *Hugh Owen Thomas: A Personal Study.* Oxford University Press, Oxford.

The Heritage of Oswestry (1961). Privately published by the Robert Jones and Agnes Hunt Hospital, Oswestry.

Useful Organisations

Arthritis and Rheumatism Council for Research
41 Eagle Street
London WC1R 4AR   01–405 8572

ATLAS
5 Akenside Court, Belsize Crescent
London NW3 5QT   01–435 3309

Back Pain Association Limited
Grundy House, Somerset Road
Teddington, Middlesex TW11 8TD   01–977 1171

Biological Engineering Society
c/o Royal College of Surgeons of England
Lincoln's Inn Fields
London WC2A 3PN   01–242 7750

British Polio Fellowship
Bell Close, West End Road
Ruislip, Middlesex HA4 6LP   Ruislip 75515

Arthritis Care
6 Grosvenor Crescent
London SW1X 7ER   01–235 0902

Brittle Bone Society
c/o 112 City Road
Dundee DD2 2PW   0382 67603

Disabled Living Foundation
380–384 Harrow Road
London W9 2HU   01–289 6111

The Haemophilia Society
PO Box 9, 16 Trinity Street
London SE1 1DE   01–407 1010

The Mathilda and Terence Kennedy Institute of Rheumatology
Bute Gardens, Hammersmith
London W6 7DW   01–748 9966

National Ankylosing Spondylitis Society
6 Grosvenor Crescent
London SW1X 7ER   01–235 9585

The Psoriasis Association
7 Milton Street
Northampton NN2 7JG   0604 711129

Rehabilitation Engineering Movement Advisory Panels (REMAP)
Thames House North, Millbank
London SW1P 4QG   01–834 4444

Riding for the Disabled Association
Avenue R, National Agricultural Centre
Kenilworth, Warwickshire CV8 2LY   0203 56107

Royal Association for Disability and Rehabilitation (RADAR)
25 Mortimer Street
London W1N 8AB   01–637 5400

Spinal Injuries Association
5 Crowndale Road
London NW1 1TU   01–388 6840

Scoliosis Self-Help Group
20 Prince Edward Mansions, Moscow Road
London W2 4EN   01-229 1674

PROFESSIONAL ORGANISATIONS

Association of Orthopaedic Chartered Physiotherapists
c/o 25 Mortimer Street
London W1N 8AB

The following are Specific Groups of the Chartered Society of Physiotherapy.
Anyone interested should write to the secretary of the relevant group c/o the
Chartered Society of Physiotherapy, 14 Bedford Row, London WC1E 4RD.

Association of Chartered Physiotherapists in Sports Medicine

Manipulation Association of Chartered Physiotherapists

Riding for the Disabled

Rheumatic Care Association of Chartered Physiotherapists

Index